Werner Hacke   Gregory J. del Zoppo
Matthias Hirschberg (Eds.)

Thrombolytic Therapy in Acute Ischemic Stroke

With 35 Figures and 54 Tables

Springer-Verlag Berlin Heidelberg GmbH

Prof. Dr. WERNER HACKE
Klinikum der Universität Heidelberg
Neurologische Klinik
Im Neuenheimer Feld 400
W-6900 Heidelberg, FRG

GREGORY J. DEL ZOPPO, MD
Department of Molecular and Experimental Medicine
and Division of Hematology/Medical Oncology
Scripps Clinic and Research Foundation
10666 North Torrey Pines Road
La Jolla, CA 92037, USA

Dr. MATTHIAS HIRSCHBERG
Klinikum der Universität Heidelberg
Neurologische Klinik
Im Neuenheimer Feld 400
W-6900 Heidelberg, FRG

ISBN 978-3-540-53680-2   ISBN 978-3-642-76439-4 (eBook)
DOI 10.1007/ 978-3-642-76439-4

© Springer-Verlag Berlin Heidelberg 1991
Originally published by Springer-Verlag Berlin Heidelberg New York in 1991

The use of general descriptive names, registered names, trademarks, etc. in this publication does not imply, even in the absence of a specific statement, that such names are exempt from the relevant protective laws and regulations and therefore free for general use.

Product liability: The publisher can give no guarantee for information about drug dosage and application thereof contained in this book. In every individual case the respective user must check its accuracy by consulting other pharmaceutical literature.

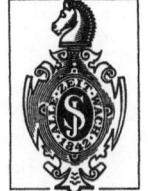

Preface

During the last decade scientists in both basic and clinical research have renewed their interest in the potential role of thrombolytic therapy in the treatment of acute ischemic stroke. The reevaluation of this approach was kindled by our growing knowledge of the pathogenesis of thrombotic and embolic stroke and by the development of new thrombolytic agents. With no proven therapy for acute ischemic stroke available, the potential value of early pharmacologic recanalization of occluded vessels in the management of acute stroke patients – an approach that has been supported by animal experiments and a limited number of uncontrolled clinical pilot studies – is again under scrutiny. A symposium on "Thrombolysis in Acute Cerebral Ischemia" was held in Heidelberg, Germany, in May 1990 to summarize and discuss the pathophysiological background for thrombolysis in acute ischemic stroke and the recent experimental and clinical experience with the new generation of thrombolytic agents.

The editors are fortunate to be able to include authoritative manuscripts from almost all the speakers at the symposium. These include reports of work by the most active investigators in this challenging field. The editors wish to express their gratitude to all the contributors for the additional work they have undertaken. Additionally, we would like to thank Springer-Verlag, Heidelberg, for its generous assistance in the preparation and rapid publication of this volume.

Heidelberg, August 1990

WERNER HACKE
GREGORY J. DEL ZOPPO
MATTHIAS HIRSCHBERG

Contents

IV. Future Directions

V. Open Communications

List of Contributors

Addresses are given at the beginning of the respective contribution.

I. Acute Cerebral Ischemia and Thrombolysis

Natural History of Atherothromboembolic Occlusion of Cerebral Arteries: Carotid Versus Vertebrobasilar Territories

A.J. FURLAN

Although natural history studies are often used as "historical controls" for evaluating new therapeutic modalities, their proper role is to help determine sample size for prospective, randomized trials. These studies can also provide important insights into variables impacting on prognosis following stroke. Unfortunately, natural history data pertinent to thrombolytic therapy for acute stroke are scant since we are most interested in *lesion-specific* outcome rather than outcome related solely to clinical parameters. Clinical and computed tomography (CT) data alone cannot be used to localize precisely the site of arterial occlusion in patients with acute cerebral infarction, and virtually all studies of acute stroke therapy lack angiographic or even non-invasive data. Furthermore, thrombolytic trials carry out treatment in the very early stages of evolving infarction, i.e., less than 8 h from onset, making it even more difficult to use existing data related to outcome since the average time from onset to stroke therapy in most trials exceeds 24 h [25].

Complicating matters further, we have yet to define which arterial lesions are potentially treatable with thrombolytic therapy. Most would agree that cardioembolic occlusion of the middle cerebral artery (MCA) trunk or perhaps its smaller branches is the best clinical model. Fortunately, there are natural history data based on angiographic studies available for MCA lesions, whereas there are virtually no data on embolic occlusion of other cerebral vessels. There have been several studies of the natural history of atherothrombotic occlusion of the internal carotid artery (ICA) origin. However, isolated atherothrombotic occlusion of the ICA origin may not be particularly amenable to thrombolytic therapy. Data are even more scant for lesion-specific posterior circulation infarcts. Indeed, the best "natural history" data on acute atherothrombosis of the basilar artery, another favored lesion for thrombolytic therapy, have come from early clinical treatment trials. Prior series of basilar artery thrombosis have generally indicated a dire prognosis or are isolated case series marvelling at the exceptional patient who survives and recovers. Exactly how often patients survive acute basilar artery thrombosis with good neurologic recovery is unclear, although this seems infrequent. Finally, it is unknown whether certain high-grade stenoses (as opposed to complete occlusion) might be treatable with thrombolytic therapy.

Department of Neurology, Cleveland Clinic Foundation, Cleveland, OH, USA.

Hacke et al (Eds.)
Thrombolytic Therapy in Acute Ischemic Stroke
© Springer-Verlag Berlin Heidelberg 1991

Beyond linking the acute stroke syndrome with the arterial lesion and outcome, we need to address the natural history of the occlusive lesion per se. Several studies have now documented a fairly high spontaneous recanalization rate for MCA occlusion using serial angiography, generally spaced days apart [1, 15, 24, 25]. The overall spontaneous recanalization rate approaches 40%–50% within 3 days of occlusion. Exactly when or how early spontaneous recanalization occurs is unclear, although this probably takes at least several hours. New studies employing transcranial Doppler scan, such as those reported at this symposium by the Giessen group, suggest that spontaneous recanalization may occur in up to 75% of MCA occlusion survivors, but the exact time sequence is again unclear. However, it would appear that in most patients spontaneous recanalization of the MCA trunk occurs too late in the course to have a favorable impact on outcome. We, and others, have documented angiographic changes in atherothrombotic lesions of the carotid artery siphon, or the basilar artery in patients on warfarin or antiplatelet therapy [3, 18]. Again, the frequency, time course, and relationship to outcome of these arterial lesion changes are unclear.

In turning to specific arterial lesions that might be amenable to treatment with thrombolytic therapy, I would like to confine my comments to MCA occlusion and basilar artery occlusion. Table 1 shows some data on the natural history of ICA occlusion [8].

Middle Cerebral Artery Occlusion

At least five recent angiographic studies have examined the natural history of MCA occlusion (Table 2) [2, 6, 17, 20–22]. These studies have been selected because they distinguish the site of arterial occlusion and they provide long-term follow-up. Several conclusions may be drawn from these studies:

1. Occlusion of the MCA trunk generally presents with a severe cerebral infarct, particularly when the occlusion is proximal to or at the level of the lenticulostriate vessels. Branch occlusions tend to present with minor stroke or transient ischemic attack (TIA).

   Saito et al. [22] correlated the site of MCA occlusion with the infarct patterns seen on CT. Patients with occlusion of the MCA proximal to or at the level of the lenticulostriate vessels typically present with deep basal ganglia, and extensive subcortical or major hemispheric infarction. MCA trunk occlusion distal to the lenticulostriate vessels, or involving multiple proximal branches, usually also produces large basal ganglia, and subcortical or hemispheric infarct. Distal branch MCA occlusions are associated with limited cortical/subcortical infarction or a normal CT.

2. Middle cerebral artery trunk occlusion is associated with a poor outcome in over 50% of cases. The immediate mortality rate approaches 30%, and severe long-term disability among survivors ranges from 40% to 65%.

Table 1. Prognosis of carotid artery occlusion

Reference	Number of patients	Type of study	Patient population	Mean period of follow-up	Strokes during follow-up	Deaths during follow-up
McDowell et al. [19]	38	Retrospective	Major completed strokes included	24 months	3 (8%)	5 (13%)
Hardy et al. [14]	133	Retrospective	Major completed strokes included	48 months	30 (23%)	51 (39%)
Dyken et al. [9]	43	Prospective	Half of patients with moderate to severe deficit	16.5 months	3 (7%)	6 (14%)
Fields and Lemak [10]	359	Prospective	Significant number of patients with initial severe deficit	44 months	89 (25%)	155 (43%)
Grillo and Patterson [12]	37	Retrospective	Majority having TIA or stroke	36 months	6[a] (16%)	10 (27%)
Samson et al. [23]	7	Prospective	TIA or minor stroke	17 months	2[b] (28%)	0
Barnett [4]	25	Prospective	TIA or minor stroke	24 months	7[b] (28%)	–
Furlan et al. [11]	138	Retrospective	TIA or minor stroke	60 months	11[b] (8%) 6[a] (4%)	30 (21%)
Heyman, O, personal communication	13	Prospective	TIA	24 months	7[b] (54%)	2 (15%)
Bogousslavsky et al. [5]	23	Retrospective	Majority having TIA or minor stroke	27 months	0	0
Cote et al. [8]	47	Prospective	TIA or minor stroke	34 months	7[b] (15%) 4[a] (8.5%)	4 (8.5%)

Modified from [8].
[a] Stroke in other vascular distribution.
[b] Ipsilateral stroke.

Table 2. Middle cerebral artery occlusion: acute mortality and long-term disability

	Trunk (n)	Branch (n)	Short-term Mortality (%)	Long-term disabled (%)	Follow-up (months)
Kaste and Waltimo [18]	23	55		28	30
Ogawa et al. [22]	120	68	14	65	2
Andreoli et al. [2]	127	–	27	46	60
Moulin et al. [21]	17	7	21 (all trunk)	37	54
Saito et al. [23]	24	19	30	38	3

3. Branch MCA occlusions have a generally good prognosis, with a very low acute mortality rate and a severe long-term disability rate of less than 30%.
4. In addition to site of MCA occlusion, effective collateral circulation on angiography and the degree of initial neurologic deficit have been correlated with long-term outcome. Although this has not held true in all studies, good angiographic collateral circulation is generally associated with a better long-term prognosis. A depressed level of consciousness is the single most important clinical factor associated with poor outcome.

Basilar Artery Occlusion

The prognosis of most patients with acute occlusion of the basilar artery appears to be poor. However, there are no large series of patients with angiographically documented basilar artery thrombosis who have been followed over time. This is partly because of the initial high mortality rate, and also due to cerebral angiography not being routinely performed in these patients. That some patients can survive basilar artery occlusion, or even bilateral distal vertebral artery occlusion, is well documented, but is probably a rare event [6, 7].

Hacke et al. [13] provided some insight into the "natural history" of acute basilar thrombosis in their studies of intraarterial thrombolytic therapy (Table 3). In 22 patients with acute vertebral basilar thrombosis treated with anticoagulants or antiplatelet therapy, the outcome was unfavorable in 19 (86%), all of whom died. Similarly, there was a 100% fatal outcome among 24 patients given thrombolytic therapy who did not recanalize. In contrast, 10 of 19 patients (53%) with acute vertebral basilar occlusions undergoing thrombolytic therapy who recanalized had a favorable outcome. These data, although imperfect, indicate that acute thrombosis of the vertebral basilar vessels is associated with a high mortality rate and very poor neurologic outcome.

Table 3. Clinical outcome in patients with vertebrobasilar artery thrombosis by treatment group. (Modified from Hacke et al. [13])

| | | Outcome | | | |
| | | Category | | Category | |
	n	Favorable	Unfavorable	Survival	Death
Antiplatelet/ anticoagulant therapy	22	3	19	3	19
Thrombolytic (recanalization)	19	10	9	13	6
Thrombolytic (no recanalization)	24	0	24	0	24

Implications for Study Design

Occlusions of the MCA trunk or of the basilar artery are most predictably associated with massive infarction and a poor neurologic outcome. "Silent" occlusion of the MCA trunk or basilar artery is rare whereas carotid artery occlusion may be silent, may produce a TIA or minor stroke, or may result in a major neurologic deficit. MCA branch occlusion typically results in a TIA or minor stroke and carries an overall excellent prognosis.

Future studies of thrombolytic therapy for acute stroke should be stratified according to the degree of neurologic deficit and site of arterial occlusion. It will be easiest to demonstrate a benefit, or lack thereof, from thrombolytic therapy in patients presenting with a major deficit due to occlusion of the MCA trunk, basilar artery, and internal carotid artery (with distal MCA trunk occlusion). Relatively small sample sizes will be required for these patients and lesions, particularly basilar artery thrombosis, where the long-term poor outcome probably exceeds 90%. On the other hand, it will be difficult (perhaps impossible) to show a *clinical* (as opposed to angiographic recanalization) benefit of thrombolytic therapy for MCA branch occlusion syndromes or internal carotid occlusion and minor stroke.

References

1. Allcock JM (1967) Occlusion of the middle cerebral artery: serial angiography as a guide to conservative therapy. J Neurosurg 27:353 ff.
2. Andreoli A, Limoni P, DeCarolis P, Benericem E, Benrenuti L, Gagliardi R, Giombini S, Parenti G, Piazza J, Reale F (1985) Prognosis of middle cerebral artery occlusion. Cooperative study on 178 cases. In: Spetzler R, Selman W, Carter LP, Martin MA

(eds) Cerebral revascularization for stroke. Thieme/Grune and Stratton, New York, pp 53–56

3. Awad I, Furlan AJ, Little JR (1984) Changes in intracranial stenotic lesions after extracranial-intracranial bypass surgery. J Neurosurg 60:771 ff.

4. Barnett HJM (1978) Delayed cerebral ischemic episodes distal to occlusion of major cerebral arteries. Neurology 28:769 ff.

5. Bogousslausky J, Regli F, Hungerbühler J-P, Chrzanowski R (1981) Transient ischemic attacks and external carotid artery. A retrospective study of 23 patients with an occlusion of the internal carotid artery. Stroke 12:627 ff.

6. Caplan LR (1979) Occlusion of the vertebral or basilar artery. Stroke 10:277 ff.

7. Caplan LR (1983) Bilateral distal vertebral artery occlusion. Neurology 33:552 ff.

8. Cote R, Barnett HJM, Taylor DW (1983) Internal carotid occlusion: a prospective study. Stroke 14:898 ff.

9. Dyken M, Klatte E, Kolar OJ, Spurgeon C (1974) Complete occlusion of common or internal carotid arteries. Clinical significance. Arch Neurol 30:343 ff.

10. Fields WF, Lemak NA (1976) Joint study of extracranial arterial occlusion. X. Internal carotid artery occlusion. JAMA 235:2734 ff.

11. Furlan AJ, Whisnant JP, Baker HL Jr (1986) Long-term prognosis after carotid artery occlusion. Neurology 30:986 ff.

12. Grillo P, Patterson RH Jr (1975) Occlusion of the carotid artery: prognosis (natural history) and the possibilities of surgical revascularization. Stroke 6:17 ff.

13. Hacke W, Zeumer H, Ferbert A (1988) Intra-arterial thrombolytic therapy improves outcome in patients with acute vertebrobasilar occlusive disease. Stroke 19:1216 ff.

14. Hardy WG, Lindner DW, Thomas LN, Gurdjian ES (1962) Anticipated clinical course in carotid artery occlusion. Arch Neurol 6:64 ff.

15. Irino T, Tandeda M, Minami T (1977) Angiographic manifestations in postrecanalized cerebral infarction. Neurol 27:471 ff.

16. Ito Z, Suzuki A, Hen R, Vemura K (1983) Prognostic factors in spontaneous recanalization of middle cerebral artery occlusion. In: Ito Z, Kutsuzawa T, Yasui N (eds) Cerebral ischemia – an update. Excerpta Medica, Amsterdam, pp 159–166

17. Kaste M, Waltimo O (1976) Prognosis of patients with middle cerebral artery occlusion. Stroke 7:482 ff.

18. Little JR, Furlan AJ (1985) Resolving occlusive lesions of the basilar artery. J Neurosurg 17:811 ff.

19. McDowell FH, Potes J, Groch S (1961) The natural history of internal carotid and vertebral-basilar artery occlusion. Neurology 11:153 ff.

20. Moulin DE, Lo R, Chiang J, Barnett HJM (1985) Prognosis in middle cerebral artery occlusion. Stroke 16:282 ff.

21. Ogawa A, Kogure T, Yoshimoto T, Fukaoa N, Seki H, Suzuki J (1985) Prognosis of middle cerebral artery occlusion. Analysis of the nationwide cooperative study in Japan. In: Spetzler R, Selman W, Carter LP, Martin NA (eds) Cerebral revascularization for stroke. Thieme-Grune and Stratton, New York, pp 57–62

22. Saito I, Segawa H, Shiokawa Y, Taniguchi M, Tsutsumi K (1987) Middle cerebral artery occlusion: correlation of computed tomography and angiography with clinical outcome. Stroke 18:863 ff.

23. Samson D, Watts C, Clark K (1977) Cerebral revascularization for transient ischemic attacks. Neurology 27:767 ff.

24. Sindermann F, Dichgans J, Bergleiter R (1965) Occlusion of the middle cerebral artery and its branches: angiographic and clinical correlates. Brain 92:607 ff.

25. Sterman AB, Furlan AJ, Pessin M, Kase C, Caplan L, Williams G (1987) Acute stroke therapy trials: an introduction to recurring design issues. Stroke 18:524 ff.

Fibrinolysis: Thrombolytic Agents, Mechanisms, and New Developments

D. Collen[1] and H.R. Lijnen

Introduction

Mammalian blood contains an enzymatic system, called the fibrinolytic system, which is schematically represented in Fig. 1. It contains a proenzyme, plasminogen, which by the action of plasminogen activators is converted to the active enzyme plasmin, which in turn digests fibrin to soluble degradation products. Two distinct physiological plasminogen activators have been identified in blood: tissue-type plasminogen activator (t-PA) and single-chain urokinase-type plasminogen activator (scu-PA). Inhibition of the fibrinolytic system occurs both at the level of the plasminogen activators, mainly by plasminogen activator inhibitor-1 (PAI-1), and at the level of plasmin, mainly by α_2-antiplasmin. The plasminogen molecule contains structures, called lysine-binding sites, which mediate its binding to fibrin and accelerate the interaction between plasmin and its physiological inhibitor α_2-antiplasmin. The lysine-binding sites play a crucial role in the regulation of fibrinolysis as discussed in detail elsewhere [6]. The current knowledge of the fibrinolytic system is reviewed elsewhere [7, 15].

Thrombolytic Agents

Thrombotic complications of cardiovascular disease are a major cause of death and disability and, consequently, thrombolysis can favorably influence the outcome of such life-threatening diseases as myocardial infarction, cerebrovascular thrombosis, and venous thromboembolism. Thrombolytic therapy has become an established procedure for the treatment of acute myocardial infarction. If given early, coronary arterial thrombolysis recanalizes occluded coronary arteries, salvages myocardial infarction, and reduces mortality.

---

[1] Center for Thrombosis and Vascular Research, Katholieke Universiteit Leuven, Herestraat 49, 3000 Leuven, Belgium.

Hacke et al. (Eds)
Thrombolytic Therapy in Acute Ischemic Stroke
© Springer-Verlag Berlin Heidelberg 1991

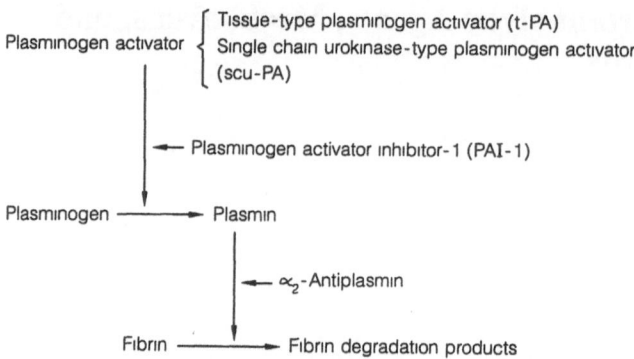

Fig. 1. Schematic representation of the fibrinolytic system

Thrombolytic agents are plasminogen activators that convert plasminogen, the inactive proenzyme of the fibrinolytic system in blood, to the proteolytic enzyme plasmin. Plasmin dissolves the fibrin of a blood clot, but may also degrade normal components of the hemostatic system and predispose to bleeding. Currently, there are five thrombolytic agents that are either approved for clinical use or are under clinical investigation in patients with acute myocardial infarction. These include streptokinase, urokinase, recombinant tissue-type plasminogen activator (rt-PA), anisoylated plasminogen streptokinase activator complex (APSAC), and single-chain urokinase-type plasminogen activator (scu-PA, prourokinase). This review will deal with the molecular mechanism of action of these plasminogen activators, with their pharmacokinetic profile and their therapeutic potential.

Mechanism of Action of Plasminogen Activators

Streptokinase

Streptokinase is a nonenzyme protein produced by several strains of hemolytic streptococci; it consists of a single polypeptide chain with an M_r of 47000–50000. Streptokinase cannot directly cleave peptide bonds; it activates plasminogen to plasmin indirectly following a three-step mechanism. In the first step, streptokinase forms an equimolar complex with plasminogen. This complex undergoes a conformational change resulting in the exposure of an active site in the plasminogen moiety. In the second step, this active site catalyzes the activation of plasminogen to plasmin and, in a third step, plasminogen-streptokinase molecules are converted to plasmin-streptokinase complex (for references see [40]).

Anisoylated Plasminogen Streptokinase Activator Complex

Anisoylated plasminogen streptokinase activator complex (APSAC) is an equimolar noncovalent complex between human plasminogen and streptokinase. It has a catalytic center located in the COOH-terminal region of the molecule, whereas the lysine-binding sites are found within the NH_2-terminal region of plasminogen. Reversible acylation of the catalytic center would thus not affect the fibrin-binding capacity of the complex [42]. The plasmin (ogen)-streptokinase complex is an efficient activator of plasminogen. APSAC binds to fibrin via the lysine-binding sites of plasminogen, although the affinity of plasminogen for fibrin is very weak. Deacylation of APSAC uncovers the catalytic center, which converts plasminogen to plasmin. Deacylation of APSAC does, however, occur both in the circulation and at the fibrin surface, and the fibrin specificity of thrombolysis with APSAC is, at best, only marginal.

Tissue-Type Plasminogen Activator

Native tissue-type plasminogen activator (t-PA) is a serine proteinase with an M_r of about 70 000, composed of a single polypeptide chain. t-PA is converted by plasmin to a two-chain form by hydrolysis of the Arg^{275}-Ile^{276} peptide bond. t-PA for clinical use is presently produced by recombinant DNA technology (Activase, Genentech Inc., or Actilyse, Boehringer Ingelheim GmbH, FRG) and consists mainly of the single-chain form.

The NH_2-terminal region of t-PA is composed of several domains with homologies to other proteins: residues 1–43 are homologous to the "finger domains" in fibronectin, residues 44–91 are homologous to human epidermal growth factor, and residues 92–173 and 180–261 are both homologous to the "kringle" regions of plasminogen. The region comprising residues 276–527 is homologous to that of other serine proteinases and contains the catalytic site, which is composed of His^{322}, Asp^{371}, and Ser^{478} [39]. t-PA has a specific affinity for fibrin. The structures involved in the fibrin-binding of t-PA are fully contained within the A-(heavy) chain. Evidence obtained with deletion mutants suggests that binding of t-PA to fibrin is mediated both via the finger domain and via the second kringle region. A lysine-binding site is involved in the interaction of the kringle-2 domain with fibrin, but not in the interaction of the finger domain with fibrin. The structures required for the enzymatic activity of t-PA are fully contained within the B-chain.

The activation of plasminogen by t-PA, both in the presence and in the absence of fibrin, follows Michaelis-Menten kinetics [27]. Although different kinetic constants were obtained by several investigators, there is a consensus that the presence of fibrin enhances the efficiency of plasminogen activation by t-PA by 2–3 orders of magnitude. The kinetic data of Hoylaerts [27] support a mechanism in which fibrin provides a surface to which t-PA and plasminogen adsorb in a sequential and ordered way, yielding a cyclic ternary complex. Fibrin essentially increases the local plasminogen concentration by creating an additional interaction between t-PA and its substrate. The high affinity of t-PA for plasminogen in the presence of fibrin thus allows efficient activation on the fibrin clot, while no efficient plasminogen activation by t-PA occurs in plasma.

Plasmin formed on the fibrin surface has both its lysine-binding sites and active site occupied and is thus only slowly inactivated by α_2-antiplasmin (half-life of about 10–100 s); free plasmin, when formed, is rapidly inhibited by α_2-antiplasmin (half-life of about 0.1 s) [46]. The fibrinolytic process thus seems to be triggered by and confined to fibrin.

Urokinase-Type Plasminogen Activator

Two-chain urokinase-type plasminogen activator (tcu-PA), a trypsin-like serine proteinase composed of two polypeptide chains (M_r 20 000 and 34 000), has been isolated from human urine and from cultured human embryonic kidney cells. Over recent years, several groups have isolated a single-chain form of urokinase with M_r 54 000 (scu-PA) from urine, plasma, or conditioned cell culture media. Recently, it was also obtained by recombinant DNA technology and prepared from the translation product in *Escherichia coli* of an expression plasmid coding for human urokinase. Upon limited hydrolysis by plasmin or kallikrein of the Lys[158]-Ile[159] peptide bond, scu-PA is converted to tcu-PA. The catalytic center is located in the COOH-terminal chain and is composed of Asp[255], His[204], and Ser[356]. The NH$_2$-terminal chain contains regions homologous to human epidermal growth factor and one region homologous to the plasminogen kringles.

Two-chain urokinase-type plasminogen activator activates plasminogen directly following Michaelis-Menten kinetics, but has no specific affinity for fibrin and activates fibrin-bound and circulating plasminogen relatively indiscriminately. Extensive plasminogen activation and depletion of α_2-antiplasmin may occur following treatment of thromboembolic diseases with tcu-PA, leading to degradation of several plasma proteins including fibrinogen, factor V, and factor VIII. We have observed that scu-PA also has some intrinsic plasminogen-activating potential. Initially refolded scu-PA expressed in *E. coli* was found to be fully active. However, preparations obtained from natural sources or expressed in mammalian cell systems were subsequently found to have less than 1% of the activity of tcu-PA [30]. A low intrinsic activity of scu-PA was confirmed by others, whereas some authors have claimed that scu-PA has no enzymatic activity and is a genuine proenzyme (for references see [29]).

Single-chain urokinase-type plasminogen activator, in contrast to tcu-PA, has significant fibrin specificity. A hypothetical mechanism of action has been proposed [30] on the basis of the observations that scu-PA has some intrinsic plasminogen-activating potential, that scu-PA does not significantly activate plasminogen in plasma in the absence of fibrin, and that fibrin reverses the inhibition exerted by plasma, although not via direct binding of scu-PA to fibrin. These findings suggest that plasma components interfere with plasminogen activation and that the fibrin specificity of the activation of plasminogen by scu-PA is due to reversal by fibrin of the inhibited state. Alternatively, the presence of fibrin may enhance the activation rate of fibrin-bound plasminogen [38]. In clot lysis systems in human plasma in vitro, conversion of scu-PA to tcu-PA has been shown to constitute a major positive feedback mechanism for fibrinolysis [30]. The molecular interactions which regulate the fibrin-specific activation of the fibrinolytic system by scu-PA remain to be further detailed.

Plasminogen Activators
in the Treatment of Coronary Artery Disease

Reduction of infarct size, preservation of ventricular function, and/or de-creased mortality have been demonstrated in patients with acute myocardial infarction following administration of streptokinase, APSAC, and rt-PA (for references see [15]). This beneficial effect of thrombolysis will probably also hold for other plasminogen activators.

Coronary reperfusion is very likely the most important, if not the only, significant contributor to preservation of ventricular function and to reduction in mortality, although the magnitude of the effect appears to be time dependent. Indeed, subgroup analyses of patients with and without successful reperfusion with streptokinase or rt-PA have consistently demonstrated a lower mortality rate in successfully reperfused patients, and a better outcome if reperfusion is obtained early. The most rational treatment of patients with acute myocardial infarction is therefore likely to be thrombolytic therapy with agents that reperfuse the highest number of coronary arteries as rapidly as possible.

The two comparative trials to date which have examined the reperfusion efficacies of rt-PA and streptokinase have been evaluated by meta-analysis [5]. These results show that rt-PA appears more effective than streptokinase for the early recanalization of occluded coronary arteries, both when given within 3 h of the onset of symptoms and when given later. Comparable effects on the preservation of left ventricular function have been demonstrated for rt-PA and streptokinase in two comparative trials, but further studies would assist in determining whether differences in early coronary reperfusion rates translate into a comparably better outcome. Much larger, direct comparative studies are needed before scientifically valid statements can be made regard-ing the relative efficacy of the available thrombolytic agents on both morbidity and mortality.

If the clinical benefit of thrombolytic therapy in patients with acute myocardial infarction were proportional to the efficacy for coronary thrombolysis, the size of randomized clinical trials required to establish differences between thrombolytic agents can be calculated. On the basis of controlled clinical trials of streptokinase versus placebo, in over 35 000 patients with acute myocardial infarction, the reduction in hospital mortality in the treatment group was found to be approximately 25%. A thrombolytic agent, such as rt-PA, with a 50% higher efficacy of coronary thrombolysis than streptokinase, would thus be anticipated to reduce early mortality by 37.5%. Assuming a control mortality of 9% in the absence of thrombolytic therapy, mortality with streptokinase treatment would be reduced by 25% to 6.75%, and that with the more potent agent by 37.5% to 5.6%. In order to establish such a difference with a statistical power of 0.8 and a significance level of 0.05, more than 10 000 patients would have to be entered into a randomized trial (D. Finkelstein, personal communication). These numbers illustrate the tremendous task to be undertaken in order to translate efficacy for coronary thrombolysis into reduction of mortality.

Two large prospective comparative clinical trials in patients with acute myocardial infarction, GISSI-2 comparing streptokinase and rt-PA in 20 000 patients, and ISIS-3, comparing streptokinase, APSAC, and rt-PA in 30 000 patients, are presently being carried out. Both trials, in a factorial design, are also investigating the effect of heparin. However, heparin is administered by subcutaneous injection and starts only 12 h and 3 h after the infusion of thrombolytic agent, respectively. This is most unfortunate, because the recent studies by Bleich et al. [1] and Ross et al. (unpublished work; presented at the American Heart Association meeting) have reported a significantly lower patency rate, determined by coronary angiography after mean times of 55–59 h and 7–24 h respectively, when rt-PA was administered without heparin. Actually the patency rates obtained with rt-PA in the absence of heparin relative to those obtained with rt-PA and heparin were similar to those previously obtained with streptokinase and heparin. On the other hand it has been claimed that streptokinase, because of the profound hypocoagulable state which it produces in the blood stream for many hours, does not require adjuvant heparin therapy for coronary recanalization [41]. If the previously established higher reperfusion rates of rt-PA relative to streptokinase require the concomitant use of heparin, with rt-PA but not with streptokinase, the GISSI-2 and ISIS-3 trials, because of their design, can no longer be expected to resolve the crucial question of whether efficacy for coronary recanalization translates into clinical benefit. Indeed, with administration schemes that produce comparable rates of recanalization, clinical outcomes are expected to be comparable, unless the reduced viscosity and hypotension induced with streptokinase would confer an additional benefit [33, 34].

In the meantime, it might be of interest to review the available data from the small comparative trials with streptokinase and rt-PA [4, 32, 44, 45] and with urokinase and rt-PA [2, 37] carried out to date with the simultaneous use of heparin anticoagulation. Statistical evaluation of the homogeneity of these studies revealed a X^2 value of 1.34 ($p = 0.85$) allowing meta-analysis of the data. Cumulative inhospital mortalities were 38/757 (5.0%) in patients randomized to rt-PA and 54/755 (7.2%) in patients allocated to the non-fibrin-specific agents streptokinase or urokinase (Table 1). The odds of death ratio, determined as described by Yusuf [48], is 0.64, with 95% confidence intervals of 0.4–1.0. The difference in mortality between rt-PA and SK/UK has a p value of 0.052. These results are derived from small studies, albeit randomized, which were not prospectively designed for a mortality end point. However, they agree remarkably well with the values calculated on the basis of the hypothesis that the clinical outcome is primarily determined by the efficacy of the thrombolytic agent, which is estimated to be 50% higher for rt-PA than for streptokinase or urokinase.

New Trends in Thrombolytic Therapy

Thrombolytic therapy for acute myocardial infarction, in its present form, is based on the premise that dissolution of the fibrin component of a coronary thrombus is necessary and sufficient for recanalization. However, this approach, even with the most potent thrombolytic agents presently available, fails in approximately 25% of patients. In addition, large doses are required and the treatment is associated with unpredictable bleeding and with recurrent posttreatment ischemic events. Therefore the quest for further improved thrombolytic agents or alternative therapeutic regimens continues.

Acute ischemic coronary syndromes occur nearly always in patients with atherosclerotic coronary artery disease and in association with plaque rupture

Table 1. In hospital mortality in randomized studies with rt-PA versus streptokinase or urokinase (SK/UK) in patients with acute myocardial infarction

Study	Reference	rt-PA	SK/UK
ECSG-1	[44]	3/64	3/65
TIMI-I	[4]	12/157	14/159
New Zealand	[45]	5/135	10/135
PAIMS	[32]	4/86	7/85
TAMI-5	[2]	8/191	15/190
GAUS	[37]	6/124	5/121
		38/757	54/755
		5.0%	7.2%

Homogeneity index: X^2, 1.34; $p = 0.85$.
Odds ratio rt-PA vs. streptokinase/urokinase, 0.64 (95% CI, 0.4–1.0).
p value of the difference, 0.0523.

[16, 19], which triggers intraluminal thrombosis [17]. The composition of the intraluminal thrombus formed in association with the rupture of an athero-sclerotic plaque is heterogeneous, consisting of platelet-rich material con-tiguous to the area of plaque rupture, and erythrocyte-rich material extending both proximally and distally. This suggests two alternative and potentially complementary targets for coronary thrombolysis: the erythrocyte-rich whole blood clot and the platelet-rich thrombus. While the potential and limitations of fibrinolytic agents for the dissolution of whole blood clots are well known, the potential of pharmacological dispersion of platelet clumps and platelet-rich thrombus has not been fully explored. Furthermore, the mechanism of bleeding and strategies to reduce it need to be elucidated.

Attempts to Improve the Fibrin-Dissolving Potency of Fibrinolytic Agents

Present research in this area is being carried out along several lines. In addition to the studies described below, several groups have reported in vitro data on synergism of thrombolytic agents, mutants of t-PA or scu-PA, and hybrids of t-PA and scu-PA at the Congress of the International Society on Thrombosis and Haemostasis, Brussels, Belgium, 1987, with abstracts published in *Thrombosis and Haemostasis*, vol. 58(1), 1987, and at the International Congress on Fibrinolysis, Amsterdam, the Netherlands, with abstracts published in *Fibrinolysis*, vol. 2(Suppl. 1), 1988, and at the recent Congress of the International Society on Thrombosis and Haemostasis, Tokyo, Japan, 1989, with abstracts published in *Thrombosis and Haemostasis*, vol. 62(1), 1989.

Synergism

The intrinsic fibrin selectivity of t-PA and scu-PA is mediated by entirely different molecular mechanisms. It is therefore not unreasonable to expect that, if administered in combination, the effect on clot dissolution would be more than additive. Synergism, if significant, would also allow a reduction of the total dose while obtaining a therapeutic effect that is equal to that achieved with higher doses of either agent alone. As a result, the potential for hemostatic side effects may be significantly reduced. In vivo, in a jugular vein thrombosis model in the rabbit, significant synergism between t-PA and scu-PA and between t-PA and urokinase for thrombolysis was observed [9, 10]. When t-PA and scu-PA were infused in a molar ratio of approximately 1:3, the specific thrombolytic activity of the mixture was approximately threefold higher than was anticipated on the basis of additive effects of both agents. The synergistic effect of t-PA and urokinase was only of borderline sig-nificance. A synergistic effect of at least a factor of 2 between t-PA and scu-PA was also found on coronary arterial thrombolysis in dogs [49].

Preliminary results in patients with acute myocardial infarction [8–10] suggest that t-PA acts synergistically with scu-PA and urokinase in humans as well. Indeed, combining t-PA and scu-PA at approximately one-fifth of their individual thrombolytic doses produced coronary artery reperfusion in patients with acute myocardial infarction without associated systemic fibrinogen breakdown. Although these results are still preliminary and need to be confirmed in larger studies, they are potentially of significant clinical importance. The synergistic effect of t-PA and urokinase on coronary reperfusion has, however, not been confirmed in a large-scale study, although the use of the combination was associated with a significant reduction of the frequency of reocclusion [43].

Mutants of t-PA and scu-PA

We have attempted to produce mutants of t-PA and scu-PA with improved fibrin selectivity with the use of recombinant DNA techniques. Deletion of specific domains of the t-PA molecule has been achieved. One of these t-PA mutants, called t-PA-ΔFE3X, a truncated t-PA molecule without the finger-like and growth factor domains and without carbohydrate side chains, appears to have an extended half-life and a slower plasma clearance rate in vivo and has retained most of its thrombolytic potency [3]. Since scu-PA has intrinsic albeit limited plasminogen-activating potential, attempts were made using recombinant DNA technology to prevent its conversion to two-chain urokinase. Two new constructs were produced by replacement of the lysine at position 158 with either glycine or glutamic acid. The kinetics of plasminogen activation with these mutants have been reported [35, 36]. Although these mutants do activate plasminogen to plasmin, their catalytic efficiency is only about 10% of that of the natural form of scu-PA. A clear dose-response relationship was seen when such mutants were injected in rabbits with an experimental jugular vein thrombus [12]. However, the specific thrombolytic activity of these mutants in vivo is also reduced severalfold. Thus, engineering of the scu-PA molecule, in order to prevent its conversion from a one-chain to a two-chain molecule, has not yielded improved molecules for thrombolysis.

Chimeras of t-PA and scu-PA

Another approach has been to construct chimeric (hybrid) molecules that contain domains of both the t-PA and scu-PA molecules. The resultant molecule might combine the fibrin affinity of t-PA (which is responsible for its concentration at the clot surface) with both the enzymatic properties of scu-PA (which is responsible for its stability in plasma) and the fibrin selectivity of scu-PA. One such chimer consisting of amino acids Ser1 through Thr263 of t-PA, fused to amino acids Leu144 to Leu411 of scu-PA, has been studied in detail [35, 36]. Although this chimer has a higher fibrin affinity than scu-PA, its affinity is not as high as that of intact t-PA. Studies of the chimer in vivo indicate that it has maintained most of the thrombolytic potential of scu-PA, but does not appear to be a superior agent for thrombolysis [13]. The chimeric approach remains promising, however, because it might enable the development of an agent that has increased fibrin selectivity at a reduced dose.

Antibody-Targeted Thrombolytic Therapy

Several alternatives to target the action of thrombolytic agents toward the thrombus with the use of fibrin-specific antibodies are presently being investigated [23]. These include chemical conjugates of fibrin-specific antibodies with thrombolytic agents or recombinant fusion proteins comprising a fibrinspecific antibody site and the B-chain of t-PA. Alternatively, chemical conjugates between a fibrin-specific and a t-PA-specific antibody, and biosynthetically produced heteroduplex antibodies that are both fibrin and t-PA specific, could bind to fibrin and localize endogenous or exogenous t-PA. These conjugates display significantly enhanced clot-specific lysis in vitro and, in an animal model, in vivo.

We have recently constructed a conjugate of rscu-PA with a murine monoclonal antibody directed against human fibrin fragment D-dimer that had an eightfold increased specific thrombolytic activity in vitro [18] and an eightfold higher thrombolytic potency in a rabbit jugular vein thrombosis model [12].

Attempts to Interfere with Platelet-Rich Thrombus

The role of platelet aggregation in the pathogenesis of intraluminal coronary arterial thrombosis in patients with acute cardiac ischemic syndromes appears firmly established as reviewed above. Indeed, pathological examination has consistently revealed platelet-rich zones contiguous with plaque rupture in patients with acute myocardial infarction, unstable angina, and sudden ischemic death. In addition aspirin appears to be efficient in the primary and secondary prevention of ischemic coronary events [26].

Platelet Disaggregation

Although the mechanisms of platelet aggregation and pharmacological approaches to interfere with the process are well known [20], no efficient means are available to disperse preformed platelet-rich thrombus. In a plasma milieu in vitro, concentrations of thrombolytic agents that will rapidly dissolve whole blood clots are virtually inactive toward preformed platelet aggregates [31] unless the platelets are pretreated with aspirin. rt-PA disaggregates platelet clumps but only at very high concentrations, an order of magnitude higher than those currently achievable by intravenous infusion. This suggested to us that platelet-rich regions of coronary clot might be more resistant to lysis than erythrocyte-rich zones and that predominance of platelet-rich zones would limit the efficacy of intravenous thrombolytic therapy. Consequently, one approach to increased efficacy and speed of coronary artery reperfusion might consist of the pharmacological dispersion of platelet-rich thrombus, in combination with fibrin-dissolving therapy. Alternatively, specific interference with platelet deposition during fibrinolysis might accelerate thrombolysis and prevent reocclusion.

At present three approaches toward platelet disaggregation appear feasible. The first consists of the use of high-dose intracoronary administration of plasminogen activators capable of disaggregating platelets. However, the logistic restrictions to intracoronary administration preclude its widespread use. The second approach involves the use of combinations of plasminogen activators with potent antiplatelet agents [47]. Thus, the combination of plasminogen activators with the antiplatelet GPIIb/IIIa antibody in animal models has resulted in accelerated lysis and elimination of reoccclusion at markedly reduced doses of the fibrinolytic agent. In a third approach, the thrombolytic agent could be targeted to platelet aggregates by means of specific monoclonal antibodies.

Prevention of Platelet Aggregation

Platelet aggregation clearly contributes to and may be the primary mechanism underlying reocclusion. This is supported by our findings that monoclonal antibodies against platelet GPIIb/IIIa efficiently abolish reocclusion in animal models with intensive thrombogenic stimulus [22]. Finally, preliminary studies have indicated that arterial occlusion by platelet-rich thrombus cannot be prevented by heparin, but that it is efficiently prevented by local infusion of a synthetic thrombin inhibitor [28]. These results confirm and extend recent observations with a synthetic chloromethyl ketone [25].

Attempts to Reduce the Bleeding Tendency

The observation that bleeding also occurs in association with fibrin-specific thrombolytic agents has led to the hypothesis that these agents cannot distinguish between the fibrin of a pathologic thrombus and that of a hemostatic plug [33, 34]. However, in a recent study with rt-PA in 50 patients with acute myocardial infarction, resulting in coronary artery patency in 83%, serial template bleeding times remained normal throughout the infusion period in 60% of the patients, despite full heparin anticoagulation. No correlation was observed between the template bleeding time and success or failure or reperfusion of the occluded coronary artery [21]. These observations are indicative of significant discrimination between hemostatic plugs and occlusive thrombi. The residual hemorrhagic tendency associated with the use of rt-PA despite its fibrin specificity might relate to its interference with platelets [31] or with the endothelial cells [24] which may mediate enhanced local activation of plasminogen. Consequently, mutants of rt-PA with reduced affinity for endothelial cells might be associated with a reduced bleeding tendency. Elimination of the structures in rt-PA responsible for the interaction with endothelial cells, while maintaining those mediating the fibrin-specific enzymatic properties, might be possible with the use of recombinant DNA technology.

Conclusions

The beneficial effect of thrombolytic therapy in acute ischemic coronary syndromes, and particularly in acute myocardial infarction, is now well established. The limited efficacy and potentially life-threatening side effects of thrombolytic agents remain a major problem. The present limitations of thrombolytic therapy can be explained on the basis of the heterogeneity of coronary arterial thrombus, consisting of both erythrocyte-rich and platelet-rich zones, and knowledge of the mechanism of fibrin dissolution and platelet disaggregation. This unified concept suggests alternative and complementary pharmacological approaches to coronary artery recanalization. Available evidence suggests that the efficacy of coronary thrombolysis may be augmented either by improvement of the potency and specificity of fibrin-dissolving agents, by dispersion of aggregated platelets, or by a combination of both. An at least partial discrimination between a pathologically occlusive thrombus and a physiologically hemostatic plug has been achieved with rt-PA and may be accessible to further modification. Continuing investigations along several new research lines will provide new insights and promote progress toward the development of the ideal thrombolytic therapy, characterized by maximized stable coronary arterial thrombolysis with minimized bleeding.

References

1. Bleich SD, Nichols T, Schumacher R, Cooke D, Tate D, Steiner C, Brinkman D (1989) The role of heparin following coronary thrombolysis with tissue plasminogen activator. Circulation 80(II):113 (abstract 455)
2. Califf RM, Topol EJ, George BS Kerieakes DJ, Samaha JK, Worley SJ, Anderson J, Sasahara A, Lee K, Stack RS (1989) TAMI-5: a randomized trial of combination

thrombolytic therapy and immediate cardiac catheterization. Circulation 80(II):418 (abstract 1660)

3. Cambier P, Werf F van de, Larsen GR, Collen D (1988) Pharmacokinetics and thrombolytic properties of a nonglycosylated mutant of human tissue-type plasminogen activator, lacking the finger and growth factor domains, in dogs with copper coil-induced coronary artery thrombosis. J Cardiovasc Pharmacol 11:468–472

4. Chesebro JH, Knatterud G, Roberts R (1987) Thrombolysis in myocardial infarction (TIMI) trial, phase I: a comparison between intravenous tissue plasminogen activator and intravenous streptokinase. Circulation 76:142–154

5. Chesebro JH, Knatterud G, Braunwald E (1988) Thrombolytic therapy. N Engl J Med 319:1544–1545

6. Collen D (1980) On the regulation and control of fibrinolysis. Edward Kowalski Memorial Lecture. Thromb Haemost 43:77–89

7. Collen D (1988) Plasminogen activators and thrombolytic therapy. ISI Atlas of Science. Pharmacology 3:116–120

8. Collen D, Werf F van de (1987) Coronary arterial thrombolysis with low-dose synergistic combinations of recombinant tissue-type plasminogen activator (rt-PA) and recombinant single-chain urokinase-type plasminogen activator (rscu-PA) for acute myocardial infarction. Am J Cardiol 60:431–444

9. Collen D, Stassen JM, Stump DC, Verstraete M (1986) Synergism of thrombolytic agents in vivo. Circulation 74:838–842

10. Collen D, Stump DC, Werf F van de (1986) Coronary thrombolysis in patients with acute myocardial infarction by intravenous infusion of synergic thrombolytic agents. Am Heart J 112:1083–1084

11. Collen D, Lijnen HR, Todd PA, Goa KL (1989) Tissue-type plasminogen activator. A review of its pharmacology and therapeutic use as a thrombolytic agent. Drugs 38:346–388

12. Collen D, Mao J, Stassen JM, Breeze R, Lijnen HR, Abercrombie D, Puma P, Almeda S, Vovis GF (1989) Thrombolytic properties of Lys-158 mutants of recombinant single chain urokinase-type plasminogen activator in rabbits with jugular vein thrombosis. J Vasc Med Biol 1:46–49

13. Collen D, Stassen JM, Demarsin E, Kieckens L, Lijnen HR, Nelles L (1989) Pharmacokinetics and thrombolytic properties of chimaeric plasminogen activators consisting of the NH₂-terminal region of human tissue-type plasminogen activator and the COOH-terminal region of human single chain urokinase-type plasminogen activator. J Vasc Med Biol 1:234–240

14. Collen D, Dewerchin M, Stassen JM, Kieckens L, Lijnen HR (1989) Thrombolytic and pharmacokinetic properties of conjugates of urokinase-type plasminogen activator with a monoclonal antibody specific for cross-linked fibrin. Fibrinolysis 3:197–202

15. Collen D, Lijnen HR, Verstraete M (1990) The fibrinolytic system and its disorders. In: Handin RI, Lux SE, Stossel JP (eds) Blood: principles and practice of hematology. Lippincott, Philadelphia (in press)

16. Davies MJ, Thomas AC (1985) Plaque fissuring – the cause of acute myocardial infarction, sudden ischaemic death, and crescendo angina. Br Heart J 53:363–373

17. Wood MA de, Spores J, Notske R, Lowell T, Mouser T, Burroughs R, Golden MS, Lang HT (1980) Prevalence of total coronary occlusion during the early hours of transmural myocardial infarction. N Engl J Med 303:897–902

18. Dewerchin M, Lijnen HR, Hoef B van, Cock F de, Collen D (1989) Biochemical properties of conjugates of urokinase-type plasminogen activator with a monoclonal antibody specific for crosslinked fibrin. Eur J Biochem 185:141–149

19. Friedman M (1971) The coronary thrombus: its origin and fate. Human Pathol 2:81–128

20. Fuster V, Badimon L, Badimon J, Adams PC, Turitto V, Chesebro JH (1987) Drugs interfering with platelet functions: mechanisms and clinical relevance. In: Verstraete, M, Vermylen J Lijnen R. Arnout J (eds) Thrombosis and haemostasis. Leuven University Press, pp 349–418

21. Gimple LW, Gold HK, Leinbach RC, Uasuda T, Johns JA, Eiskind AA, Collen D (1988) Bleeding time measurement predicts spontaneous bleeding during thrombolysis with recombinant tissue-type plasminogen activator (rt-PA). J Am Coll Cardiol 11:231A

22. Gold HK, Coller BS, Yasuda T, Saito T, Fallon JT, Guerrero JL, Leinbach RC, Eiskind AA, Collen D (1988) Rapid and sustained coronary artery recanalization with combined bolus injection of recombinant tissue-type plasminogen activator and monoclonal antiplatelet GPIIb/IIIa antibody in a canine preparation. Circulation 77:670–677

23. Haber E, Quertermous T, Matsueda GR, Runge MS (1989) Innovative approaches to plasminogen activator therapy. Science 243:51–56

24. Hajjar KA, Hamel NM, Harpel PC, Nachman RL (1987) Binding of tissue plasminogen activator to cultured human endothelial cells. J Clin Invest 80:1712–1719

25. Hanson SR, Harker LA (1988) Interruption of acute platelet-dependent thrombosis by the synthetic antithrombin D-phenylalanyl-L-prolyl-L-arginyl chloromethyl ketone. Proc Natl Acad Sci 85:3184–3188

26. Harker LA (1986) Clinical trials evaluating platelet-modifying drugs in patients with atherosclerotic cardiovascular disease and thrombosis. Circulation 73:206–223

27. Hoylaerts M, Rijken DC, Lijnen HR, Collen D (1982) Kinetics of the activation of plasminogen by human tissue plasminogen activator. Role of fibrin. J Biol Chem 257:2912–2919

28. Jang IK, Ziskind AA, Gold HK, Leinbach RC, Fallon JT, Collen D (1988) Prevention of arterial platelet occlusion by selective thrombin inhibition. Circulation 78(II):311

29. Lijnen HR, Stump DC, Collen D (1987) Single-chain urokinase-type plasminogen activator: mechanism of action and thrombolytic properties. Sem Thromb Haemost 13:152–159

30. Lijnen HR, B Hoef van, De Cock F, Collen D (1989) The mechanism of plasminogen activation and fibrin dissolution by single chain urokinase-type plasminogen activator in a plasma milieu in vitro. Blood 73:1864–1872

31. Loscalzo J, Vaughan DE (1987) Tissue plasminogen activator promotes platelet disaggregation in plasma. J Clin Invest 79:1749–1755

32. Magnani B, for the PAIMS Investigator (1989) Plasminogen activator Italian multicenter study (PAIMS): group comparison of intravenous recombinant single-chain human tissue-type plasminogen activator (rt-PA) with intravenous streptokinase in acute myocardial infarction. J Am Coll Cardiol 13:19–26

33. Marder VJ, Sherry S (1988a) Thrombolytic therapy: current status (first of two parts). N Engl J Med 318:1512–1520

34. Marder VJ, Sherry S (1988b) Thrombolytic therapy: current status (second of two parts). N Engl J Med 318:1585–1595

35. Nelles L, Lijnen HR, Collen D, Holmes WE (1987) Characterization of a fusion protein consisting of amino acids 1 to 263 of tissue-type plasminogen activator and amino acids 144 to 411 of urokinase-type plasminogen activator. J Biol Chem 262:10855–10862

36. Nelles L, Lijnen HR, Collen D, Holmes WE (1987) Characterization of recombinant human single chain urokinase-type plasminogen activator mutants produced by site-specific mutagenesis of lysine 158. J Biol Chem 262:5682–5689

37. Neuhaus TL, Tebbe U, Gottwick M, Weber MAJ, Feuerer W, Niederer W, Haerer W, Praetorius F, Grosser KD, Huhmann W, Hoepp HW, Alber BG, Sheikhzadeh A, Schneider B (1988) Intravenous recombinant tissue plasminogen activator (rt-PA) and urokinase in acute myocardial infarction: results of the German activator urokinase study (GAUS). J Am Coll Cardiol 12:581–587

38. Pannell R, Black J, Gurewich V (1988) Complementary modes of action of tissue-type plasminogen activator and pro-urokinase by which their synergistic effect on clot lysis may be explained. J Clin Invest 81:853–859

39. Pennica D, Holmes WE, Kohr WJ, Harkins RN, Vehar GA, Ward CA, Bennett WF, Yelvérton E, Seeburg PH, Heyneker HL, Goeddel DV, Collen D (1983) Cloning and

expression of human tissue-type plasminogen activator cDNA in *E. coli.* Nature 301:214–221

40. Reddy KNN (1988) Streptokinase – biochemistry and clinical application. Enzyme 40:78–89

41. Sherry S (1988) Unresolved clinical pharmacological questions in thrombolytic therapy for acute myocardial infarction. J Am Coll Cardiol 12:519–525

42. Smith RAG, Dupe RJ, English PD, Green J (1981) Fibrinolysis with acyl-enzymes: a new approach to thrombolytic therapy. Nature 290:505–508

43. Topol EJ, Califf RM, George BS, Kereicakes DJ, Rothbaum D, Candela RJ, Abbotsmith CW, Pinkérton CA, Stump DC, Collen D, Leekl, Pitts S, Kine EM, Boswick JM, O'Neill WW, Stack RS (1988) Coronary arterial thrombolysis with combined infusion of recombinant tissue-type plasminogen activation and urokinase in acute myocardial infarction. Circulation 77:1100–1107

44. Verstraete M, Bernard R, Bory M, Brower RW, Collen D, de Bono DP, Erbel R, Huhmann W, Lennane RJ, Lubsen J, Mathey D, Meyer J, Michels HR, Rutsch W, Schartl M, Schmidt W, Uebis R, von Essen R (1985) Randomised trial of intravenous recombinant tissue-type plasminogen activator versus intravenous streptokinase in acute myocardial infarction. Lancet 1:842–847

45. White HD, Rivers JT, Maslowski AH, Ormiston JA, Takayama M, Hart HH, Sharpe DN, Whitlock RML, Norris RM (1989) Effect of intravenous streptokinase as compared with that of tissue plasminogen activator on left ventricular function after first myocardial infarction. N Engl J Med 320:817–821

46. Wiman B, Collen D (1978) Molecular mechanism of physiological fibrinolysis. Nature 272:549–550

47. Yasuda T, Gold HK, Leinbach RC, Saito T, Fallon JT, Guerrero JL, Coller BS, Collen D (1988) Tissue plasminogen activator (t-PA) resistant platelet rich white thrombus (WT) and combination treatment of t-PA and antiplatelet antibody to GPIIb/IIIa receptor (7E3). Circulation 78(II):15

48. Yusuf S, Collins R, Peto R, Furberg C, Stampfer MJ, Goldhaber SZ, Hennekens CH (1985) Intravenous and intracoronary thrombolytic therapy in acute myocardial infarction: overview of results on mortality, reinfarction and side effects from 33 randomized clinical trials. Eur Heart J 6:556–685

49. Ziskind AA, Gold HK, Yasuda T, Kanke M, Guererro JL, Fallon JT, Collen D (1987) Coronary thrombolysis in dogs with synergistic combinations of human tissue-type plasminogen activator (t-PA) and single urokinase-type plasminogen activator (scu-PA). Clin Res 35:337A

Fibrinolysis in Myocardial Infarction:
Lessons for Cerebrovascular Disease

J. MEYER

Until about 15 years ago the prevailing view of the pathogenesis of acute myocardial infarction was that it was based on total or subtotal atherosclerotic coronary obstructions causing a major decrease in antegrade flow. Fresh thrombi, which were often found during autopsy, were thought to be the result rather than the cause of the infarction [4]. With the increasing availability of coronary arteriography for acute myocardial infarction came a major change in the understanding of the pathophysiology of the disease. DeWood et al. [9], using serial coronary arteriograms, showed that a fresh, occluding coronary thrombus is the cause and can be found in the majority of acute myocardial infarctions. While within the first 6 h the rate of total occlusions was 85%, this fell to 68% in the 6th–12th h – and to 64% in the 12th–24th h. These results also demonstrated that spontaneous thrombolysis occurs in about 20% of all patients within the 1st day.

Chazov et al [7] and Rentrop et al [23] were the first to draw clinical conclusions from these findings. They started thrombolytic therapy of acute myocardial infarction by injecting streptokinase directly into the occluded vessel [3, 14, 24, 27]. This mode of application, however, depended on the availability of a team to perform complete catheterization as soon as the patient reached hospital. Since then it has been shown by several authors that the intravenous administration of thrombolytic agents is also able to dissolve the intracoronary clot in a high percentage of cases [1, 5, 8, 11–13, 15–18, 20, 21, 26, 28–31, 33].

Besides streptokinase and urokinase, which for several years were also used for deep venous thrombi and other thrombotic diseases, most recently APSAC (anisylated plasminogen streptokinase activator complex), rt-PA (recombinant tissue-type plasminogen activator), and pro-urokinase (saruplase) have been developed especially for thrombolysis in acute myocardial infarction.

The main goals in the early treatment of acute myocardial infarction are reduction of mortality and vessel patency, and improvement of left ventricular function. Since reopened coronary vessels have a high tendency toward early reocclusion, this problem also has to be tackled [19, 24, 32].

Second Medical University Clinic, Langenbeckstraße 1, W-6500 Mainz 1, FRG.

Hacke et al (Eds)
Thrombolytic Therapy in Acute Ischemic Stroke
© Springer-Verlag Berlin Heidelberg 1991

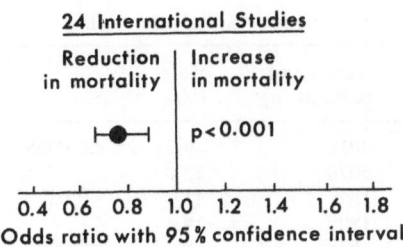

24 International Studies

Reduction in mortality	Increase in mortality
⊢●⊣	p< 0.001

0.4 0.6 0.8 1.0 1.2 1.4 1.6 1.8
Odds ratio with 95 % confidence interval

Fig. 1. Effect of thrombolytic treatment on mortality in 24 international studies [34]

On the other hand, severe adverse effects of thrombolysis such as bleeding complications, especially cerebrovascular bleeding, allergic reactions, and a decrease in blood pressure have to be considered. In addition, the practicability of the administration either as a single-shot administration or as an infusion for up to 3 h and the cost of treatment and adjunctive therapy are important factors. From experimental studies and from autopsy findings it is known that the ischemic tolerance of human myocardium is limited to a fairly short period. If recanalization of the occluded vessel occurs too late, the ischemic or stunned myocardium may deteriorate to irreversible necrosis [6, 25].

Yusuf et al [34] have demonstrated a significant reduction in mortality from an analysis of 24 international studies (Fig. 1). Several studies have shown that early treatment with streptokinase leads to a reduction of mortality compared with nonthrombolytic treatment [1, 11, 13, 16, 18, 20, 21, 28–30].

The Italian infarction study [GISSI] [11] has shown that hospital mortality is linearly correlated to the time between infarct onset and start of thrombolytic treatment (Table 1). Based on these and other findings, thrombolysis is mostly restricted to the first 6 h after onset of the typical cardiac symptoms.

The intravenous infusion of APSAC and urokinase has shown similar results [1, 18]. Several studies have been conducted in which different thrombolytic treatment regimes were compared (Table 1). Many studies have compared streptokinase with rt-PA [16, 28, 29]; only one so far has compared streptokinase with saruplase [21].

The short-term benefit of thrombolysis is often shown by the angiographically controlled patency of the infarct-related vessel (Table 2). Several short-term studies have shown that the spontaneous recanalization of the vessel is about 20%. By intracoronary administration of streptokinase, patency rates of between 60% and 79% can be achieved within 90 min [3, 14, 27]. With intravenous administration the short-term patency 60–90 min after treatment varies between 40% and 75% [5, 17, 20, 21, 28, 31]. Higher patency rates have also been documented when the control angiogram has been performed much later. It is, however, doubtful as to whether these late openings really contribute to the reduction of mortality and the improvement of ventricular wall motion. The late reopened vessel may only perfuse to a

Table 1. Hospital mortality rates after thrombolysis in acute myocardial infarction

Study	Treatment	Time after onset (h)	Number of patients (n)	Rate (%)	p
GISSI	SK	<3	3016	9.2	<0.0005
[11]	Control		3078	12.0	
	SK	>3–6	1849	11.7	<0.03
	Control		1800	14.1	
	SK	<1	635	8.2	<0.0001
	Control		642	15.4	
	SK	0–12	5860	10.7	<0.0002
	Control		5852	13.0	
ISIS II	SK	<24	8592	9.2	<0.00001
[13]	Control		8595	12.0	
GAUS	UK	<6	121	4.1	NS
[20]	rt-PA		124	4.8	
AIMS	APSAC	<6	502	6.4	$p = 0.0016$
[1]	Control		502	12.2	
APSAC MTG	APSAC	<4	162	5.6	$p = 0.032$
[18]	Control		151	12.6	
PAIMS	SK	<3	85	8.2	NS
[16]	rt-PA		86	4.6	
TIMI I	SK	<7	147	8.0	NS
[28]	rt-PA		143	5.0	
TIMI II	rt-PA	<4	1626	4.7	
[29]					
	rt-PA	<5	355	2.8	NS
[30]	Control		366	5.7	
PRIMI	SK	<4	203	4.9	NS
[21]	Saruplase		198	3.5	

SK, streptokinase; *rt-PA*, recombinant tissue-type plasminogen activator.

completely ischemic myocardial area, which on longer benefits from this reperfusion.

In the PRIMI study, comparison between the intravenous administration of saruplase (scu-PA) and streptokinase showed that, as soon as 60 min after the onset of treatment in the saruplase group, 71.8% of the vessels were open compared with 48.0% in the streptokinase group [21]. After 90 min the rates were 71.2% vs. 63.9%. After 34–36 h, however, the patency rates were very high and not different between groups (91.2% vs. 92.0%).

Many factors may influence the patency rate:

1. Definition of patency
2. Recanalization versus patency
3. Thrombolytic agent
4. Time to treatment start
5. Time to angiography
6. Repetitive coronary injections
7. Severity of underlying stenosis
8. Platelet-rich thrombi
9. Anterior > inferior infarctions

We also have to differentiate between patency and recanalization. Patency is the demonstration of an open vessel, be it spontaneous or caused by the thrombolytic agent. Recanalization, on the other hand, requires the reopening of a previously occluded vessel to be recorded. There is clearly a difference in the ability of different thrombolytic drugs to open the vessels (Table 2). The patency rate is not only dependent on the type of medication but also on the time of start of treatment, the time of angiographic control, and probably also the interference of repetitive coronary injections into the occluding thrombus. Not only the contrast medium but also the injection pressure may contribute to the reopening. If a highly obstructive atherosclerotic lesion is below the coronary thrombus, the recanalization rate may be lower than in vessels with only a flat atheroma. Further differences exist between the platelet-rich, white, and red thrombi. The results of the PRIMI study have also shown that the opening rate is higher in anterior than in inferior infarctions [21].

Despite initial success in the treatment of thrombosis, there is always a threat of early rethrombosis [19, 21, 24, 25, 27, 29, 32]. Many factors have been analyzed which are responsible for such rethrombosis:

1. Pathologic substrate

    a) Deep injury of ruptured plaque
    b) Exposure of collagen and fatty gruel
    c) Injured endothelium
    d) Lack of endothelium-derived vasodilators: prostacyclin and endothelium-derived relaxation factor
    e) Platelets activated by collagen and thrombin
    f) Thrombogenic surface of residual thrombosis

2. Rheology

    a) Residual stenosis
    b) Increase in shear rate
    c) Dead water zones

Table 2. Patency and Recanalization rates after thrombolysis in acute myocardial infarction

Study	Mode	No. of patients	Patency rate (%)	Treatment delay (min)	Dosage	Time of angiography
[27]	SK i.c.	269	79	195	250 000 U	−90 min
West. Wash [14]	SK i.c.	134	68	274	250 000–350 000 U	−90 min
[3]	SK i.c.	111	60	204	160 000 U	90 min
TIMI I [28]	SK i.v.	147	40	285	1.5	90 min
[31]	SK i.v.	65	55	156	1.5	75–90 m
PRIMI I [21]	SK i.v.	203	63.9	140	1.5	90 min
[5]	APSAC i.v.	42	64	150	30 U	15–90 m
[17]	UK i.v.	50	60	120	2	66 min
GAUS [20]	UK i.v.	117	65.8	?	3	90 min
[31]	rt-PA i.v.	64	70	180	0.75 mg/kg	75–90 m
TIMI I [28]	rt-PA i.v.	143	60	285	80 mg	90 min
TIMI II [29]	rt-PA i.v.	1626	84.7/84.6	162	150/100 mg	32.5 h
PRIMI [21]	Saruplase i.v.	197	71.2	139	80 mg	90 min

SK, streptokinase; *UK*, urokinase; *rt-PA*, recombinant tissue-type plasminogen activator.

Pathological and rheological features may contribute to vascular flow and the interference between the blood stream, the coagulation system, and the endothelium. Several studies have shown that the thrombolytic drugs have different capacities to keep the vessels open [21, 29].

The dynamic balance between thrombosis and thrombolysis can be influenced by optimization of the thrombolysis on the one hand and the subsequent antithrombotic therapy on the other hand (Table 3).

The major drawback and threat to thrombolytic treatment of acute myocardial infarction is bleeding complications (Table 4), which may occur because of the thrombolytic agent itself or because of additional therapy with heparin, acetylsalicylic acid, and other drugs [5, 11–13, 14–18, 20–22,

Table 3. Treatment for prevention of early and late rethrombosis after thrombolytic treatment in acute myocardial infarction

Heparin 100 IU/kg at start of lysis + ca. 1000 IU/h for at least 24 h
100 mg ASS for >3 months
3 × 10 − 20 mg/day nifedipine
Nitroglycerin i.v./oral nitrates
Sodium warfarin (Coumadin)?

Table 4. Bleeding complications in thrombolytic therapy of acute myocardial infarction

Study	Substance	Bleeding complications		
		No. of patients	Total bleedings (%)	Cerebral bleedings (%)
GISSI [11]	SK	5860	3.7	<1
TIMI I [28]	SK	147	31	0
PRIMI [28]	SK	203	24.6	0.5
[17]	UK	50	0	0
GAUS [20]	UK	121	22.3	0
[3]	APSAC	123	33	0
AIMS [1]	APSAC	503	5	0.4
[31]	rt-PA	64	26.6	0
TIMI I [28]	rt-PA	143	33	0
[30]	rt-PA	355	29.3	1.7
PAIMS [16]	rt-PA	86	9.0	0
TIMI II [29]	rt-PA	1626	12.9/12.6	1.9/0.5
PRIMI [21]	Saruplase	198	14.1	1.0

SK, streptokinase; *UK*, urokinase; *rt-PA*, recombinant tissue-type plasminogen activator.

26–31]. The definition of "bleeding" is different in the studies published so far [5, 15, 18, 21, 28, 29, 31]. While some authors count only the bleedings which needed transfusions or which have led to cerebrovascular damage, others have also mentioned minor hemorrhages. Especially in patients with acute catheterization, bleedings at the site of puncture are quite frequent and to be expected. Because of the age of the patients and previous hypertensive diseases, spontaneous bleedings may also occur, not only in the cerebrum but also in the retroperitoneal area and the abdomen.

The risk factors for bleeding in thrombolysis may be divided into general risk factors, already damaged vessels, and disturbances in the hemostaseologic system:

---

1. General risk factors

   a) Hypertension
   b) Aged vessels
   c) Proliferative diabetic retinopathy
   d) Liver/renal diseases
   e) Pericarditis sicca

2. Bleeding from already damaged vessels and lysis of previously formed thrombus

   a) Gastroduodenal ulcers
   b) Previous operation
   c) Previous vessel puncture
   d) Recent CNS tranma
   e) Urogenital disease

3. Hemostatic reasons

   a) Hemorrhagic diathesis
   b) Previous anticoagulation
   c) Adjuvant and subsequent anticoagulation

In the PRIMI study [21] the beginning rate was compared between the groups treated with saruplase and streptokinase. This showed that severe bleedings were not very frequent and often related to the puncture site. The administration of streptokinase has led to a significantly higher bleeding rate than that of saruplase.

The advantages of thrombolysis have to be balanced against the risk of cerebral bleedings as the most severe complication. There seems to be a relationship to the age of patient, male disease, previous hypertension, and rate of cerebral bleedings. The cerebral bleeding rate is between 0.5% and 1%. It has been shown in the TIMI study that higher doses of thrombolytic agents may lead to a higher rate of cerebrovascular bleeding. The lysis of an intracoronary clot by the intravenous administration of a thrombolytic substance can only take place via a general activation of the thrombolytic system. In this way, all thrombolytic agents bring about a decrease in fibrinogen, plasminogen, and α-2-antiplasmin, and a rise in fibrinogen degradation products and of D-dimer [21, 31]. Figure 2 shows the drop in fibrinogen after the administration of streptokinase and saruplase in the PRIMI study [21].

The substances available and tested for thrombolytic treatment at the moment are quite different (Table 5). They show individual fibrin enhancement and interference with the hemostatic state of plasma. While some drugs

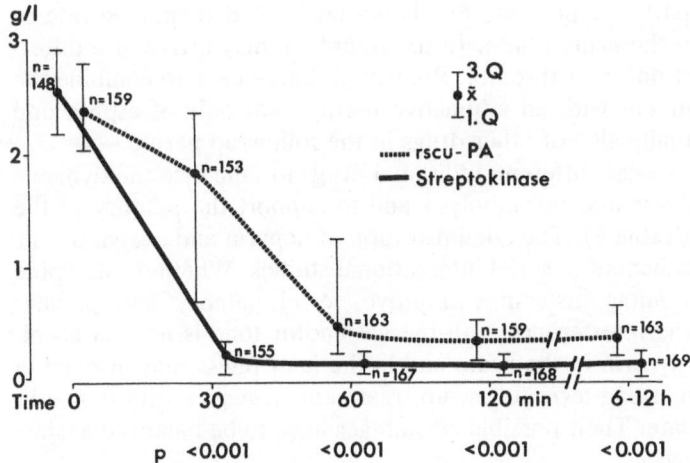

Fig. 2. Degradation of fibrinogen after treatment with streptokinase and saruplase (rscu-PA) in the PRIMI study. [21]

Table 5. Special features of thrombolytic drugs

	SK	APSAC	UK	rt-PA	Saruplase
Fibrin enhancement	+	+	++	+++	+++
Plasma proteolytic state	+++	+++	++	+	+
Simultaneous heparin	No	No	No	Yes	Yes
Bleedings	++	++	++	+	+
Allergic reactions	Yes	Yes	No	No	No
Pressure drop	Yes	Yes	No	No	No
Expense	+	++	++	+++	Not yet defined

SK, streptokinase; *UK*, urokinase; *rt-PA*, recombinant tissue-type plasminogen activator.

need additional treatment with heparin, others do not. Not only the rate of bleedings, but also the rate of allergic reactions and of decrease in arterial pressure are of importance. The indication for the use of thrombolytic therapy is finally also influenced by the availability of the drug, the ease of the administration mode, and the expenses. Up to now the drugs developed by gene technology seem not only to be the most effective but also the most expensive ones.

Despite the many advances over the past 10 years in the thrombolytic treatment of acute myocardial infarction, there are still unresolved questions. One of the major problems is to find drugs which show a high clot selectivity and have as few systemic actions as possible. There seem to be differences in the treatment of red and white, platelet-rich thrombi. Probably, different lytic substances have to be used in fresh versus old thrombi. The platelet-rich thrombi may be partly responsible for the so far limited reopening rate of only 70%–80% in the acute phase. In the future we may arrive at a differential treatment of different thrombi. We will probably have to combine the thrombolytic treatment with an adjunctive therapy not only of aspirin and heparin but eventually also of other drugs in the follow-up period.

In cardiology we use different additional drugs to influence the dynamic balance of thrombosis and thrombolysis and to support the patency of the reopened vessels (Table 3). The administration of heparin and acetylsalicylic acid has proven its benefit in serial international studies. Whether nifedipine or other calcium antagonists may improve vessel patency and prevent rethrombosis by the interference with the vasomotor tone is not yet absolutely clear. Nitroglycerin in the acute and in the later phase may also act in a similar direction. Long-term follow-up treatment strategies with oumadin are still under debate. Their possible advantages have to be balanced against the risk of bleeding.

New developments such as antifibrin monoclonal antibodies, and the increased importance of free radicals, superoxide dismutase, and catalase require analysis. In the coronary artery system we also need to deal with the underlying coronary atherosclerosis and the sometimes severe coronary obstruction in the area of the previous occlusion [10, 19, 29]. In some cases mechanical intervention with guidewires or intracoronary balloons is feasible [10, 19, 24].

Despite there being many differences between the thrombosis of cerebrovascular vessels and thrombosis in the coronary artery system, such as ischemic tolerance, collateral flow, danger of bleeding into the jeopardized area and others, there are also some similarities. In both cases the question of optimal treatment time arises. The opening rate has to be balanced against the danger of reocclusion. The severity of the underlying atherosclerotic disease not only in the involved vessel but also in other areas of the body may interfere with the indication to start treatment in the individual patient. Since any thrombolytic treatment and the additional medical and also angiographic and instrumental measures may be harmful to the patient, we have to decide,

Table 6. Contraindications for Thrombolysis [2]

Not eligible for thrombolysis	76%
Age >75 years	31%
Nondiagnostic ECG	50%
Pain >6 h	25%
Hypertension >180/100 mmHg	19%
Cerebrovascular disease	12%
Recent surgery/trauma	9%
Coma	4%
Bleeding	3%
Renal failure	3%
Other reasons	4%

in each situation, whether it will be of advantage of the patient to use such drugs. The study by Althouse et al. [2] has demonstrated that because of several contraindications only a fraction of the patients admitted to hospital can be treated with thrombolysis (Table 6).

References

1. AIMS Trial Study Group (1988) Effect of intravenous APSAC on mortality after acute myocardial infarction. Lancet i:545–549
2. Althouse R, Maynard C, Olsufka M, Kennedy JW (1988) Incidence of contraindications to thrombolysis in patients with myocardial infarction. Circulation 78(Suppl II) 211
3. Anderson JL, Marshall HW, Bray BE dute JR, Frederick PR, Yanowite FG, Date FL, Klausner SC, Hagan AD (1983) A randomized trial of intracoronary streptokinase in the treatment of acute myocardial infarction. N Engl J Med 308:1312–1318
4. Baroldi G (1976) Coronary thrombosis:facts and beliefs. Am Heart J 91:683–688
5. Bonnier HJRM, Visser RF, Klamps HC, Hoffmann HJML (1988) Comparison of intravenous anisoylated plasminogen streptokinase activator complex and intracoronary streptokinase in acute myocardial infarction. Am J Cardiol 61:25–30
6. Braunwald E, Kloner RA (1982) The stunned myocardium:prolonged, postischemic ventricular dysfunction. Circulation 66:1146–1149
7. Chazov EJ, Mateeva LS, Mazaev AV, Sargin KE, Sadovskaya GV, Ruda MY (1976) Intracoronary administration of fibrinolysin in acute myocardial infarction. Ter Arkh 48:8–19
8. Chesebro JH, Knatterud G, Roberts R Borery, Cohen LS, Dalen J, Dodge HT, Francis CK, Hillis D, Ludbrook P, Markis JE, Huellerth, Passamani ER, Powers ER, Rao AK, Robertson T, Ross A, Ryan TJ, Sobel E, Willerson J, Williams DO, Qaret BL, Brannwald E (1987) Thrombolysis in myocardial infarction (TIMI) trial, phase I:a comparison between intravenous tissue plasminogen activator and intravenous streptokinase. Circulation 76:142–154
9. Wood MA de, Spores J, Notske R, Mouser LT, Burroughs R, Golden MS, Lang HT (1980) Prevalence of total coronary occlusion during the early hours of transmural myocardial infarction. N Engl J Med 303:897–902
10. Erbel R, Pop T, Meinertz T, Kasper W, Schreiner G, Henkel B, Henrichs KJ, Pfeiffer C, Rupprecht HJ, Meyer J (1985) Combined medical and mechanical recanalization in acute myocardial infarction. Cathet Cardiovasc Diagn 11:361–377
11. Gruppo Italiano per lo Studio della Streptochinasi nell Infarto Miocardico (GISSI) (1986) Effectiveness of intravenous thrombolytic treatment in acute myocadial infarction. Lancet i:397–402
12. ISIS Steering Committee (1987) Intravenous streptokinase given within 0–4 hours of onset of myocardial infarction reduced mortality in ISIS-2. Lancet i:502
13. ISIS-2 Collaborative Groups (1988) Randomised trial of intravenous streptokinase, oral aspirin, both, or neither among 17187 cases of suspected acute myocardial infarction. Lancet ii:349–360
14. Kennedy JW, Ritchie JL, Davis KB, Fritz JK (1983) Western Washington randomized trial of intracoronary streptokinase in acute myocardial infarction. N Engl J Med 309:1477–1481
15. Kennedy JW, Martin GV, Davis KB, Maynard C, Stadius M, Sheehan FH, Ritchie JL (1988) The Western Washington intravenous streptokinase in acute myocardial infarction randomized trial. Circulation 77:345–352
16. Magnani B, for the PAIMS Investigastors (1989) Plasminogen activator Italian multicenter study (PAIMS) comparison of intravenous recombinant single-chain human

tissue-type plasminogen activator (rt-PA) with intravenous streptokinase in acute myocardial infarction. J Am Coll Cardiol 13:19–26

17. Mathey DG, Schofer J, Sheehan FH, Becker H, Tilsner V, Dodge HT (1985) Intravenous urokinase in acute myocardial infarction. Am J Cardiol 55:878–882

18. Meinertz T, Kasper W, Schumacher M, Just H, for the APSAC Multicenter Trial Group (1988) The German multicenter trial of anisoylated plasminogen streptokinase activator complex versus heparin for acute myocardial infarction. Am J Cardiol 62:347–351

19. Meyer J, Merx W, Schmitz H, Erbel R, Kiesslich T, Dörr R, Lambertz H, Bethge C, Krebs W, Bardos P, Minale C, Messmer BJ, Effert S (1982) Percutaneous transluminal coronary angioplasty immediate after intracoronary streptolysis of transmural myocardial infarction. Circulation 66:905–913

20. Neuhaus KL, Tebbe U, Gottwik M, Weber MAJ, Feurer W, Niederer W, Haerer W, Praetorius F, Grosser KD, Huhmann W, Hoepp HW, Alber G, Sheikhzadeh JA, Schneider B (1988) Intravenous recombinant tissue plasminogen activator (rt-PA) and urokinase in acute myocardial infarction:results of the German activator urokinase study (GAUS). J Am Coll Cardiol 12:581–587

21. Primi Trial Study Group (1989) Randomized double-blind trial of recombinant prourokinase against streptokinase in acute myocardial infarction. Lancet i:863–868

22. Rao AK (1988) Thrombolysis in myocardial infarction (TIMI) trial phase I: hemorrhagic manifestations and changes in plasma fibrinogen and the fibrinolytic system in patients treated with recombinant tissue plasminogen activator and streptokinase. J Am Coll Cardiol 11:1–11

23. Rentrop P, Blanke H, Karsch KR, Wiegand V, Köstering H, Rahlf G, Oster H, Leitz K (1979) Wiedereröffnung des Infarktgefäßes durch transluminale Rekanalisation und intrakoronare Streptokinase-Applikation. Dtsch Med Wochenschr 104:1438–1440

24. Rutsch W, Schartl M, Mathey D, Kuck K, Merx W, Dörr R, Rentrop P, Blanke H, Karsch K (1982) Perkutane, transluminale, koronare Rekanalisation: Methodik, Ergebnisse und Komplikationen. Z Kardiol 71:7–13

25. Santoro GM, Bisi G, Sciagra R, Leoncini M, Fazzini PF, Meldolesi V (1990) Single photon emission computed tomography with technetium-9 m hexakis 2-methoxyisobutyl isonitrile in acute myocardial infarction before and after thrombolytic treatment – assessement of salvaged myocardium and prediction of late functional recovery. J Am Coll Cardiol 15:301–314

26. Schröder R, Biamino G, von Leitner ER, Linderer T (1981) Intravenöse Streptokinase-Infusion bei akutem Myokardinfarkt. Dtsch Med Wochenschr 106:294–301

27. Simoons ML, van den Brand M, de Zwan C, Verhengt FWA, Remme WJ, Serruys PW, Bär F, Res J, Krauss XH, Vermeer F, Lubsen J (1985) Improved survival after early thrombolysis in acute myocardial infarction. Lancet ii:578–581

28. TIMI Study Group (1985) The thrombolysis in myocardial infarction (TIMI) trial phase I findings. N Engl J Med 312:932–936

29. TIMI Study Group (1989) Comparison of invasive and conservative strategies after treatment with intravenous tissue plasminogen activator in acute myocardial infarction. Results of the thrombolysis in myocardial infarction (TIMI) phase II trial. N Engl J Med 320:618–627

30. van de Werf F, Arnold AER (1988) Intravenous tissue plasminogen activator and size of infarct, left ventricular function, and survival in acute myocardial infarction. Br Med J 297:1374–1379

31. Verstraete M, Bernard R, Bory M, Brower RW, Collen D, deBono DP, Erbel R, Huhmann W, Lennane RJ, Lubsen J, Mathey D, Meyer J, Michels HR, Rutsch W, Schartl M, Schmidt W, Uebis R, von Essen R (1985) Randomised trial of intravenous recombinant tissue-type plasminogen activator versus intravenous streptokinase in acute myocardial infarction. Lancet ii:842–847

32. White CW (1989) Recurrent ischemic events after successful thrombolysis in acute myocardial infarction. Circulation 80:1482–1485

33. White HD, Norris RM, Brown MA (1987) Effect of intravenous streptokinase on left ventricular function and early survival after acute myocardial infarction. N Engl J Med 317:850–855
34. Yusuf S, Collins R, Peto R, Furberg C, Stampter MJ, Goldhaber SZ, Hennekens CH (1985) Intravenous and intracoronary fibrinolytic therapy in acute myocardial infarction: overview of results on mortality, reinfarction and side effects from 33 randomized controlled trials. Eur Heart J 6:556–585

Reperfusion of Ischemic Brain: Why and Why Not!

L.R. CAPLAN

Since the time of William Harvey, physiologists, anatomists, and clinicians alike have viewed the heart and circulatory system as supporting actors whose role it was to provide blood to the various organs of the body. Arguably the principal organ supplied is the brain, which controls the perceptions, thoughts, and actions of the body. Clearly, the raison d'etre of the arteries coursing to the brain is to supply blood which carries fuel, mainly sugar and oxygen, to nervous system structures which cannot function without it. When an artery is blocked, even temporarily, the brain is deprived of fuel and stops working just as a car would without gas. If fuel is lacking for long enough, the brain wilts, softens, and dies. Some components seem more vulnerable to the lack of fuel supply and die before others.

Although I am confident that neurologists and neuroscientists now accept this interpretation as indisputable fact, this was not always the case. Not until the work of Rudolph Virchow in the mid-nineteenth century was the relationship between brain softenings (also called encephalomalacia or ramollissements) and vascular disease clarified [9, 31]. Virchow showed that blockage of arteries, either because of in situ clotting provoked by intimal disease or an embolus from another site, caused the softenings. The terms "ischemia," "lack of blood," and "infarction" replaced the purely descriptive nonetiological terms "softenings" or "encephalomalacias." Before Virchow, some had thought the organ lesion caused the vascular process, or that the organ and vascular lesions were simply fellow travelers.

Ischemia and Ischemic Thresholds

More recently, it has become possible to quantitate the brain's need for blood. This can be done in experimental animals by blocking arteries, and measuring the residual blood flow, electrical activity and functions, and the chemical nature of the tissues within the region supplied. Heiss and Rosner showed, in cats with reversible middle cerebral artery occlusion, that spon-

Department of Neurology, Tufts University, New England Medical Center Hospitals, 750 Washington Street, Boston, MA 02111, USA.

Hacke et al. (Eds)
Thrombolytic Therapy in Acute Ischemic Stroke
© Springer-Verlag Berlin Heidelberg 1991

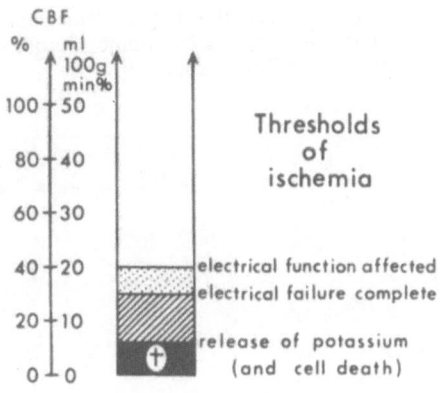

CBF

% ml
100g
min%

Thresholds
of
ischemia

electrical function affected
electrical failure complete

release of potassium
(and cell death)

Fig. 1. Ischemic thresholds for electrical failure and for release of cellular potassium ion. (From [20])

taneous electrical activity ceased at flow values on average of 18 ml/100 g per minute [16]. Neurons exposed to a residual flow of 14 ml/100 g per minute or less for more than 45 min usually did not recover function even after reperfusion [16]. Electrical activity (baseline EEG, evoked responses, or central conduction time) is diminished at flow levels below 15 ml/100 g per minute [2, 13]. The cerebral metabolic rate for oxygen (CMRO$_2$) begins to fall when the cerebral blood flow (CBF) goes below 20 ml/100 g per minute and energy exchange is also altered below this level of blood flow [20]. Below 10 ml/100 g per minute there is outpouring of potassium ions from the cells, and calcium ions move into cells through ischemic membranes and irreversible cell death results [20]. Figure 1 from Jafar and Crowell [20] graphically depicts these ischemic thresholds.

The effects of reperfusion have been studied in experimental models. The duration of time that flow is diminished and the severity of the decreased perfusion, of course, are very important variables. How long does flow need to be diminished to cause infarction? Sundt and colleagues, in 1969, temporarily occluded the middle cerebral artery with a ligature in 100 squirrel monkeys and 30 cats [30]. Camera pictures of the brain surface effects of reperfusion showed that, immediately after removal of the ligature, the arteries distal to the ligature dilated to their normal size and were filled with bright red blood instead of the previous darker "venous blood." The cortex quickly regained its normal color and shape. Restoration of blood flow after 3 h in the monkey and 6 h in the cat reduced the size of infarction in Sundt's model [30]. Crowell and colleagues more recently showed, in a middle cerebral artery ligature study in monkeys, that deficits from ischemia were commonly reversible after 30 min and 4 h of occlusion but rarely reversed if the ligature was placed for 8 h or more [5]. Figure 2 shows the relationship of time and severity of reduced CBF to infarction in their study. Reperfusion, i.e., bringing in more blood into the temporarily ischemic zone, usually allowed the limping brain to recover when the length of ischemia was less than 4 h. These results are just what Virchow and naive, unsuspecting neuro-

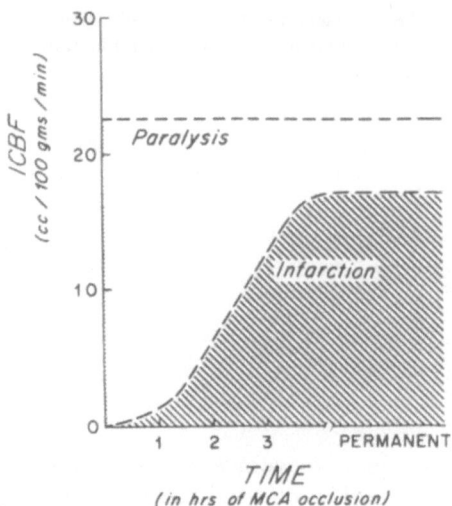

Fig. 2. Ischemia thresholds. Time and severity of ischemia determine morphologic reversibility. (From [20]).

scientists and clinicians should expect. After all if the problem is too little blood, more blood surely should help. Intuitively, the longer and more severe the ischemia, the less likely would be recovery. The title I was given for today was why reperfuse the brain? The material presented so far should stimulate the intelligent listener to turn the question. Surely why *not* reperfuse the ischemic brain seems an eminently more sensible and practical query. I will devote the rest of my time to the issue of why not reperfuse?

Delayed Neurological Deterioration After Hypoxia and Ischemia: Reperfusion Injury

The first clinical clue that bringing fuel to a previously deprived brain might not always be beneficial was the report by Plum et al. in 1962 describing delayed neurological deterioration after anoxic insults [25]. In this report five patients were described. Three had had pure anoxic insults (two had carbon monoxide exposure and one crawled into a tank of pure nitrogen gas) and the other two had prolonged hypotension possibly with poor ventilation during or after surgery. The anoxic insults were severe; all patients were immediately comatose but awakened within 24 h. All patients resumed activities within a few days. After a delay of up to 13 days (4- to 13-day range; average, 9 days), mental changes developed and motor abnormalities were prominent. The delayed deterioration was severe and, in fact, fatal in two patients. The other three patients had some degree of recovery after their delayed neurological deterioration. Necropsy in the two fatal cases showed extensive cerebral hemispheric white matter changes with demyelination. One patient had degeneration of pallidal neurons. The demyelination was severe and involved nearly the entire hemispheric white matter except for subcortical arcuate fibers. There were no important vascular changes. Later, Protass reported a similar instance of delayed deterioration in a 16-year-old boy who had been found cyanotic and comatose after a heroin overdose [27]. He awakened on the 2nd hospital day but on day 5 deteriorated and became unresponsive and decorticate. Recovery began after 3 weeks. Dooling and Richardson described a tragic case of delayed neurologic deterioration in an 11-year-old boy who had been assaulted and strangled. A week after the assault he developed cognitive and behavioral changes and very abnormal motor signs, including episodic posturing and abnormal limb movements. Autopsy showed cavitating lesions in the caudate nuclei, putamen, and globus pallidus bilaterally with sparing of the white matter and cerebral cortex [7].

In an experimental model of forebrain ischemia in rats, Pulsinelli and colleagues were able to show histological evidence of delayed neuronal changes [28]. After permanent bilateral vertebral artery occlusions, the carotid arteries were temporarily occluded for 10, 20, or 30 min and the animals were killed at various later intervals. The number of damaged neurons increased significantly between the 24- and 72-h specimens. In both the clinical situations and the experimental models, it was difficult to know if the delayed neurologic deterioration and morphologic abnormalities were set in motion by the original insult but merely took time to mature (that is, deterioration despite restitution of blood flow and oxygenation) or whether the restitution of oxygen and blood flow somehow promoted the changes.

Another hint that some blood flow might be worse than none also came from animal experiments [24]. Hossman and Kleihues showed that animals exposed to 60 min of ischemia fared worse if a low level of blood flow remained than if circulation was absent [17]. In their model of global ischemia, reperfusion was often followed by poor recirculation. Rehncrona et al. showed that there was poorer biochemical recovery in rat brains after 30 min of partial ischemia than in brains with the same period of complete ischemia [29]. However, all of these situations are those of global brain ischemia, or hypoxia, or hypoxia and ischemia. Though they might mimic cardiac arrest or shock, they do not resemble infarcts caused by occlusion of cerebral arteries which are focal ischemic processes. Brain hypoxia without reduction in blood flow as induced by hypoxemia does not reproduce the cellular consequences of ischemia [29] and the brain pathology after cardiac arrest is quite different from thrombotic or embolic brain infarcts.

The concept of "reperfusion injury" after focal infarction has been much discussed but evidence of its occurrence has been scanty. Babbs, in a paper reviewing his theory of reperfusion injury, cites a study of reperfusion in rat hearts [1]. Creatinine kinase release occurred only after oxygen was restored, leading the authors to conclude that myocardial injury occurred during the period of reperfusion. deCourten-Myers and colleagues recently showed that, in hyperglycemic rats subjected to 4 h of middle cerebral artery (MCA) clipping, reperfusion usually reduced the size of infarction but some animals showed augmented tissue damage [6]. There was a bimodal distribution of results in the reperfused hyperglycemic animals, either no or little infarction or very large fatal infarcts. The larger infarcts were characterized by massive edema in contrast to nonreperfused specimens [6].

How Might Reperfusion Be Harmful?

Although reperfusion has not been shown conclusively to harm nerve cells, there are ways that introduction of blood could potentially injure tissues that had previously been ischemic. The influx into the ischemic region could:

1. Cause bleeding from previously damaged capillaries
2. Cause edema because of breakdown of membranes and capillary functions
3. Bring particles into the region such as platelet aggregates, platelet-fibrin nidi, cholesterol crystals, or thrombin clots that had formed during the period of ischemia
4. Carry substrates into the region such as sugar and oxygen that might be metabolized suboptimally or abnormally by the ischemic tissue leading to the accumulation of lactate or free radicals
5. Cause increased circulation of chemicals formed within the ischemic zone such as glutamate and other potential excitotoxins, oxygen-free radicals, potassium, calcium
6. Bring calcium and potassium into the region causing influx of these substances into cells through damaged membranes

There is evidence that hemorrhagic infarction and edema can be potentiated by reperfusion so I will concentrate on these topics. The other theoretical biochemical concerns will be touched on briefly but will be discussed further by others.

Hemorrhage into the Region of the Infarction

In 1950, Fisher and Adams presented their theory of the mechanism of hemorrhagic infarction to the American Association of Neuropathologists. The full text was published 37 years later, probably giving this paper the longest gestation of any paper I know of [10]. Simply stated, Fisher and Adams related hemorrhagic infarction to reperfusion of ischemic zones. The major evidence cited related to the location of hemorrhagic infarction, and the absence of thrombi that could explain the extent of the infarction. They presented several specimens in which hemorrhagic infarction occurred in deep zones fed by penetrating arteries or branches proximal to a thrombus found at necropsy. The brain regions distal to the thrombus had bland infarction without evidence of hemorrhage. The authors posited that an embolus had blocked an artery proximally leading to capillary damage. The embolus had moved distally allowing blood to course into the proximal region and to leak through damaged capillaries causing hemorrhagic infarction. The distal region was still blocked so that it escaped bleeding. Since the time of Fisher and Adams' original report, hemorrhagic infarction is most often seen after embolism, and after infarction due to systemic hypotension and later restoration of blood flow. In some cases hemorrhagic infarction is seen in zones where the feeding arteries are still occluded.

Garcia and colleagues studied the response of capillaries and reperfusion in an experimental model of focal ischemia [12]. The MCA was occluded for 30, 60, and 120 min and the ultrastructure of capillaries was examined after reperfusion. He found expansion of capillaries often with rupture and interruption of the endothelial linings of capillaries. The severity of the capillary changes paralleled the duration of ischemia. Garcia believed that the changes in the capillaries explained hemorrhagic infarction. Crowell and colleagues, also using an experimental model of MCA temporary ischemia, showed that hemorrhagic infarction correlated with longer duration of clipping and presumably with the severity of ischemia [4].

Edema Augmented by Reperfusion

There is now considerable evidence that, in some experimental animals and patients, reperfusion causes an increase in edema within the zone of ischemia. Plum et al. in an early study of experimental ischemia in 1963 showed, in a model of focal ischemia produced by ligation of an artery, that edema correlated with cell necrosis and breakdown of the blood-brain barrier as shown by trypan-blue staining [26]. Sundt and colleagues in their large study (130 animals) already cited of focal ischemia showed that edema was slightly worse in the zone of infarction in those animals that had restoration of blood flow (30). The proposed mechanism was disruption of the blood-brain barrier with passage of osmotically active particles and fluid into the ischemic region.

Kuroiwa and colleages, in two experimental studies [21, 22], examined the function of the blood-brain barrier to test this hypothesis. In their first study they analyzed ischemia in cats caused by temporary 3-h clipping followed by 3 h of reperfusion and compared the results with animals that had 6-h clipping of the MCA without reperfusion [21]. They measured edema by specific gravity measures of tissue samples taken from coronal brain sections of the ischemic zone. The severity of the blood-brain barrier disruption was determined by measuring the amount of extravasated serum albumin labeled with [125]I. Edema was more severe in animals with 3 h of temporary ischemia followed by reperfusion than in animals put to death after 6 h of ischemia without reperfusion. In areas with blood-brain barrier disruption, edema was more extensive than in those with an intact barrier. The degree of edema correlated with the extent of extravasation of radioisotope-labeled protein [21].

In their second study of the blood-brain barrier in a focal temporary ischemia model, Kuroiwa and colleagues showed that the barrier opening was biphasic [22]. In this study, the authors used both an Evans-blue tracer and an immunohistochemical method of examining the barrier and vascular endothelia. They stained the tissues with a peroxidase-antiperoxidase immune serum. The initial opening of the blood-brain barrier occurred shortly after reperfusion. Opening occurred only in animals in which rCBF had been below 15 ml/100 g per minute and occurred during the phase of reactive hyperemia. There was then a phase of resistance to opening of the blood-brain barrier at 3 h after the reperfusion. A second opening of the blood-brain barrier occurred between 5 and 72 h after recirculation and was again limited to animals with rCBF below 15 ml/100 g per minute flow during the ischemia. At the time of the second opening, cerebrovascular endothelial linings including tight junctions looked normal. The authors concluded that the first opening was related to hemodynamic factors; the drastic increase in rCBF rushing through maximally dilated blood vessels led to outpouring of fluids. To explain the second opening, they invoked some hypothetical tissue factor derived from the ischemic zone that led to an opening of the blood-brain barrier [22]. They emphasized that there were two types of edema within the tissues, cytotoxic edema, related to swelling of cells and caused by cell ischemia, and vasogenic edema, related to interstitial fluid caused by breakdown of the blood-brain barrier [21].

Other authors [15, 32] concentrated on quantifying the effects of arterial pressures and hydrostatic pressure gradients on edema in animal models of focal ischemia. Both studies used permanent occlusion models without reperfusion. Hatashita and Hoff varied arterial pressures in a permanent MCA occlusion model in cats [15]. The duration and depth of ischemia were important factors in edema formation. Increased intraarterial pressure causing a hydrostatic pressure gradient led to more edema formation. Yamaguchi et al. analyzed edema formation in the core and periphery of a permanent MCA occlusion model in cats [32]. The severity of decreased rCBF correlated with cytotoxic edema in the core of the lesion and a hydrostatic pressure gradient induced edema formation in the peripheral zone. Maintenance of high perfusion pressure soon after ischemia somewhat suppressed edema formation in the core of the lesion by decreasing the severity of the ischemia.

Turning to human patients, Irino and colleagues studied the effects of reperfusion by analyzing the angiographic findings showing recanalization of previously blocked arteries [18, 19]. Using serial angiography, they selected patients in whom initial angiography showed occlusion and later films showed opening of the previously occluded area. Some of the arteries showed persistent narrowing of the arterial caliber in the area of previous occlusion. Capillary blush was common and correlated with mass effect produced by edema formation.

The studies cited lead me to conclude that reperfusion can enhance edema formation. Edema probably develops early after reperfusion due to rapid influx into zones with decreased blood-brain barrier and is associated with hyperemia. Edema can also occur later when the blood-brain barrier opens a second time. Edema formation probably only occurs when the initial ischemia has been severe (rCBF less than 15 ml/100 g per minute) and/or prolonged. The degree of edema probably correlates with hydrostatic pressure gradients between intraarterial pressure and tissue pressures.

Other, More Hypothetical Sequelae of Reperfusion

Some have speculated that reperfusion might wash into the ischemic zone particulate matter that could block distal vessels. The vascular occlusive process might lead to release of coagulation factors and factors that promote platelet aggregation and agglutination. Petito showed, in an experimental model of carotid occlusion in rats, that platelet thrombi form in association with infarcts [23]. In a gerbil model, Dougherty and colleagues showed that circulating platelet aggregates formed after carotid occlusion [8]. Conceivably, both red thrombi and platelet aggregates formed proximal to the opened artery could wash into the ischemic zone during reperfusion. Cholesterol crystals or calcified plaque material could also go into the zone but I cannot think why reperfusion would augment their influx.

Other putative hazards of reperfusion center around chemical and metabolic changes within the ischemic zone. Sugar metabolism is considered a very important factor. In reperfused infarcts, Hakim et al. showed with positron emission tomography (PET) that, despite an adequate supply of oxygen, reperfused tissue preferentially used glucose [14]. Spontaneous reperfusion enhanced anaerobic glycolysis. Plum, in his Wartenberg lecture of 1982, emphasized the potential hazards of anaerobic glycolysis [24]. A continued blood supply or reperfusion could lead to entry of glucose while oxygenation was poor. Enhanced anaerobic glycolysis would lead to the formation of lactate. Local lactic acidosis could harm tissues. The blood sugar level and extent of continued perfusion and reperfusion would be important factors in the extent of lactate formation [24]. Babbs, among others, has emphasized the possibility of free radical formation [1]. In this theory, partially reduced oxygen species, including superoxide radicals, hydrogen peroxide, and hydroxyl radicals, initiate lipid peroxidation and other deleterious oxidative reactions after reperfusion has brought oxygen into the ischemic zones [1]. Excitotoxins such as glutamate from within ischemic tissues [3] might be circulated widely during reperfusion. Calcium entering the tissue might enter cells through damaged membranes and augment cell death [11]. Although unquestionably these metabolic changes occur within ischemic zones, their relative importance, and the effect of reperfusion on these factors, is still in a rather early phase of investigation.

References

1. Babbs C (1988) Reperfusion injury of postischemic tissues. Ann Emerg Med 17:1148–1157
2. Branston NM, Symon L, Crockard HA, Pasztar E (1974) Relationship between the cortical evoked potential and local cortical blood flow following acute middle cerebral artery occlusion in the baboon. Exp Neurol 45:195–208
3. Collins RC, Dobkin B, Choi DW (1989) Selective vulnerability of the brain: new insights into the pathophysiology of stroke. Ann Int Med 110:992–1000
4. Crowell RM, Olsson Y, Klatzo I, Ommaya A (1970) Temporary occlusion of the middle cerebral artery in the monkey: clinical and pathological observations. Stroke 1:439–448
5. Crowell RM, Marcoux FW, deGirolami U (1981) Variability and reversibility of focal cerebral ischemia in unanesthetized monkeys. Neurol 31:1295–1302
6. de Courten-Myers G, Kleinholz M, Wagner K, Myers R (1989) Fatal strokes in hyperglycemic cats. Stroke 20:1707–1715
7. Dooling EC, Richardson EP (1976) Delayed encephalopathy after strangling. Arch Neurol 33:196–199
8. Dougherty JH, Levy DE, Weksler BB (1979) Experimental cerebral ischemia produces platelet aggregates. Neurol 29:1460–1465
9. Fisher CM (1987) The history of cerebral embolism and hemorrhagic infarction. In: Furlan AJ (ed) The heart and stroke. Springer, Berlin Heidelberg, New York, pp 2–16
10. Fisher CM, Adams RD (1951) Observations on brain embolism with special reference to hemorrhagic infarction. J Neuropathol Exp Neurol 10:92–94; also published (1987) In: Furlan AJ (ed) The heart and stroke. Springer, Berlin, Heidelberg, New York, pp 17–36
11. Garcia J, Anderson M (1989) Physiopathology of cerebral ischemia. CRC Crit Rev Neurobiol 4:303–24
12. Garcia JH, Lowry SL, Briggs L, Mitchem HL, Morawetz R, Halsey JH, Conger KA (1983) Brain capillaries expand and rupture in areas of ischemia and reperfusion. In: Reivich M, Hurtig H (ed) Cerebrovascular diseases. Raven, New York, pp 169–179
13. Hagardine JR, Branston NM, Symon L (1980) Central conduction time in primate brain ischemia – a study in baboons. Stroke 11:637–642
14. Hakim A, Pokrupa R, Villaneuva J, Diksic M, Evans AC Thompson CJ, Meyer E, Yamamoto YL, Feindel WH (1987) The effect of spontaneous reperfusion on metabolic function in early human cerebral infarcts. Ann Neurol 21:279–289
15. Hatashita S, Hoff JT (1986) Role of a hydrostatic pressure gradient in the formation of early ischemic brain edema. J Cereb Blood Flow Metab 6:546–552
16. Heiss W-D, Rosner G (1983) Functional recovery of cortical neurons as related to degree and duration of ischemia. Ann Neurol 14:294–301
17. Hossman K-A, Kleihues P (1973) Reversibility of ischemic brain damage. Arch Neurol 29:375–384
18. Irino T, Minami T, Taneda M, Hara K (1977) Brain edema and angiographic hyperemia in postrecanalized cerebral infarction. Acta Neurol Scand (Suppl) 64:134–35
19. Irino T, Taneda M, Minami T (1977) Angiographic manifestations in post recanalized cerebral infarction. Neurol 27:471–475

20. Jafar J, Crowell RM (1987) Focal ischemic thresholds. In: Wood JW (ed) Cerebral blood flow. McGraw-Hill, New York, pp 449–457
21. Kuroiwa T, Ting P, Martinez H, Klatzo I (1985) The biphasic opening of the blood-brain barrier to proteins following temporary MCA occlusion. Acta Neuropathol 68:122–129
22. Kuroiwa M, Shibutani M, Okeda R (1988) Blood-brain barrier disruption and exacerbation of ischemic brain edema after restoration of blood flow in experimental focal cerebral ischemia. Acta Neuropathol 76:62–70
23. Petito C (1979) Platelet thrombi in experimental cerebral infarction. Stroke 10:192–196
24. Plum F (1983) What causes infarction in ischemic brain: the Robert Wartenberg Lecture. 33:222–233
25. Plum F, Posner JB, Hain RF (1962) Delayed neurological deterioration after anoxia. Arch Neurol 110:18–25
26. Plum F, Posner JB, Alvord EC (1963) Edema and necrosis in experimental cerebral infarction. Arch Neurol 9:563–570
27. Protass LM (1971) Delayed postanoxic encephalopathy after heroin use. Ann Int Med 74:738–739
28. Pulsinelli WA, Brierley JB, Blum F (1982) Temporal profile of neuronal damage in a model of transient forebrain ischemia. Ann Neurol 11:491–498
29. Rehncrona S, Rosen I, Siesjo BK (1981) Brain lactic acidosis and ischemic cell damage I. Biochemistry and neurophysiology. J Cereb Blood Flow Metabol 1:297–311
30. Sundt TM, Grant W, Garcia J (1976) Restoration of middle cerebral artery flow in experimental infarction. J Neurosurg 31:311–322
31. Virchow R (1847) Ueber die akute Entzuendung der Arterien. Virchows Arch [A] 1:272–378
32. Yamaguchi S, Kobayashi S, Yamashita K, Kitani M (1989) Pial arterial pressure contribution to early ischemic brain edema. J Cereb Blood Flow Metabol 9:597–602

Thrombolysis in Stroke: Timing of Recanalization and Its Clinical Consequences

K. Asplund[1] and B. Carlberg

Thrombolytic therapy of evolving brain infarction is based on the concept that ischemic neurons can be salvaged by restoring blood supply to reversibly damaged tissue. In this article, the following aspects of timing will be discussed: (a) factors that determine the delay to start of treatment, (b) the time from onset of treatment to clot lysis, and (c) the impact of delay on recanalization, clinical outcome, and cost.

Since clinical data on thrombolytic therapy in stroke patients are very limited, this presentation relies to a large extent on data from experimental studies and thrombolytic therapy in patients with myocardial infarction. Emphasis will be on tissue plasminogen activator (t-PA), the thrombotic agent presently used in most clinical trials of cerebral thromboembolism.

What Factors Determine the Delay to Onset of Treatment?

In the ASSET trial of t-PA in myocardial infarction, a 5-h upper time limit was used for inclusion of patients. Of all subjects considered for the study, 45% had to be excluded because of too long delay [49]. In detailed studies of the reasons for delay in patients with myocardial infarction, time to hospital admission and in-hospital delays account for about equal proportions [41]. Approximately 50% of the delay in reaching the hospital is due to patient indecision about how to interpret the symptoms [48].

To explore what factors determine the delay to hospital admission, we have analyzed 803 consecutive patients admitted to our stroke unit. The patients are admitted directly from the emergency room of the single hospital serving a well-defined geographical district. We have documented that home care for stroke is rare and few patients are seen by a general practitioner before they seek hospital care for stroke [1].

Only a third of the total stroke patient population enters the hospital within the first 3 h after onset of symptoms (Fig. 1A). The delay is not dependent on patient age (Fig. 1B), but it is clearly determined by the

---

[1] Department of Medicine, University Hospital, 901 85 Umeå, Sweden.

Hacke et al. (Eds)
Thrombolytic Therapy in Acute Ischemic Stroke
© Springer-Verlag Berlin Heidelberg 1991

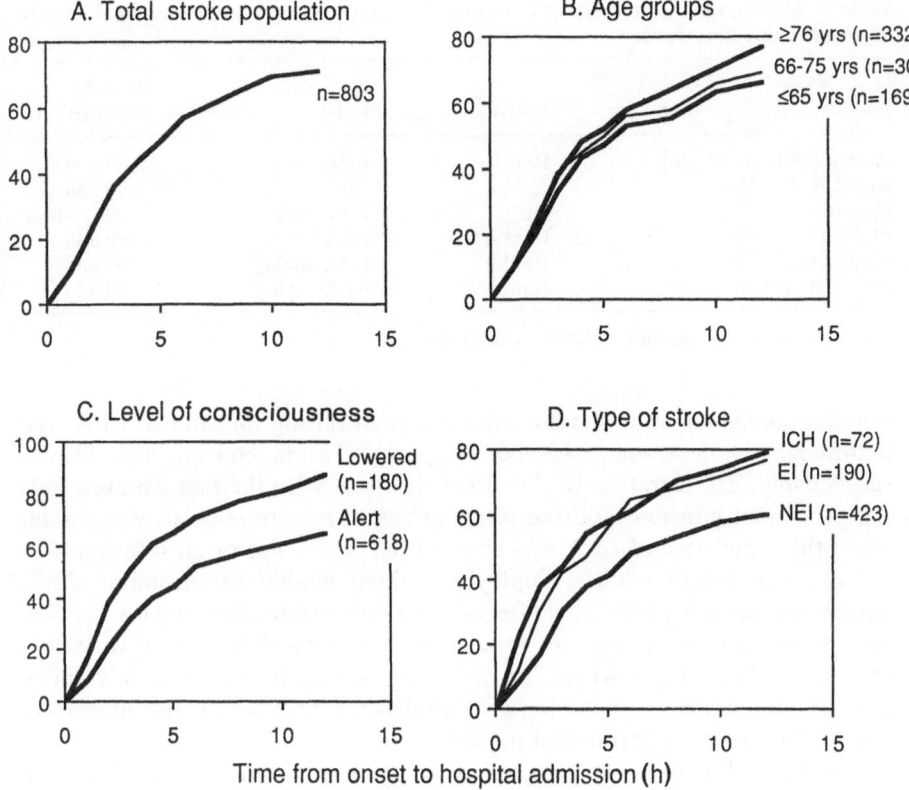

Fig. 1A–D. Delay from onset of symptoms to admission to hospital in subsets of a population-based sample of 803 consecutive patients with acute cerebrovascular disease. For each patient category, the accumulated proportion of patients is shown and 100% represents all patients entering the hospital within 1 week of onset. *ICH*, intracerebral hemorrhage; *EI*, embolic infarction; *NEI*, nonembolic infarction

severity of symptoms (Fig. 1C). Patients with intracerebral hemorrhage seek medical attention earlier than those with ischemic lesions (Fig. 1D). Of the patients with ischemic lesions and severe symptoms, 47% arrive at the hospital within the first 3h after onset of symptoms; this subset, a possible target group for early thrombolytic intervention, represents only 12% of all patients admitted to hospital for stroke.

How Rapid Is Recanalization Achieved After Start of Treatment?

In a rabbit jugular vein thrombosis model, Clozel et al. [6] found the effect of t-PA to be dependent on dose and mode of administration. Initial throm-

Table 1. Median time from onset of thrombolytic therapy to reperfusion in animal models
of thromboembolic stroke

Authors	Species	Drug	Time to reperfusion
Papadopoulos et al. [36]	Rat	t-PA	>30 min
Kissel et al. [25]	Rabbit	t-PA	>90 min
Hirschberg et al. [19]	Dog	Urokinase	30–55 min[a]
Phillips et al. [37]	Rabbit	t-PA	90 min
Phillips et al. [38]	Rabbit	t-PA analog	60 min
Fisher et al. [15]	Rabbit	t-PA analog	70 min

[a] Dependent on the duration of artery occlusion.

bolysis was higher after a bolus injection than during infusion of t-PA: the
half-maximal effect was achieved at approx. 15 min and approx. 30 min,
respectively. The duration of the effect was limited to the first 2 h even during prolonged infusion, and the ultimate extent of thrombolysis was similar
when the same dose of t-PA was given either as a bolus or an infusion [6].

In some recent studies employing animal models of thromboembolic
stroke and reporting beneficial effects of various thrombolytic agents, median
time from onset of therapy to reperfusion has ranged from <30 to 90 min
(Table 1). It should, however, be noted that not all investigators have been
able to demonstrate reperfusion of occluded cerebral vessels during thrombolytic therapy in experimental models.

In clinical studies of patients with acute myocardial infarction, the
average time to recanalization is 45–50 min even with the highest doses of
thrombolytic therapy [35]. In most studies of t-PA, the maximum proportion
of acute infarct vessel patency is approximately 75% [44, 46]; this plateau
is not reached until 90–120 min after onset of therapy [9]. In direct comparisons, the effect of rt-PA on coronary reperfusion was considerably faster
than that of streptokinase in one study [5] but not in another [32]. New, enhanced clot-selective agents have the potential to lyse thrombi more rapidly
[8].

In series of stroke patients subjected to thrombolytic therapy and repeated angiography the median time to clot lysis has generally been below

Table 2. Time from onset of thrombolytic therapy to angiographically verified reperfusion
in recent studies of patients with ischemic stroke

Authors	Vascular territory	Time to reperfusion in >50% of patients
del Zoppo et al. [12]	Carotid	<1–4 h
von Kummer et al. [47]	Carotid + vertebrobasilar	<90 min
Ikeda et al. [21]	Carotid	<60 min
Zeumer et al. [51]	Vertebrobasilar	<2 h

2h (Table 2), although the exact time relationships have not been possible to establish. When the experiences from experimental studies and clinical studies on patients with myocardial infarction and ischemic stroke are combined, it seems reasonable to assume that clot lysis occurs within 45–90 min of the start of treatment in the majority of cases.

Does Early Treatment Increase the Chance of Reperfusion?

In experimental vein thrombosis, clots can still be lysed after 24h [7] or even 7 days [29] of aging. Prolonging the t-PA infusion may increase the extent of lysis of old thrombi [24]. In animal stroke models, autologous [31, 37] or human blood clots [36] aged 18–24h are readily dissolved and internal carotid arteries are reperfused by t-PA or a t-PA analogue.

When data from the European Cooperative Study Group trial and the TIMI trial of patients with acute myocardial infarction were combined [30], the proportion of patients with patent coronary arteries decreased modestly with time; this was apparent for both t-PA and streptokinase (Fig. 2). On the other hand, in the TAMI trial involving 386 patients with acute myocardial infarction treated with t-PA, no relationship was found between the time interval from symptom onset to treatment and reperfusion after adjustment for confounding variables [4].

There are several reports on successful recanalization in acute thromboembolic stroke despite relatively long intervals from onset of symptoms to start of treatment. In patients with occlusions in the carotid vascular territory, complete recanalization following local intraarterial treatment

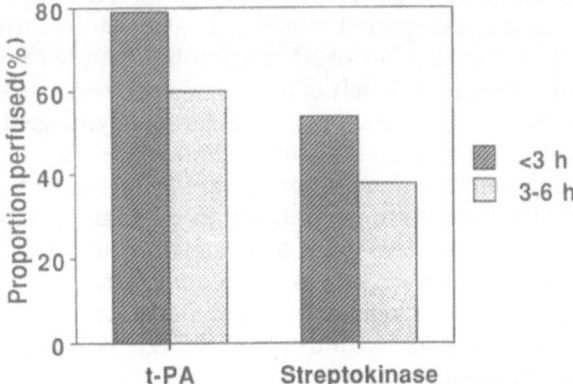

Fig. 2. Proportion of patients with angiographically verified patent coronary arteries in relation to delay to start of treatment. Combined data from the European Cooperative Study Group trial and the TIMI trial of patients with acute myocardial infarction as calculated by Loscalzo and Braunwald [30]

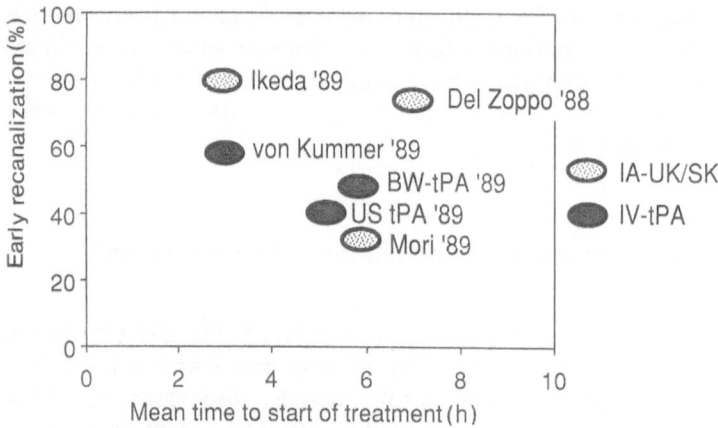

Fig. 3. Rate of recanalization as reported in series of patients with carotid territory occlusions undergoing thrombolytic treatment in relation to the mean interval from onset of symptoms to start of treatment. First author and year of publication are given. *IA-UK/SK*, intraarterial urokinase or streptokinase; *IV-tPA*, intravenous tissue plasminogen activator

with streptokinase or urokinase was obtained in 15 out of 20 patients despite a relatively long delay (mean 7.6 h) from onset of symptoms to start of therapy [12]. Locally administered urokinase has been reported to lyse clots in the vertebrobasilar territory as late as 8 h [51] after onset of symptoms. In other reported cases of basilar artery occlusions, Zimmermann et al. [52] noted complete resolution in a patient with 96 h of symptoms before start of treatment with urokinase, and Zeumer et al. [50] achieved recanalization when intraarterial streptokinase treatment was started 7 days after onset of symptoms.

In Fig. 3, the effect of thrombolytic therapy on recanalization rates in patients with carotid artery stroke, as reported in articles or abstracts by early 1990, have been summarized. There is no overt relationship between the delay and the proportion of recanalized vessels in these studies. It seems that factors other than time, such as patient selection, type of thrombolytic agent, doses, and mode of administration, account for a major share of the variation in recanalization rates. The results are given as group means and it is possible that analyses based on individual cases are more informative. Also, in none of the patient series has the mean time to onset of treatment been shorter than 3 h. The most recent series of stroke patients undergoing thrombolytic therapy in the Federal Republic of Germany and United States suggest that there may, after all, be a modest time dependency on the rate of recanalization (see elsewhere in this volume).

Interpretation of the time-dependent rate of recanalization is complicated by the fact that spontaneous thrombolysis and recanalization appears to be common in the cerebral arteries. Based on positron emission tomography studies, Hakim et al. [18] concluded that the ischemic cortex may be reperfused in a third of patients within 48 h of clinical onset of stroke. Signs of very early reperfusion in a substantial proportion of stroke patients investigated within 6 h have been documented by Fieschi et al. [14].

To summarize these observations, it seems that, as the clot ages, the possibility to lyse it may be somewhat reduced, but this probably plays only a minor role in view of the importance of other time factors that decide the ultimate clinical outcome after thrombolytic therapy.

What Are the Consequences of the Delay in Patient Survival and Function?

Experiences from the three largest randomized studies of thrombolytic therapy in acute myocardial infarction indicate that the beneficial effects on survival are time dependent but that they extend to at least 5 h after onset in all three trials [17, 22, 49]. In one of the two streptokinase studies, a significant treatment effect was still present in the 12- to 24-h interval [22], whereas the GISSI study [17] showed a gradual reduction of therapeutic effects with increasing time to onset of treatment. The ASSET trial, involving t-PA, did not include patients later than 5 h after onset of symptoms, but within this time frame, late treatment (3–5 h) reduced the risk to the same extent as early treatment [49]. Early (versus late) treatment has also been associated with improved myocardial function (assessed as ejection fraction) in survivors in one study [45].

Any conclusions about the effect of timing of thrombolytic therapy on outcome in acute ischemic stroke must rely on case reports and data from animal studies. In published patient series, the lack of consistent time relationships is apparent. At one end of the spectrum, del Zoppo et al. [12] reported on three patients who had carotid artery embolic events during angiographic procedures and received thrombolytic therapy within 1 h. Complete recanalization was observed in all three patients but none showed clinical improvement. At the other extreme, Zimmermann et al. [52] induced nearly full remission in a comatose patient with occlusion of the basilar artery in whom urokinase was administered 96 h after onset of symptoms. Complete or nearly complete restitution of neurological symptoms or "excellent outcome" has been reported in some of the patients with carotid artery ischemic events treated 4–10 h [17] and vertebrobasilar occlusion treated 4–6 h [51] after onset of ischemic stroke. Within these time frames, there is no apparent relationship between onset-treatment interval and clinical outcome [12]. Surgical intervention against carotid artery occlusions approx. 6 h after onset of symptoms has been associated with good clinical outcome when compared with a group of similar patients that were not operated upon [16]. The effect of very early treatment with t-PA (within 90 min) as used by Brott et al. [2] is difficult to assess in the absence of a control group. These investi-

Table 3. Time to onset of thrombolytic treatment versus outcome in experimental stroke models

Authors	Species	Delay	Recanalization	Infarction	Neurology
Zivin et al. [53]	Rabbit	2 min	NA	Not reduced	Improved
Kissel et al. [25]	Rabbit	30 min	Yes	Reduced	Improved
Phillips et al. [37]	Rabbit	15 min	Yes	Not reduced	NA
Zivin et al. [54]	Rabbit	45 min	NA	Not reduced	Improved
Zivin et al. [54]	Rabbit	60 min	NA	Not reduced	Not improved
Lee et al. [28]	Rabbit	0–30 min	Yes	NA	Reduced mortality
Lyden et al. [31]	Rabbit	15/90 min	Yes	Not reduced	NA
Papadopoulos et al. [36]	Rat	2 h	Yes	NA	Improved EEG
De Ley et al. [11]	Dog	30 min	Yes	Not reduced	NA
Del Zoppo et al. [10]	Monkey	3 h	(Yes)	Reduced	Improved

Reported changes that have not achieved statistical significance have been considered as negative results. *NA*, data not available in the article.

gators treated only patients with mild or moderate neurological deficits, and the outcome in such patients is often excellent [39].

Hakim et al. [18] demonstrated that spontaneous reperfusion within the first 48 h was associated not only with hyperemia but also with a marked improvement in cerebral metabolic rate for glucose and partial recovery of neurological deficits. The improvement in glucose metabolic rate occurred despite the appearance of hypodense lesions on CT scan. These observations indicate that reperfusion may be clinically meaningful even if it does not salvage all ischemic brain tissue [14].

The experiences of experimental studies are equally conflicting. As shown in Table 3, very early thrombolytic treatment (with documented recanalization in most cases) was often not associated with an effect on infarct size or neurological outcome. The most encouraging results were obtained by del Zoppo et al. [11] in a primate model: they demonstrated reduced cerebral infarct size and improved neurology when urokinase treatment was started 3 h after embolization. Others have reached more dismal conclusions from animal studies: ischemic changes are reversible only when thrombolytic therapy is started within 30 min [28].

Thus, the limited information available supports the contention that thrombolytic treatment may be beneficial in some patients as late as 6–8 h after onset of symptoms. In this regard, the time relationships for ischemic stroke seem to be similar to those for myocardial ischemia. However, other stroke patients do not benefit even from very early treatment and animal studies suggest that, under some circumstances, recanalization within the first ½ h does not salvage brain tissue. The reasons for these discrepancies have not been established, but restoration of blood flow to partly hypoperfused areas surrounding a core of ischemic brain tissue is the most apparent explanation for the partial success of thrombolytic therapy started several hours after the index event. It may also be that some of the reported improvements are not related to reperfusion but to delayed neuronal recovery analogous to the late functional recovery of "stunned" myocardium [13].

Are Hemorrhagic Complications and Brain Edema Dependent on Delay?

Serial CT scans indicate that spontaneous hemorrhagic transformation occurs in 11%–42% of patients whose initial examination showed nonhemorrhagic lesions [20, 40]. Among the factors influencing the tendency of infarcts to bleed are infarct size, cerebral perfusion pressure, and altered clotting mechanisms [42]. Exposure of damaged vessels to the full force of re-established perfusion pressure is one of several underlying pathophysiological mechanisms, and endothelial damage seems to increase with time of ischemia [23, 33].

A few controlled experimental studies have addressed the question of time delay in hemorrhagic transformation during treatment with thrombolytic agents. In a rabbit stroke model, treatment 1 h after occlusion caused no excess intracerebral bleedings, whereas streptokinase or t-PA given after 24 h produced gross hemorrhage in a substantial proportion of animals [42]. Lyden et al. [31], also using a rabbit cerebral embolism model, observed a tendency toward a higher frequency of macroscopic brain hemorrhages in animals treated with t-PA 24 h after occlusion (64% in treated versus 38% in nontreated animals). No excess in hemorrhages was found if treatment was started 8 h after the occlusion. Treated animals with reperfusion did not have more intracerebral bleedings than those that did not reperfuse [31]. In other stroke models, no excess gross hemorrhages were present after early treatment (within 0–5 h) with urokinase in baboons [11], t-PA in rats [36], a t-PA analogue in rabbits [38], streptokinase in dogs [10], or urokinase in dogs [19]. Thus, from animal studies it appears that early thrombolytic treatment (within the first few hours) does not substantially increase the risk for intracerebral hemorrhage, but late onset of treatment may increase the risk. It must, however, be remembered that atherosclerotic cerebral arteries in stroke patients may be more vulnerable to ischemia than the vessels of experimental animals and that this could increase the risk for rupture and gross intracerebral hemorrhage.

In clinical studies of thrombolytic therapy in patients with ischemic stroke, hemorrhagic transformation and intracerebral hematomas have often been observed. Bleedings have been reported in patients treated both very early [2] and late [12] after stroke. Hemorrhages after late reperfusion may possibly be related to the use of anticoagulants [11]. Since thrombolysis is not associated with an exceedingly high risk of bleeding (Hacke, this volume), only controlled trials with large patient series will establish whether the risk for hemorrhage increases with time or not. However, in view of the results from animal experiments (see above), it seems advisable to be cautious with thrombolytic therapy in patients with a delay of more than 8 h to reduce the risk of severe intracranial hemorrhages.

Koudstaal et al. [26] reported the death from massive brain edema of two patients treated with t-PA. They concluded that delay of reperfusion of damaged tissue by 3–4 h after onset of a major ischemic stroke may have caused fatal edema. From other published series of stroke patients treated with thrombolytic agents there is little to support this contention. In experimental cerebral infarction, recanalization in the 6- to 24-h interval has been associated with increased brain edema, although mortality or neurological outcome was not affected [43].

What Is the Impact of Delay on Cost-Effectiveness?

Using published data on the effects of thrombolytic therapy in different subsets of patients with acute myocardial infarction, Laffel et al. [27] developed a cost-effectiveness model. The delay to start of treatment was one of four major factors determining cost in relation to effectiveness (the other three being infarct size, treatment procedure, and reocclusion management strategy). In these calculations, delaying the onset of therapy by 2 h meant a two- or three fold increase in the cost per additional survivor. More complicated procedures for recanalization (such as intracoronary administration of the thrombolytic agent, primary angioplasty, or immediate surgery) have a con-siderable procedural delay. Since the cost-effectiveness ratios increase with time from onset, the more aggressive protocols are outperformed by simple intravenous protocols in this model [27]. It should, however, be noted that recently published data on the effect of t-PA show smaller detrimental effects of delay than the background data used by Laffel et al.

Corresponding analyses of cost-effectiveness in patients with stroke must await solid background data. However, the experiences from the studies of myocardial infarction suggest that complicated and time-consuming thrombolytic procedures using angiography and intraarterial drug administration must be much superior to intravenous protocols in efficacy to be cost-effective.

Conclusions

Even in acute myocardial infarction, the exact role of the delay to start of thrombolytic treatment has not been settled, despite the large number of patients that have been studied. It is not surprising then that the impact of delay on the outcome after thrombolytic therapy in patients with ischemic stroke has been difficult to establish so far. Based on the limited clinical experience of thrombolytic therapy in patients with stroke, on the results from animal models of stroke, and on deductions from clinical trials of thrombolytic therapy in myocardial infarction, the following conclusions, tentative and some of them necessarily vague, are drawn:

1. The time from onset of symptoms to hospital admission is an important determinant of the total delay. Unless radical measures, including extensive population education, are initiated, early thrombolytic treatment will remain restricted to a small minority of patients with acute stroke.
2. Once thrombolytic therapy is started, the time to partial or total recanalization is in the 30- to 90-min range in the great majority of patients with eventual successful thrombolysis.
3. Time from onset of symptoms to start of treatment is probably not a major determinant of the proportion of patients with successful recanalization; it seems that other factors are more important.
4. Theoretical considerations and results from animal studies suggest better neuronal survival and/or reduced neurological deficits after very early recanalization. However, improved clinical outcome (reduced case fatality rate, improved functional outcome in survivors) by very early treat-

ment in patients with stroke has not yet been documented. Large series
of patients and controlled studies are needed to establish a time-effect
relationship.
5. A delay longer than 6–8 h is possibly associated with an increased risk of
    intracerebral hemorrhagic complications.

References

1. Asplund K, Tuomilehto J, Stegmayr B, Wester PO, Tunstall-Pedoe H (1988) Diagnostic criteria and quality control of the registration of stroke events in the MONICA
   Project. Acta Med Scand (Suppl) 728:26–39
2. Brott T, Haley C, Levy D, Barsan B, Sheppard G, Broderick J, Rea R, Marler J
   (1990) Safety and potential efficacy of tissue plasminogen activator (tPA) for stroke.
   Stroke 21:181 (abstract)
3. BW-tPA Acute Stroke Study Group (1989) An open multicenter trial of rt-PA in
   acute stroke. Abstracts from the 1st International Congress, 15–19 Oct 1989, Kyoto.
   (abstract no PS-12-17)
4. Califf RM, O'Neil W, Stack RS, Aronson L, Mark DB, Mantell S, Geonge BS, Candel
   RJ, Kereiakes DJ, Abbottsmith C, Topol EJ (1988) Failure of simple clinical measurements to predict perfusion status after intravenous thrombolysis. Ann Intern Med 108:
   658–662
5. Chesebro JH, Knatterud G, Roberts R, Borer J, Cohen L, Dalen J, Dodge H, Francis
   CK, Hillis D, Ludbrook P, Markis JE, Mueller H, Passamaui ER, Powers ER, Rao
   AK, Robertson T, Ross P, Ryan TJ, Sobel BE, Willerson J, William DO, Zaret BL,
   Braumuald E (1987) Thrombolysis in myocardial infarction (TIMI) trial, phase I: a
   comparison between intravenous tissue plasminogen activator and intravenous streptokinase. Circulation 76:142–154
6. Clozel J-P, Tschopp T, Luedin E, Holvoet P (1989) Time course of thrombolysis
   induced by intravenous bolus of infusion of tissue plasminogen activator in a rabbit
   jugular vein thrombosis model. Circulation 79:125–133
7. Collen D, Stassen JM, Verstraete M (1983) Thrombolysis with human extrinsic (tissue-
   type) plasminogen activator in rabbits with experimental jugular vein thrombosis. J
   Clin Invest 71:368–376
8. Collen D, Stassen J, Larsen G (1988) Pharmacokinetics and thrombolytic properties
   of deletion mutants of human tissue-type plasminogen activator in rabbits. Blood
   71:216–219
9. de Bono DP for the European Cooperative Study Group (1988) The European Cooperative Study Group trial of intravenous recombinant tissue-type plasminogen
   activator (rt-PA) and conservative therapy versus rt-PA and immediate coronary
   angioplasty. J Am Coll Cardiol 12:20A–23A
10. De Ley G, Weyne J, Demeester G, Stryckmans K, Goethals P, van de Velde E,
    Leusen I (1988) Experimental thromboembolic stroke studied by positron emission
    tomography: immediate versus delayed reperfusion by fibrinolysis. J Cereb Blood
    Flow Metab 8:539–545
11. Del Zoppo GJ, Copeland BR, Waltz TA, Zyroff J, Plow EF, Harker LA (1986) The
    beneficial effect of intracarotid urokinase on acute stroke in a baboon model. Stroke
    17:638–643
12. Del Zoppo GJ, Ferbert A, Otis S, Brückmann D, Hacke W, Zyroff J, Harker LA,
    Zeumer H (1988) Local intra-arterial fibrinolytic therapy on acute carotid territory
    stroke. A pilot study. Stroke 19:207–313
13. Ellis SG, Henschke CI, Sandor T (1983) Time course of functional and biochemical
    recovery of myocardium salvaged by reperfusion. J Am Coll Cardiol 1:1047–1055

14. Fieschi C, Argentino C, Lenzi GL, Sacchetti ML, Toni D (1989) Clinical and instrumental evaluation of patients with ischemic stroke within the first six hours. J Neurol Sci 91:311–21
15. Fisher M, Phillips DA, Davis MA, Smith TW, Pang RHL (1989) Delayed treatment with a t-PA analog and streptokinase in a rabbit embolism stroke model. Abstracts from the 1st International Stroke Congress, 15–19 Oct 1989, Kyoto. (abstract no PS-12-13)
16. Gagliardi R, Benvenuti L, Guizzardi G, Briani S (1983) Acute focal cerebral ischaemia: revascularization or not? Neurosurg Rev 6:13–17
17. GISSI (1986) Effectiveness of intravenous thrombolytic treatment in acute myocardial infarction. Lancet ii:397–402
18. Hakim AM, Pokrupa RP, Villanueva J, Diksic M, Evans AC, Thompson CJ, Meyer E, Yamamoto H, Feinder WH (1987) The effect of spontaneous reperfusion on metabolic function in early human cerebral infarcts. Ann Neurol 21:279–289
19. Hirschberg M, Wiesmann W, Korves M, Koc I, Hofferberth B (1988) Experimentelle Thrombolyse von Thrombembolien im Arteria-cerebri-media-Stromgebiet. Fortschr Röntgenstr 148:117–120
20. Hornig CR, Dorndorf W, Agnoli AF (1986) Hemorrhagic cerebral infarction: a prospective study. Stroke 17:179–185
21. Ikeda S, Muraishi K (1989) Intraarterial urokinase infusion therapy for the superacute intracranial major artery occlusion. Abstracts from the 1st International Stroke Congress, 15–10 Oct 1989, Kyoto. (abstract no OS-12-08)
22. ISIS-2 (Second International Study of Infarct Survival) Collaborative Group (1988) Randomised trial of intravenous streptokinase, oral aspirin, both, or neither among 17 187 cases of suspected acute myocardial infarction: ISIS-2. Lancet ii:349–360
23. Jorgensen L, Torvik A (1969) Ischemic cerebrovascular diseases in an autopsy series. Part 2. Prevalence, location, pathogenesis, and clinical course of cerebral infarcts. J Neurol Sci 9:285–320
24. Kanamasa K, Watanabe I, Cercek B, Yano J, Fishbein ME, Ganz W (1989) Selective decrease in lysis of old thrombi after rapid administration of tissue-type plasminogen activator. J Am Coll Cardiol 14:1359–1364
25. Kissel P, Chehrazi B, Seibert JA, Wagner FC Jr (1987) Digital angiographic quantification of blood flow dynamics in embolic stroke treated with tissue-type plasminogen activator. J Neurosurg 67:399–405
26. Koudstaal PJ, Stibbe J, Vermeulen M (1988) Fatal ischaemic brain oedema after early thrombolysis with tissue plasminogen activator in acute stroke. Br Med J 297:1571–1574
27. Laffel GL, Fineberg HV, Braunwald E (1987) A cost-effectiveness model for coronary thrombolysis/reperfusion therapy. J Am Coll Cardiol 10:79B–90B
28. Lee BCP, Brock JM, Fan T, Seibert A, Moonen C, Kissel P, Chehrazi B, Bradbury EP (1989) ^{31}P spectroscopy in thrombolytic treatment of experimental cerebral infarct. Am J Roentgenol 152:623–628
29. Loren M, Garcia Frade LJ, Torrado MC, Navarro JL (1989) Thrombus age and tissue plasminogen activator mediated thrombolysis in rats. Thromb Res 56:67–76
30. Loscalzo J, Braunwald E (1988) Tissue plasminogen activator. N Engl J Med 319:925–931
31. Lyden PD, Zivin JA, Clark WA, Madden K, Sasse KC, Mazzarella VA, Terry RD, Press GA (1989) Tissue plasminogen activator-mediated thrombolysis of cerebral emboli and its effect on hemorrhagic infarction in rabbits. Neurology 39:703–708
32. Magnani B, for the PAIMS Investigators (1989) Plasminogen activator Italian multicenter study (PAIMS): comparison of intravenous recombinant single-chain human tissue-type plasminogen activator (rt-PA) with intravenous streptokinase in acute myocardial infarction. J Am Coll Cardiol 13:19–26
33. Meyer JS (1958) Importance of ischemic damage to small vessels in experimental cerebral infarction. J Neuropathol Exp Neurol 17:571–585

34. Mori E, Tabushi M, Ohsumi Y (1989) Intraarterial urokinase infusion therapy in acute thromboembolic stroke. Abstracts from the 1st International Stroke Congress, 15–19 Oct 1989, Kyoto. (abstract no PS-08-04)
35. Mueller HS, Rao AK, Forman SA, and the TIMI Investigators (1987) Thrombolysis in myocardial infarction (TIMI): comparative studies of coronary reperfusion and systemic fibrinogenolysis with two forms of recombinant tissue-type plasminogen activator. J Am Coll Cardiol 10:479–90
36. Papadopoulos SM, Chandler WF, Salamat MS, Topol EJ, Sackellares JC (1987) Recombinant human tissue-type plasminogen activator therapy in acute thromboembolic stroke. J Neurosurg 67:394–398
37. Phillips DA, Fisher M, Smith TW, Davis MA (1988) The safety and angiographic efficacy of tissue plasminogen activator in a cerebral embolization model. Ann Neurol 23:391–394
38. Phillips DA, Fisher M, Smith TW, Davis MA, Pang RHL (1989) The effects of a new tissue plasminogen activator analogue, Fb-Fb-CF, on cerebral reperfusion in a rabbit embolic stroke model. Ann Neurol 25:281–285
39. Scandinavian Stroke Study Group (1988) Multicenter trial of hemodilution in acute ischemic stroke. Results of subgroup analyses. Stroke 19:464–471
40. Seto H, Nonaka N, Kuratsu I (1984) Clinical feature of hemorrhagic cerebral infarction. Neurol Med Chir 24:706–711
41. Sharkey SW, Brunette DD, Ruiz E, Hession WT, Uysham DE, Goldenberg F, Hodges M (1989) An analysis of time delays preceding thrombolysis for acute myocardial infarction. JAMA 262:3171–3174
42. Slivka A, Pulsinelli W (1987) Hemorrhagic complications of thrombolytic therapy in experimental stroke. Stroke 18:1148–1156
43. Sundt TM, Grant WC, Garcia JH (1976) Restoration of middle cerebral artery flow in experimental infarction. J Neurosurg 31:311–322
44. Topol EJ, Califf RM (1989) Tissue plasminogen activator: why the backlash? J Am Coll Cardiol 13:1477–1480
45. Topol EJ, Bates ER, Walton JA, Baumann G, Wolfe S, Maino J, Bayer L, Gorman L, Kline EM, O'Neill WW, Pitt B (1987) Community hospital administration of intravenous tissue plasminogen activator in acute myocardial infarction: improved timing, thrombolytic efficacy and ventricular function. J Am Coll Cardiol 10:1173–1177
46. Topol EJ, Califf RM, George BS, Kereiakes DJ, Lee KL, for the TAMI Study Group (1988) Insights from the thrombolysis and angioplasty in myocardial infarction (TAMI) trials. J Am Coll Cardiol 12:24A–31A
47. von Kummer R, Forsting M, Hutschenreuter B, Wildemann B, Hacke W (1989) Angiography in acute stroke due to occlusions of intracerebral arteries before and after treatment with intravenous recombinant tissue plasminogen activator. Abstracts from the 1st International Stroke Congress, 15–19 Oct 1989, Kyoto. (abstract no OS-12-03)
48. Weaver WD, Martin JS, Litwin PE (1988) Prehospital thrombolytic therapy: preliminary report on feasibility. Circulation 78 (Suppl II): 111 (abstract)
49. Wilcox RG, von der Lippe G, Olsson CG, Jensen G, Skene AM, Hampton JR (1988) Trial of tissue plasminogen activator for mortality reduction in acute myocardial infarction. Anglo-Scandinavian study of early thrombolysis (ASSET). Lancet 2:525–530
50. Zeumer H, Hacke W, Ringelstein EB (1983) Local intraarterial thrombolysis in vertebrobasilar thromboembolic disease. Am J Neuroradiol 4:401–404
51. Zeumer H, Freitag H-J, Grzyska U, Neuzig H-P (1989) Local intraarterial fibrinolysis in acute vertebrobasilar occlusion. Technical developments and recent results. Neuroradiology 31:336–340
52. Zimmermann R, Heuck CC, Harenberg J (1981) Fibrinolytische Therapie einer schweren Arteria-basilaris-Thrombose. Dtsch Med Wochenschr 106:464–467

53. Zivin JA, Fisher M, DeGirolamo U, Hemenway CC, Stashak JA (1985) Tissue plasminogen activator reduces neurological damage after cerebral embolism. Science 230: 1289–1292
54. Zivin JA, Lyden P, DeGirolami U, Kochbar A, Mazzarella V, Hemenway CC, Johnston P (1988) Tissue plasminogen activator: reduction of neurological damage after experimental embolic stroke. Arch Neurol 45:387–391

The Ischemic Penumbra: Fact or Fiction?*

B.K. Siesjö[1] and H. Memezawar[2]

Stroke due to occlusion of a middle cerebral artery (MCA), or another major artery in the brain, causes incomplete ischemia which varies from severe to mild (e.g., [19, 26, 34, 35]). A major dividing line is between tissues which are severely ischemic and which, therefore, quickly become infarcted, and tissues which are underperfused but essentially viable. Following experimental MCA occlusion the lateral part of the caudoputamen and some of the overlying neocortex usually belong to the first category, while other neocortical areas and the medial part of the caudoputamen constitute areas "at risk." In baboons, an ischemic threshold exists at flow rates of about 0.12 ml/g per minute, below which ischemic periods of 1–2 h invariably cause infarction [20]. One major problem in stroke research is to assess the revival time of cells existing in the focus, i.e., the longest periods of ischemia which can be tolerated without causing permanent functional deficits, or histological cell damage. Thus, if methods become available to restore flow in an occluded vessel, the revival times are of crucial importance. As we will discuss below, the revival times vary with the actual flow rates. The second major problem is to define ischemia of intermediate degrees, and to assess its functional and histopathological effects. Or, expressed otherwise, it is of crucial importance to explore events in the perifocal tissue ("infarct rim"), as contrasted to those in the focus. This is because the perifocal tissue is potentially salvageable even if the vascular occlusion is permanent.

Symon and colleagues, working in baboons, defined two thresholds of cerebral blood flow (CBF), which are useful in making the division between dying tissues, and tissues at risk ([1–4] see also [10, 33]). One threshold, at CBF values of about 0.15 ml/g per minute, is functional since it marks ischemia of sufficient severity to cause cessation of electrical activity (EEG and somatosensory evoked potentials). Transgression of another threshold, at CBF values of about 0.12 ml/g per minute, leads to membrane failure and loss of ion homeostasis. The twilight zone in-between, characterized by

*This study was supported by grants from the Swedish Medical Research Council, and from the United States Public Health Service (via the NIH).

[1] Laboratory for Experimental Brain Research, Lund University Hospital, 22185 Lund, Sweden.

[2] On leave of absence from the Second Department of Internal Medicine, Nippon Medical School, Tokyo, Japan.

Hacke et al (Eds)
Thrombolytic Therapy in Acute Ischemic Stroke
© Springer-Verlag Berlin Heidelberg 1991

electrical silence but retaining membrane polarization, has been called the ischemic penumbra [2, 8]. The term thus stands for tissues which are energetically sufficiently deprived to lose their capacity of electrical communication, yet sufficiently nourished to maintain gross energy and ion homeostasis. In small animals, like the rat, both the CBF values for the electrical and for the membrane failure thresholds are higher and infarction seems to occur at CBF values of 0.20–0.25 ml/g per minute [5, 36]. One example is provided by Jones et al. [12], who report that infarction was observed in tissues with local flows reduced below 0.10–0.12 ml/g per minute for 2–3 h, and in tissues with flow rates below 0.17–0.18 ml/g per minute during permanent occlusion. The term "penumbra," as defined, has been very useful in discussing perifocal events. However, it runs the risk of restricting the discussion to a special case rather than covering the general one. Thus whereas the penumbra in cats and monkeys, as defined, denotes an ischemic interval corresponding to CBF values in the range 0.12–0.18 ml/g per minute, tissues are probably "at risk" even if their flow rates exceed that range. In fact, it is probably of relatively little importance if flow is 0.15 ml/g per minute (with cessation of electrical activity), or 0.18 ml/g per minute (with retained function).

The important fact is that marginally perfused tissues run the risk of succumbing to the ischemia, or perhaps to the strains and stresses of living close to mortally sick neighbors. For that general reason, and particularly for the present discussion, we wish to use the term "penumbra" for the perifocal tissues which have a reduced CBF and which, at least in the long run, may be recruited in the infarction process.

The Ischemic Penumbra: CBF Versus Histopathology

Autoradiographic studies reveal that, whereas the ischemic focus is clearly discerned as an area of very low flow, the surroundings represent a whole spectrum of flow rates [5, 19, 33]. In the focus, flow rates vary between species, and between animals of the same species. These variations probably determine the revival times. Thus, even though all flow rates below about 0.12 ml/g per minute disrupt membrane homeostasis, the revival times seem directly proportional to the actual flow rates [6, 8, 17, 20]. This is probably because the flow determines how much ATP is formed per unit of time, and because ATP is required to drive some essential endergonous reactions, such as calcium efflux and/or sequestration. Clearly, if this is so even a modest rise of CBF in the focus may save time. However, "focal" tissue will be salvaged only when the ischemia is followed by relatively prompt recirculation, and provided that hyperglycemia is not present (see [22]). Since recirculation can not usually occur, interest is often directed toward the penumbra. As defined, this comprises tissues which are potentially salvageable also when the vessel occlusion is permanent.

The importance of the penumbra is that it potentially forms the nidus for an extension of the infarct. Theoretically, this can occur in one of two ways. In the first, the poorly perfused perifocal areas develop islands of necrotic tissue which subsequently coalesce and become part of the infarct. In the second, the infarct grows laterally at the very infarct rim in a relentless manner, only stopping when its edge reaches areas which have adequate flow rates. In either case, one would expect to encounter zones in which the insult has not yet given infarction but only neuronal necrosis.

It is difficult to document an increase in infarct size with time since neuronal necrosis (and infarction) requires time to mature, giving unequivocal evidence of devitalization of cells. In theory, growth of the infarct may be assessed if the tissue is reperfused after varying periods of ischemia. Practical problems arise, though, since reperfusion may exacerbate the ischemic process or lead to fulminating edema and death. In the rat, some cortical areas seem to be "penumbral" in the sense that they are initially only moderately underperfused (CBF is higher than the presumed threshold for infarction); yet, they subsequently become part of the infarct (see [5, 36]). However, the best evidence available is the amelioration of damage by N-methyl-D-aspartate (NMDA) antagonists, and by certain calcium antagonists, which may all reduce infarct size to 50%–60% that of the control (e.g., [21, 28, 29, 30]). A similar but less dramatic effect is observed when animals are given free radical scavengers [16, 18]. All these drugs salvage neocortical tissues, i.e., penumbral tissues at risk, without affecting the size of the focus, suggesting that they prevent these tissues from being recruited in the infarction process. Since the drugs lose efficacy after 3–6 h of MCA occlusion, the growth of the infarct is probably completed in that time.

In these species, disseminated neuronal necrosis has been documented in the perifocal tissue; this selective neuronal necrosis appears to have a superficial distribution [7, 11, 24]. This feature, which is particularly evident in the rat, gives the impression that the focus extends in the plane of the outer cortical layers, mainly layers 2–3. Such findings also demonstrate that the disseminated neuronal necrosis is confined to the immediate perifocal zone. One could envisage, therefore, that an extension of the infarct occurs by continuous recruitment of damaged neurons at the infarct rim, and that it is caused by events which mainly affect layers 2–3.

Unfortunately, results of studies in man or in subhuman primates fail to conform to this simple picture. In monkeys, perifocal reductions in CBF unquestionably occur [33], but data exist suggesting that such tissues only become infarcted if CBF falls below 0.12 ml/g per minute ([12], however, see also [11]). Since CBF in focal and perifocal areas may be stable for hours, there is little evidence that perifocal tissues are continuously recruited in the infarction process. Furthermore, in human autopsy material there is a sharp boundary between infarcted and essentially normal tissue, and we thus have no clear evidence of a perifocal rim or of islands of neuronal necrosis representing a penumbra (for documentation and further references, see [27]).

It may be argued that the pattern observed reflects the end stage, when all tissue "at risk" has become part of the infarct. However, it must be discussed whether pathophysiological events are dissimilar in primates and in small animal species.

Mechanisms of Cell Damage

The question must be posed: what mechanisms could lead to a gradual destruction of cells in tissues having CBF values well above flow rates which cause neither energy failure nor overt loss of ion homeostasis? It has been suggested that perifocal tissues are subjected to repeated, spontaneous waves of depolarizations [23]. These resemble spreading depressions [SDs], i.e., the propagated disturbance of electrical functions and ion homeostasis which can be elicited by stab wounds, electrical stimulation, or KCl (see [9, 13]). Since an SD involves cellular loss of K^+, and uptake of Ca^{2+}, Na^+, and Cl^-, it represents a potential threat to the tissue. However, since SDs repeated over a 5-h period do not lead to neuronal necrosis [32], such ionic perturbations can be tolerated by the normal brain. It may be agreed that, although repeated SDs do not cause neuronal necrosis in normal animals, they may do so in animals with induced hypoxia. Thus, if depolarizations of the SD type are elicited in the penumbra zone, they may well be expected to damage neurons.

Spreading depressions are believed to cause release of glutamate. If this occurs during the depolarizations affecting the perifocal tissues, an excitotoxic mechanism could be responsible for neuronal necrosis [7]. Very probably, glutamate toxicity is mediated by calcium influx via agonist-operated cation channels (see [31, 32]). One could thus envisage that the factor causing neuronal necrosis is a train of calcium transients, and that NMDA antagonists ameliorate such damage by impeding the influx of calcium. By the same token, calcium antagonists could act similarly by reducing calcium influx via voltage-dependent channels; besides, since such antagonists increase flow, they may also enhance ATP production and, thereby, aid in the efflux and/or sequestration of calcium.

While SD-like depolarizations may well be what cause sporadic neuronal necrosis in the perifocal tissue, one cannot imagine a simple scheme in which sporadic necrosis is the forerunner of infarction. Thus, although preischemic hypoglycemia increased sporadic neuronal necrosis, infarction was reduced [7]. Furthermore, although hyperglycemia reduced depolarizations and sporadic cell loss, it did not reduce infarction. These results can be most readily explained if one assumes that the mechanisms leading to sporadic neuronal necrosis are different from those leading to infarction. It would seem reasonable to assume that the former encompass calcium-related neuronal necrosis, while the latter probably cause vascular damage mediated by acidosis. The molecular mechanisms of such vascular damage could well encompass de-compartmentalization of pro-oxidant iron, and iron-induced free radical reactions [34].

One may summarize results obtained in rats (and, to some extent, in cats) by stating that the final damage following stroke probably comprises a densely ischemic focus and a variable amount of less ischemic perifocal tissue, forming the penumbra of the stroke lesion. The latter is, at least initially, salvageable, but it may be recruited in the infarct process. The mechanisms causing such slow devitalization of perifocal tissues may encompass both calcium-dependent sporadic neuronal necrosis, as well as acidosis- and free radical-dependent vascular damage. The presence of such a penumbra zone is revealed by the fact that the final size of the infarct, following permanent MCA occlusion, can be reduced by agents which block calcium influx into neurons, increase CBF, or scavenge free radicals.

At present, we do not know it if this concept applies to man. Thus, depolarizations of the spreading depression type, which could be the im-mediate cause of neuronal necrosis in the penumbra zone, may occur in cats and rats, but not in subhuman primates or man. Furthermore, although a perifocal reduction of CBF has been documented in man, it is not known if it reveals areas which are inadequately perfused from collateral channels and, therefore, "at risk," or if it reflects functional depression of neurons which are bereaved of their synaptic inputs (see [14, 15]).

In view of these uncertainties, we can conclude that a penumbral zone, amenable to treatment, exists in rats and cats. We do not yet know if it exists, as defined, in man. What seems established, though, is that, what-ever the species, reperfusion of tissues supplied by an occluded MCA may lead to the revival of tissues which have perfusion rates adequate for short-term, but not long-term, survival. In a practical sense, therefore, penumbral tissues must exist in any stroke lesion which can be ameliorated by recanal-ization of the occluded vessel.

References

1. Astrup J, Symon L, Branston NM, Lassen NA (1977) Cortical evoked potential and extracellular K^+ and H^+ at levels of brain ischemia. Stroke 8:51–57
2. Astrup J, Siesjo BK, Symon L (1981) Thresholds in cerebral ischemia – the ischemic penumbra. Stroke 12:723–725
3. Branston NM, Symon L, Crockard HA, Pasztor ED (1974) Relationship between the cortical evoked potential and local cortical blood flow following acute middle cerebral artery occlusion in the baboon. Exp Neurol 45:195–208
4. Branston NM, Symon L, Strong AJ (1978) Reversibility of ischemically induced changes in extracellular potassium in primate cortex. J Neurol Sci 37:37–49
5. Bolander HG, Persson L, Hillered L, d'Argy R, Ponten U, Olsson Y (1989) Regional cerebral blood flow and histopathologic changes after middle cerebral artery occlusion in rats. Stroke 20:930–937

6. Carter LP, Yamagata S, Erspamer R (1983) Time limits of reversible cortical ischemia. Neurosurg 12:620–623
7. Garcia JH, Mitchem HL, Briggs L, Morawetz R, Hudetz AG, Hazelrig JB, Halsey JH, Conger KA (1983) Transient focal ischemia in subhuman primates. J Neuropathol Exp Neurol 42:44–60
8. Hakim AM (1987) The cerebral ischemic penumbra. Can J Neurol Sci 14:557–559
9. Hansen AJ (1985) Effect of anoxia on ion distribution in the brain. Physiol Rev 65:101–148
10. Heiss WD, Hayakawa T, Waltz AG (1976) Cortical neuronal function during ischemia. Arch Neurol 33:813–820
11. Iizuka H, Sakatani K, Young W (1989) Selective cortical neuronal damage after middle cerebral artery occlusion in rats. Stroke 20:1516–1523
12. Jones TH, Moravetz RB, Crowell RM, Marcoux FW, FitzGibbon SJ, DeGirolami U, Ojemann RO (1981) Thresholds of focal cerebral ischemia in awake monkeys. J Neurosurg 54:773–782
13. Kraig RP, Ferreira-Filho CR, Nicholson C (1983) Alkaline and acid transients in cerebellar microenvironment. J Neurophysiol 49:831–850
14. Lassen NA (1982) Incomplete cerebral infarction – focal incomplete ischemic tissue necrosis not leading to em. Stroke 13:522–523
15. Lassen NA, Vorstrup S (1984) Ischemic penumbra results in incomplete infarction. Stroke 15:755–758
16. Liu TH, Beckman JS, Freeman BA, Hogan EL, Hsu CY (1989) Polyethylene glycol-conjugated superoxide dismutase and catalase reduce ischemic brain injury. Am J Physiol 256:H589–H593
17. Marcoux FW, Morawetz RB, Crowell RM, DeGirolami U, Halsey JH (1982) Differential regional vulnerability in transient focal ischemia. Stroke 13:339–364
18. Martz D, Rayos G, Schielke GP, Betz AL (1989) Allopurinol and dimethylthiourea reduce brain infarction following middle cerebral artery occlusion in the rat. Stroke 20:488–494
19. Mohamed AA, Gotoh O, Graham DI, Osborne KA, McCulloch JM, Mendelow AD, Teasdale GM, Harper AM (1985) Effect of pretreatment with the calcium antagonist nimodipine on local cerebral blood flow and histopathology after middle cerebral artery occlusion. Ann Neurol 18:705–711
20. Morawetz RB, Crowell RM, DeGirolami U, Marcoux FW, Jones TH, Halsey JH (1979) Regional cerebral blood flow thresholds during cerebral ischemia. Fed Proc 38: 2493–2494
21. Nakayama H, Ginsberg MD, Dietrich WD (1988) (S)-Emopamil, a novel calcium channel blocker and serotonin S2 antagonist, markedly reduces infarct size following middle cerebral artery occlusion in the rat. Neurology 38:1667–1673
22. Nedergaard M (1987) Transient focal ischemia in hyperglycemic rats is associated with increased cerebral infarction. Brain Res 408:79–85
23. Nedergaard M, Astrup J (1986) Infarct rim: effect of hyperglycemia on direct current potential and ^{14}C-2-deoxyglucose phosphorylation. 6:607–615
24. Nedergaard M, Diemer NH (1987) Focal ischemia of the rat brain, with special reference to the influence of plasma glucose concentration. Acta Neuropathol 73: 131–137
25. Nedergaard M, Hansen AJ (1988) Spreading depression is not associated with neuronal injury in the normal brain. Brain Res 449:395–398
26. Nedergaard M, Vorstrup S, Astrup J (1986) Cell density in the border zone around old small human brain infarcts. Stroke 17:1129–1137
27. Nedergaard M, Gjedde A, Diemer NH (1986) Focal ischemia of the rat brain: autoradiographic determination of cerebral glucose utilization, glucose content, and blood flow. J Cereb Blood Flow Metab 6:414–424
28. Ozyuart E, Graham DI, Woodruff GN, McCulloch JM (1988) Protective effect of the glutamate antagonist, MK-801, in focal cerebral ischemia in the cat. J Cereb Blood Flow Metab 8:138–143

29. Park CK, Nehls DG, Graham DI, Teasdale GM, McCulloch JM (1988) The glutamate antagonist MK-801 reduces focal ischemic brain damage. Ann Neurol 24:543–551
30. Park CK, Nehls GD, Graham DI, Teasdale GM, McCulloch JM (1988) Focal cerebral ischemia in the cat. Treatment with the glutamate antagonist MK-801 after induction of ischemia. J Cereb Blood Flow Metabol 8:757–762
31. Siesjo BK, Bengtsson F (1989) Calcium fluxes, calcium antagonists, and calcium-related pathology in brain ischemia hypoglycemia, and spreading depression: a unifying hypothesis. J Cereb Blood Flow Metabol 9:127–140
32. Siesjo BK, Bengtsson F, Grampp W, Theander S (1989) Calcium, excitotoxins, and neuronal death in the brain. Ann New York Acad Sci 568:234–251
33. Symon L (1980) The relationship between CBF, evoked potential and the clinical features in cerebral ischemia. Acta Neurol Scand (Suppl 78) 62:175–190
34. Symon L, Pasztor ED, Branston NM (1974) The distribution and density of reduced cerebral blood flow following acute middle cerebral artery occlusion: an experimental study by the technique of hydrogen clearance in baboons. Stroke 5:355–364
35. Tamura A, Asano T, Sano K (1980) Correlation between rCBF and histological changes following temporary middle cerebral artery occlusion. Stroke 11:487–493
36. Tyson GW, Teasdale GM, Graham DI, McCulloch JM (1984) Focal cerebral ischemia in the rat: topography of hemodynamic and histopathological changes. Ann Neurol 15:559–567

Hemorrhagic Transformation in the Natural History of Acute Embolic Stroke

M.S. Pessin

Introduction

Interest generated by the potential benefits of thrombolytic treatment (especially tissue-type plasminogen activator, t-PA) for acute stroke is tempered by the serious complication of intracranial bleeding. The risks of intracranial bleeding are presently being assessed in several United States and European pilot trials, of different design, using intravenously administered t-PA in acute stroke. Serious intracranial bleeding in these studies refers to bleeding which causes clinical neurologic deterioration not attributable to the original stroke. When the pilot phase of these investigations is complete, control groups of untreated patients will help us compare, in a scientific fashion, intracranial bleeding associated with t-PA. Meanwhile, observations on the natural incidence and clinical computed tomography (CT) features of hemorrhagic transformation (HT) in untreated patients with acute embolic stroke will have to serve as a framework for comparison with acute stroke patients treated with thrombolytic agents.

In reviewing this topic, points of major interest include: (a) the natural incidence of HT in autopsy and CT studies, (b) the timing of HT occurrence, (c) the clinical consequences, (d) the types of intracranial bleeding, whether hemorrhagic infarction (HI) or parenchymatous hematoma (PH), and (e) intracranial bleeding comparisons between thrombolytic trials and controls.

Incidence of Hemorrhagic Infarction and Parenchymatous Hematoma

Autopsy Studies

Autopsy studies [4, 5, 10, 12] have established a high incidence of HI, 50%–70%, in association with cerebral embolism (Table 1). In their report, Fisher

---

Department of Neurology, Tufts University School of Medicine, New England Medical Center, 750 Washington Street, Boston, MA 02111, USA.

Hacke et al. (Eds)
Thrombolytic Therapy in Acute Ischemic Stroke
© Springer-Verlag Berlin Heidelberg 1991

Table 1. Hemorrhagic infarcts in autopsy studies

Study	Cases of embolism	HI
Fisher and Adams [4]	123	63 (51%)
Fisher and Adams [5]	57	38 (67%)
Jorgensen and Torvik [10]	59	42 (71%)
Lodder et al. [12]	19	10 (53%)

and Adams [4] described the neuropathologic spectrum of HI and proposed their now well-known theory of migratory embolism to account for the phenomenon of bleeding within an area of ischemic infarction. In 373 brains examined with vascular occlusion, 66 (18%) had HI and all except 3 were associated with the 123 (51%) cases of brain embolism. Later Fisher and Adams [5] described HI in 38 of 57 patients (67%) with brain embolism. Similarly, Jorgensen and Torvik [10] found HI in 42 of 59 patients (71%) with embolic stroke collected from a population of 994 autopsies. Lodder et al. [12] reported HI in 10 of 19 patients (53%) with cardioembolic stroke among 48 patients dying within 15 days of supratentorial infarction. A majority of patients died of brain herniation, making large infarcts a better predictor of HI than embolism. Autopsy material suggests a high incidence of HI but obviously the nature of postmortem material, with more serious and large infarcts, biases the conclusions.

Computed Tomography Studies

In selected CT studies of nonanticoagulated patients the incidence of HI associated with cerebral embolism ranges from 5% to 43% [6, 9, 11, 14, 20] (Table 2), generally less than autopsy reports. Petechial bleeding below the sensitivity of CT may account for some of the discrepancy, but the inherent bias toward more serious, larger strokes with herniation effects may be a major factor accounting for the different incidence in the two types of study. Also, the likelihood that CT scanning is not routinely performed in a serial fashion may lead to identification of fewer HIs.

Table 2. Hemorrhagic infarcts in CT studies

Study	CTs reviewed	HI
Lodder [11]	952	48 (5.1%)
Fisher et al. [6]	193[a]	10 (5.0%)
Weisberg [20]	35	9 (26%)
Hornig et al. [9]	65	28 (43%)
Okada et al. [14]	140[a]	45 (32%)

[a] Patients on antithrombotics excluded.

Table 3. Time to HI on CT [8, 9, 15, 16]

	Hours			Days		
	24	48	72	7	14	21
Percentage patients ($n = 69$)	37	10	9	9	32	3

The studies by Lodder [11] and Fisher et al. [6] represent CT surveys of large numbers of consecutive patients with ischemic infarction of all types (not exclusively embolism) in which the incidence of HI is approximately 5%. Weisberg [20] reported HI in 9 of 35 patients (26%) with cardiogenic cerebral embolism. Hornig et al. [9] performed a prospective, serial CT scan study of 65 patients with ischemic cerebral infarction (many with cardiogenic embolism) at regular intervals over 4 weeks. The overall incidence of HI was 28 of 65 patients (43%). In a large series of patients with cardioembolic stroke, Okada et al. [14] reported HI in 45 of 140 patients (32%).

Timing of Hemorrhagic Infarction

At least three CT studies [8, 9, 15], in nonanticoagulated patients, documented that the majority of HIs are detected by day 3–4, but some as late as the 2nd week poststroke as reflected by the prospective serial CT study by Hornig et al. [9] (Table 3). HT occurred within 10 days on CT in two-thirds of 65 patients, but none later than 1 month, reported by Okada et al. [14], including 20 patients treated with antithrombotic agents.

Most authorities agree that, in the absence of anticoagulation, HI is not present immediately after the stroke but develops some time later, usually not before 6 h. In the Cerebral Embolism Study Group report [8, 16] on 28 patients with HI, no HI was present in 7 patients who had CTs before 6 h while HI was present in 45% of 11 patients between 6 and 18 h.

Clinical Consequences of Hemorrhagic Transformation

Clinicians have known that HI may be identified on CT scan when the patient is either stable or improving, but usually not worsening. Several reports [9, 15, 16] have documented this observation in non-anticoagulated patients (Table 4). In the Cerebral Embolism Study Group report [8, 16] of 47 non-anticoagulated patients with HI, only 2 of 47 (4.2%) had worsening, while 45 were stable or improving, when HI was discovered. This is in contrast to clinical deterioration noted in 15 of 17 patients (88%) with HI associated

Table 4. Hemorrhagic infarction and clinical status[a]

Study	n	Clinical status	
		Stable-improved	Worsened
CE Study Group [8, 16]	47	45	2 (4.2%)
Ott et al. [15]	24	24	0
Hornig et al. [9]	28	25	3 (10.7%)
Total	99	94	5 (5%)

[a] Nonanticoagulated patients.

with anticoagulation treatment. Similarly, Ott et al. [15] found none of 24 patients with HI had worsening, compared with 7 of 20 who deteriorated while on anticoagulation. In the study by Hornig et al. [9], only 3 of 28 patients (10.7%) had clinical worsening associated with HT, and 2 of the 3 had hematoma patterns on CT. The data suggest that the preponderance of HIs are asymptomatic.

Distinction Between Hemorrhagic Infarction and Parenchymatous Hematoma

The distinction on CT between severe HI and PH is not always possible and subjectivity affects categorization. The spectrum of HI on CT includes a myriad of patchy, petechial, and sometimes more confluent bleeding with indistinct margins affecting the gray matter of cerebral cortex and basal ganglia. Often the bleeding is gyriform in configuration. PH, in contrast, is a more solid homogeneous pattern with circumscribed borders, surrounding edema, and mass effect. PH tends to occupy a greater extent of the area of ischemic infarct than HI. An additional troubling feature is the occurrence of PH at a location remote from the original infarct.

Many reports lump all bleeding into the term "intracranial hemorrhage" and in others anticoagulation treatment has complicated the outcome. Three reports provide a CT definition of HI and PH along with sufficient numbers of nonanticoagulated patients to allow analysis (Table 5). Fisher et al. [6] in a CT survey of 193 scans in patients with ischemic stroke found only 4 of 193 (2%) with hematomas. The Cerebral Embolism Study Group report [2] focused on patients with embolic stroke and CT evidence of HT. There were 11 HIs and no PHs. The largest and most extensive study to assess the incidence of HT was reported by Okada et al. [14]. One hundred and Sixty patients were selected consecutively based on strict clinical and cardiologic criteria for cerebral embolism. Twenty patients were excluded from the analysis here because they received urokinase, heparin, or both. Angio-

Table 5. Parenchymatous hematomas in CT studies[a]

Study	Total cases	HT	HI	PH
Fisher et al. [6]	193	14 (7%)	10	4 (2%)
CE Study Group [2]	11	11	11	0
Okada et al. [14]	140	57 (40.7%)	45	12 (8.6%)

[a] Nonanticoagulated patients.

graphy was performed in 142 patients, and repeated in 59. CT defined a spectrum of intracranial bleeding which included four subtypes: petechial, diffuse, small hematomas, and massive hematomas (greater than 3). Of the 140 patients not receiving antithrombotic agents, 45 had HI, and 12 had hematomas (3 massive, 9 small). No information is provided on whether the hematomas were exclusively in the area of ischemic infarct. These three studies suggest a relatively low incidence of PH in the untreated patient with ischemic infarct.

Thrombolytic Trials

Recent Studies

Four recent trials using intraarterial urokinase or streptokinase plus heparin in acute carotid or vertebrobasilar (VB) stroke suggest that the incidence of intracranial bleeding is low. Del Zoppo et al. [3] reported four HIs without clinical worsening and no PHs in 20 patients with carotid territory stroke treated with urokinase. Hacke et al. [7] treated 43 patients with urokinase and heparin with acute VB stroke and reported one HI and three pontine hemorrhages, the latter associated with clinical deterioration. Mori et al. [13] treated 22 patients with middle cerebral artery occlusion using urokinase and heparin; one HI (asymptomatic) and three PHs occurred. Theron et al. [17] treated 12 patients with acute carotid territory stroke with either urokinase or streptokinase. There were three PHs, one of which was asymptomatic. In an aggregate analysis of the 97 patients from these 4 studies, there were 6 HIs (6%) and 9 PHs (9%).

Current Studies: t-PA

Two United States studies using intravenous t-PA to assess efficacy and safety in acute stroke are in progress (Table 6). In the NIH-sponsored study [1], patients were treated within 90 min of symptom onset, after a negative CT.

Table 6. Intracranial bleeding: current t-PA studies

Study	n	HI[a]	PH[b]
NIH t-PA Study [1]	74	3 (4%)	3 (4%)
t-PA Stroke Study Group [18]	71	25 (35%)	6 (8.4%)

[a] Only 2/28 had clinical worsening.
[b] 7/9 had clinical worsening.

In a recent progress report on 74 patients there were 3 HIs (4%) on the 24-h CT following t-PA (no additional HIs on 7-day CT), all asymptomatic, and 3 PHs (4%) associated with clinical worsening. The PHs were within the area of infarct in two, and in a previously unaffected region in one.

The t-PA Stroke Study Group report [18] is also a dose-range finding efficacy and safety trial of intravenous t-PA administered within 8 h of stroke onset, after a negative CT and angiographic documentation of an occluded cerebral artery appropriate to clinical signs. In a progress report on 71 patients, 25 (35%) had HIs, the majority on the 24-h CT following t-PA but several on later CTs, up to 14 days. Only two showed clinical deterioration. Six additional patients, (8.4%) had PHs, four of whom had clinical worsening (three died).

In a preliminary report of an ongoing European pilot study, 12 patients have been treated with intravenous t-PA for acute middle cerebral artery or VB territory stroke, and no intracranial bleeding has occurred [19].

Intracranial Bleeding: Comparisons Between Thrombolytic Studies and Historical Controls

While the selected historical control studies lack precise comparability with either the two current intravenous t-PA trials [1, 18] or the four recent intra-arterial thrombolytic studies [3, 7, 13, 17], some general statistical comparisons are possible (Table 7). At least three studies [9, 14, 20], with sufficient numbers of non-anticoagulated patients with cardioembolic stroke, reported HIs in 82 of 240 patients (34%) up to 30 days after stroke onset compared with 3 of 74 (4%) in the NIH t-PA trial [1], and 25 of 71 patients (35%) in the t-PA Stroke Study Group report [18], including HIs noted as late as 14 days post-treatment. No statistically significant difference was present comparing the historical controls and the t-PA Stroke Study ($p = 0.87$, chi-square $= 0.03$, 1 df), but there were significantly fewer HIs in the NIH t-PA trials than in controls ($p < 0.01$, chi-square 25.98, 1 df). If the 6 HIs from an aggregate analysis of the 97 patients from the 4 intraarterial studies are combined with the NIH and the t-PA Stroke Study findings, the results show significantly more HIs in the controls ($p < 0.01$, chi-square 26.68, 1 df).

Table 7. Intracranial bleeding comparisons: hemorrhagic infarcts

	Total patients	HI (%)
Controls [9, 14, 20]	240	82 (34%)
NIH t-PA Study [1]	74	3 (4%)
t-PA Stroke Study Group [18]	71	19 (27%)
Intraarterial thrombolytic Studies [3, 7, 13, 17]	97	6 (6.2%)

Table 8. Intracranial bleeding comparisons: parenchymatous hematomas

	Total patients	PH (%)
Controls [2, 14]	151	12 (8%)
NIH t-PA Study [1]	74	3 (4%)
t-PA Stroke Study Group [18]	71	6 (8.4%)
Intraarterial thrombolytic Studies [3, 7, 13, 17]	97	9 (9.2%)

The incidence of PHs (Table 8) (12 in 151 patients, 8%) in two selected historical control studies [2, 14] of nonanticoagulated patients was not statistically significant compared with either the 2 t-PA trials in which PHs occurred in 3 of 74 patients (4%) in the NIH t-PA Study and 6 of 71 patients (8.4%) in the t-PA Stroke Study Group [18], or also including the 9 PHs from the aggregate analysis of 97 patients treated with intraarterial thrombolytic agents ($p = 0.61$) (chi-square $= 1.01$, 3 df).

Conclusions

Hemorrhagic infarction occurs regularly and in substantial numbers in the natural evolution of acute embolic stroke based on the historical control studies reviewed. PHs also occur, but less frequently. The clinical features suggest that HT occurs early in the course of embolic stroke and that most HIs are asymptomatic, while PHs are associated with clinical worsening, except for the smallest ones. Only the most general and qualified statistical comparisons are possible with these uncontrolled data. Accurate assessment of intracranial bleeding must await the next phase of controlled, randomized studies. The general impression that emerges from this review, however, is that HI and PH in the recent intraarterial thrombolytic and the current intravenous t-PA studies are not excessive and further study should continue to evaluate for potential benefits.

Acknowledgement. I am grateful to Richard F. Kaplan, Ph.D., for his assistance in the statistical analyses.

References

1. Brott T, Haley C, Levy D, Barsan W, Sheppard G, Broderick J, Reed R, Marler J (1990) Safety and potential efficacy of tissue plasminogen activator (t-PA) for stroke. Stroke 21:181
2. Cerebral Embolism Study Group (1984) Immediate anticoagulation of embolic stroke: brain hemorrhage and management options. Stroke 15:779–789
3. Del Zoppo GJ, Ferbert A, Otis S, Bruckmann B, Hacke W, Zyroff J, Harker LA, Zeumer H (1988) Local intra arterial fibrinolytic therapy in acute carotid territory stroke. Stroke 19:307–313
4. Fisher CM, Adams RD (1951) Observations on brain embolism with special reference to the mechanism of hemorrhagic infarction. J Neuropathol Exp Neurol 10:92–94
5. Fisher CM, Adams RD (1987) Observations on brain embolism with special reference to hemorrhagic infarction. In: Furlan AJ (ed) The heart and stroke. Springer, Berlin Heidelberg New York, pp 17–36
6. Fisher M, Zito JL, Siva A, DeGirolami U (1984) Hemorrhagic infarction: a clinical and CT study. Stroke 15:192
7. Hacke W, Zeumer H, Ferbert A, Bruckmann H, Del Zoppo GJ (1988) Intra arterial thrombolytic therapy improves outcome in patients with acute vertebro-basilar occlusive disease. Stroke 19:1216–1222
8. Hart RG, for Cerebral Embolism Study Group (1986) Timing of hemorrhagic transformation of cardioembolic stroke. In: Stober T, Schimrigk K, Ganten D, Sherman DG (eds) Central nervous system control of the heart. Nijhoff, Boston, pp 229–232
9. Hornig CR, Dorndorf W, Agnoli AL (1986) Hemorrhagic cerebral infarction – a prospective study. Stroke 17:179–185
10. Jorgensen L, Torvik A (1969) Ischemic cerebrovascular diseases in an autopsy series, part 2. Prevalence, location, pathogenesis, and clinical course of cerebral infarcts. J Neurol Sci 9:285–320
11. Lodder J (1984) CT-detected hemorrhagic infarction; relation with the size of the infarct, and the presence of midline shift. Acta Neurol Scand 70:329–335
12. Lodder J, Krijne-Kubat B, Broekman J (1986) Cerebral hemorrhagic infarction at autopsy: cardiac embolic cause and the relationship to the cause of death. Stroke 17:626–629
13. Mori E, Tabuchi M, Yoshida T, Yamadori A (1988) Intracarotid urokinase with thromboembolic occlusion of the middle cerebral artery. Stroke 19:802–812
14. Okada Y, Yamaguchi T, Minematsu K, Miyashita T, Sawada T, Sadashima S, Fujishima, Omae T (1989) Hemorrhagic transformation in cerebral embolism. Stroke 20:598–603
15. Ott BR, Zamani A, Kleefield J, Funkenstein HH (1986) The clinical spectrum of hemorrhagic infarction. Stroke 17:630–637
16. Sherman DG, Hart RG, for the Cerebral Embolism Study Group (1986) Brain hemorrhage in embolic stroke. In: Stober T, Schimrigk K, Ganten D, Sherman DG (eds) Central nervous system control of the heart. Nijhoff, Boston, pp 249–253
17. Theron J, Courtheoux P, Casasco A, Alachkar F, Notan F, Ganem F, Maiza D (1989) Local intraarterial fibrinolysis in the carotid territory. AJNR 10:753–765
18. The tPA Acute Stroke Study Group (1990) An open multicenter study of the safety and efficacy of various doses of tPA in patients with acute stroke. Stroke 21:181
19. von Kummer R, Hutschenreuter M, Wildemann B, Hacke W (1989) Thrombolytic therapy with intravenous recombinant tissue plasminogen activator in acute occlusions of intracranial arteries. J Cereb Blood Flow Metab 9(Suppl 1):S721
20. Weisberg LA (1985) Nonseptic cardiogenic cerebral embolic stroke: clinical-CT correlations. Neurology 35:896–899

Intracranial Hemorrhage After Coronary Thrombolysis with Tissue Plasminogen Activator

C.S. KASE

The thrombolytic agent recombinant tissue-type plasminogen activator (rt-PA) produces clot lysis by catalyzing the conversion of plasminogen into plasmin [15]. In the coronary circulation, this effect is followed in 70%–89% of cases by reperfusion of occluded arteries, which in turn results in improved ventricular function and survival as compared with untreated controls [2, 31]. The relative clot-specificity of rt-PA as compared with other thrombolytic agents (such as streptokinase and urokinase) determines a lesser degree of activation of circulating plasminogen, as well as decreased degradation of factors V, VIII, and fibrinogen by this agent [32]. This property is responsible for a lower hemorrhagic potential for rt-PA. Despite this advantage over streptokinase and urokinase, rt-PA use results in hemorrhagic complications, both systemic and intracranial, that partially limit its clinical usefulness. Intracranial hemorrhage (ICH) has been reported in 0.4%–1.3% of cases in clinical trials of the predominantly single-chain agent "alteplase" (Genentech Laboratories, South San Francisco, CA) [8]. An overall rate of 0.68% was derived from the analysis of a combined experience of 5258 patients treated in the United States and European clinical trials of coronary thrombolysis [4].

The following analysis of the data on ICH in the setting of rt-PA treatment of acute myocardial infarction (MI) will focus primarily on the clinical and laboratory features of these hemorrhages, as documented in recent clinical reports in the literature [4].

Reported Rates of Intracranial Hemorrhage in Trials of rt-PA Treatment of Acute Myocardial Infarction

Many studies have reported on rates of rt-PA-related hemorrhagic complications in acute MI trials (Table 1). In most, no detailed clinical analysis of the ICH cases was attempted, thus offering little insight into the issues of

Department of Neurology, Boston University School of Medicine, 720 Harrison Avenue, Suite 600, Boston, MA 02118, USA.

Hacke et al. (Eds.)
Thrombolytic Therapy in Acute Ischemic Stroke
© Springer-Verlag Berlin Heidelberg 1991

Table 1. Rates of intracranial hemorrhage in trials of rt-PA treatment of myocardial infarction. Modified from [6]

Study	Treatment	No. patients	ICH (%)
Collen et al. [5]	rt-PA	31	0
	Placebo	14	0
Verstraete et al. [34]	rt-PA	62	0
	Placebo	62	0
Guerci et al. [9]	rt-PA	72	0
	Placebo	66	0
ASSET [1]	rt-PA	366	1.4
	Placebo	355	0.3
Topol et al. [29]	rt-PA	75	1.3
	Placebo/streptokinase	25	0
Topol et al. [28]	rt-PA and angioplasty	386	0.5
Simoons et al. [23]	rt-PA	184	0.5
	rt-PA and angioplasty	183	0.5
Mueller et al. [16]	rt-PA	305	0.3
Verstraete et al. [33]	rt-PA	64	0
	Streptokinase	65	0
TIMI [26]	rt-PA	143	0
	Streptokinase	147	0
Australian study [17]	rt-PA	73	1.4
	Placebo	71	0
Linnik et al. [14]	rt-PA	124	1.5

pathogenesis and clinical presentation. The reported data document rather low rates of major hemorrhagic complications, including ICH. Although these studies cannot be compared directly, since doses of rt-PA and concomitant medications (streptokinase, heparin, aspirin) or procedures (coronary angioplasty) differ widely among protocols, they suggest an rt-PA dose-relationship for the occurrence of ICH: 0.4% ICH rates were associated with a 100-mg rt-PA dose, whereas rates in the 1.3% range followed the use of a 150-mg dose [8]. Other factors related to increased hemorrhagic potential have included advanced age, female sex, and low body weight [30], as well as hypertension and aspirin use [20].

Data on Detailed Analysis of Intracranial Hemorrhage Cases After Thrombolysis in Acute Myocardial Infarction

A number of recent publications have dealt with a detailed analysis of ICH cases after coronary thrombolysis with rt-PA. These have resulted in the characterization of clinical and laboratory profiles for these hemorrhages. These studies have primarily come from large clinical trials on MI patients, whereas a smaller number of patients with ICH have been reported after use of rt-PA in the community.

Series of Intracranial Hemorrhage Cases Reported from Clinical Trials of rt-PA in Acute Myocardial Infarction

Most of the available information in this area comes from cases reported from the Thrombolysis in Myocardial Infarction (TIMI) II trial, in which the predominantly single-chain rt-PA "alteplase" was tested [4, 8, 24]. Additional experience with the double-chain rt-PA "duteplase" (Burroughs Wellcome Co., Research Triangle, NC) has been recently reported [11]. The main characteristics of these ICHs are shown in Table 2. The onset of symptoms of ICH occurred relatively early in the studies using "alteplase," 39% of the hemorrhages starting during drug infusion (within 6 h from rt-PA treatment onset), with an additional 26% of cases occurring within 12 h from onset of rt-PA infusion [24]. In the "duteplase" trials, the ICHs occurred between 7 and 72 h (median, 21 h) from rt-PA infusion onset. The ICHs were predominantly lobar in location: 16/23 (70%) with "alteplase," 8/9 (89%) with "duteplase"; posterior fossa (cerebellar, pontine) hemorrhages occurred rarely (12.5% for both studies combined), and putaminal varieties were not recorded. Multiple ICHs were documented in one-third of the cases reported by Kase et al. [11], in one of them with an additional subdural hematoma.

The series reported by O'Connor et al. [19] involved 13 cases of ICH among 1696 patients treated at one institution, resulting in a 0.76% rate of ICH. However, slightly less than one-half of these ICH cases occurred after use of rt-PA alone, the others having been treated with streptokinase, either alone or in combination with rt-PA. These authors found that potential risk factors for the development of ICH included advanced age, hypertension, and prior use of aspirin. They commented on the generally serious character of this complication, which had a 61% mortality, as well as on the variability of its clinical presentation, with examples of intracerebral, subdural, and subarachnoid hemorrhage in various combinations. They found an excessive prolongation of activated partial thromboplastin time (aPTT) (beyond 100) in 10 of their 13 patients (77%) at the time of ICH onset. The clinical presentation at onset of ICH included nausea and vomiting in 46%, severe headache in 15%, and agitation and confusion in 15%; presentation with unilateral facial palsy, lethargy, and coma each occurred in one patient.

The laboratory parameters associated with these ICHs were reported in detail by Carlson et al. [4] and Kase et al. [11]. The former authors found significant levels of hypofibrinogenemia (0.77 g/l, for a normal range of 2.0–3.5 g/l) in their two cases, whereas Kase et al. [11] only documented this abnormality in one of six patients tested (17%). Similarly, thrombocytopenia was present in only one of the nine patients (11%) reported by the latter authors. A more frequent coagulation abnormality reported by the latter

Table 2. Series of ICH cases reported from clinical trials of coronary thrombolysis with rt-PA

Study	Agent	No. of ICH cases	Dose	Rate of ICH %	(cases ICH/ cases treated)	Mortality
Carlson et al. [4]	Alteplase	2	150 mg 90 mg	0.44%	(2/450)	–
Sloan et al. [24]	Alteplase	23	150 mg 100 mg	1.3% 0.4%	(12/908) (11/3016)	52%
O'Connor et al. [19]	Alteplase	13	?	0.76%	(13/1696)	61%
Kase et al. [11]	Duteplase	9	0.25 – 0.66 MU/kg	0.53%	(9/1700)	44%

authors was excessive prolongation of aPTT during intravenous heparin infusion: in five of eight patients (63%) this value was prolonged beyond twice the control value at onset of ICH. Bleeding outside the nervous system was recorded in five of nine patients after use of "duteplase" [11], in subcutaneous tissues in four and in the gastrointestinal tract in one, with none requiring blood transfusion.

Intracranial Hemorrhage Cases Reported After rt-PA Use in the Community, Outside Clinical Trials

Since the Food and Drug Administration (FDA) approved the use of "alteplase" for coronary thrombolysis in the United States, a few clinical reports have stressed its intracranial hemorrhagic complications. Kase et al. [10] collected 6 such cases, 3 of which occurred among a group of 60 patients treated over a 1-year period, amounting to an unusually high frequency of 5% for this complication. All patients received the recommended 100-mg dose of "alteplase," as well as concomitant intravenous heparin for the purpose of avoiding coronary reocclusion. The hemorrhages occurred between 2 and 14 h after the end of rt-PA infusion, and 3–17 h after onset of heparin treatment. All patients had excessively prolonged aPTT (between 81 and >150 s) at the time of hemorrhage onset. The ICHs were predominantly lobar in location, were multiple in two patients, and an associated subdural hematoma was present in one patient (Fig. 1). One patient required surgical drainage of an enlarging frontal lobe hemorrhage; histologic examination of the hematoma cavity and cerebral wall was negative for vascular malformations or evidence of cerebral amyloid angiopathy on Congo red staining. Among the possible risk factors for ICH, two patients had a history of hypertension, but none was hypertensive on admission; none of these patients had either been previously treated with antiplatelet agents or developed thrombocytopenia in the setting of intravenous heparin therapy. The mortality in this series was 66% (four of six patients). No autopsy studies were conducted.

Clinical and Laboratory Profiles of Intracranial Hemorrhage After rt-PA Use

The analysis of these various clinical series, although not strictly comparable with one another, nevertheless provides a general clinical and laboratory profile of ICH complicating coronary thrombolysis with rt-PA. These features include: (a) onset of ICH in relatively close proximity to the rt-PA infusion, the majority of cases occurring either during the infusion or within a few hours of its termination; (b) frequent association (in approximately two-thirds of the cases) with excessive prolongation of aPTT at the time of ICH onset, with insignificant occurrence of hypofibrinogenemia and throm-

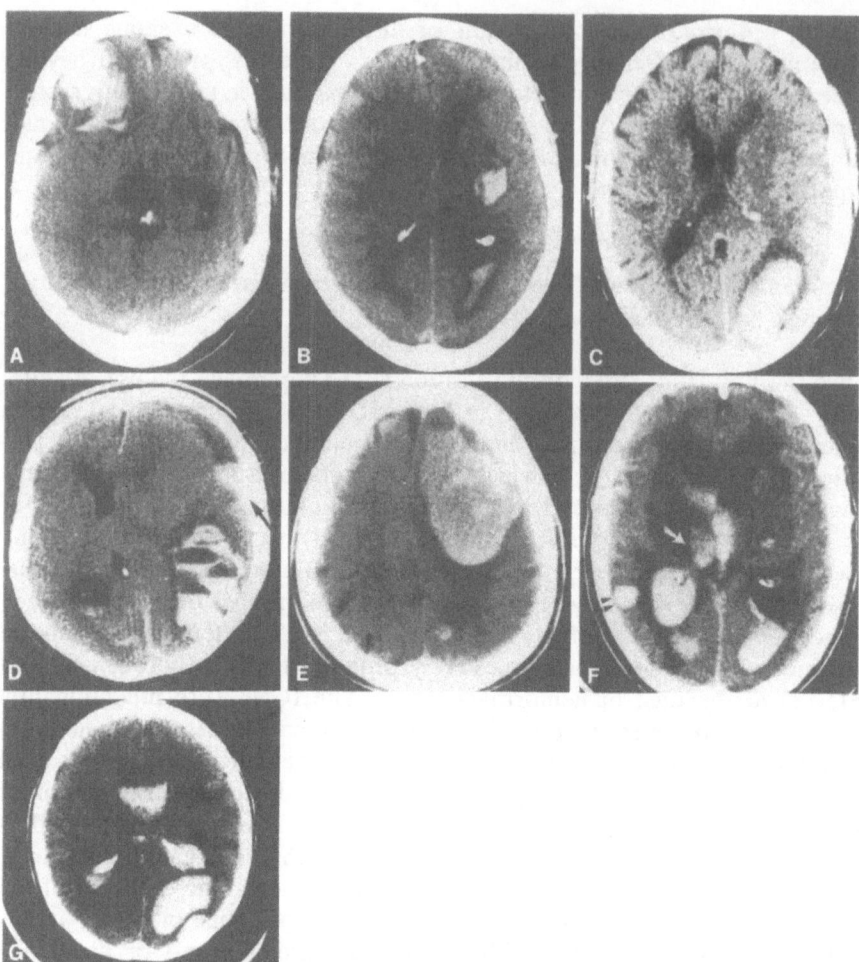

Fig. 1. A Right frontal lobe hematoma involving cortex and subcortical white matter. **B** Left putaminal-corona radiata hematoma with midline shift *from right to left* (resulting from the larger right-sided frontal hematoma shown in **A**). **C** Left occipital lobe hemorrhage with surrounding edema and anterior displacement of the lateral ventricle. **D** Large irregular left parietal lobe hematoma with extension into the subdural space (*arrow*) and marked midline shift *from left to right*. **E** Massive left frontal lobe hematoma involving the cortex and subcortical white matter, with marked midline shift. **F** Right thalamic (*arrow*) and temporo-occipital (*arrowheads*) hematomas, intraventricular hemorrhage, and generalized hydrocephalus. **G** Left temporo-occipital lobar hemorrhage with intraventricular extension. From Kase et al. [103]

bocytopenia as potential risk factors for ICH; (c) generally serious, frequently catastrophic presentation of intracerebral, subdural, or subarachnoid hemorrhage, with mortalities ranging between 44% and 66%; (d) predilection for a lobar location of ICH, with uncommon posterior fossa examples, and very rare ganglionic (i.e., putaminal) varieties, the latter being in contrast to the "spontaneous," mostly hypertensive ICHs commonly observed in clinical practice; (e) risk factor profile that may include advanced age, hypertension, low body weight, history of prior stroke, and prior or concomitant use of antiplatelet agents as features predisposing to this complication.

Possible Mechanisms of Intracranial Hemorrhage Related to rt-PA Use

The relatively common bleeding at vascular access sites after rt-PA use can be easily explained by lysis of a local vascular hemostatic plug [3]. Intracranial bleeding is unlikely to be due to a similar process, except for the rare instances in which ICH has followed an obvious concomitant cerebral event, such as head trauma. The majority of documented cases of ICH after rt-PA use remain unexplained, and most suspected mechanisms can only be regarded as speculative at the present time. A number of factors, alone or in combination, may contribute to the occurrence of ICH in the setting of thrombolytic therapy with rt-PA.

Systemic Fibrinolysis

Despite its relative fibrinspecificity, rt-PA use is followed by a dose-related systemic fibrinolytic state [27], with 20%–25% decline in serum fibrinogen levels after doses of 100 mg "alteplase." Although significant hypofibrinogenemia has been occasionally present in the setting of ICH after rt-PA [4], the majority of reported cases have shown a weak association with this factor [11]. This observation of a poor correlation between fibrinogen levels and ICH also applies to the case of systemic bleeding events, as documented in the TIMI trial [21]. These data point to a weak contribution of hypofibrinogenemia to the bleeding complications, both systemic and intracranial, of rt-PA use, and suggest it is unlikely to be a primary pathogenic factor.

Intracranial Hemorrhage as a Complication of Heparin Therapy

The concomitant use of intravenous heparin is intended to avoid coronary reocclusion after cessation of the effect of rt-PA. A role for heparin in the production of ICH and other hemorrhagic complications thus needs consideration. A hemorrhagic effect of heparin mediated through the mechanism of heparin-induced thrombocytopenia has not been documented in series of ICH: Kase et al. [11] found significant thrombocytopenia in only one of their nine patients (11%) with ICH after "duteplase" use, and in none of their six patients treated with "alteplase" [10]. On the other hand, a direct hemorrhagic effect is a well-documented side-effect of heparin and other anticoagulants, raising the possibility that the ICHs observed after rt-PA use may simply represent anticoagulant-related hemorrhages. The limited data available argue against this explanation, rather suggesting that rt-PA itself adds to the hemorrhagic potential of this thrombolytic-anticoagulant combination; these arguments include: (a) the observation that the incidence of ICH after rt-PA follows a dose relationship, with significantly higher rates of ICH (1.3%) after 150 mg than after 100 mg (0.4%) rt-PA [8]; (b) the finding of a very low rate of ICH (0.08%) after use of heparin alone in acute MI, with a threefold increase in the rate of ICH (to 0.27%) following the combined use of rt-PA and heparin [1]. Although this increase in hemorrhagic strokes with the heparin-rt-PA combination was not statistically significant, it indicates a trend toward a higher frequency of ICH, as compared with heparin alone. The strongest available evidence to implicate a heparin effect in post-rt-PA ICH is the frequent observation of excessively prolonged aPTT at the onset of ICH, with values in excess of 100 s in two-thirds of the reported cases [10, 11, 19]. However, a more definite case against a heparin effect cannot be made because of the unfortunate lack of information on aPTT values at comparable times on the patients from the same trials who did not bleed intracranially. These data should be obtained in future MI trials in order to properly evaluate the eventual causal relationship between excessively prolonged aPTT and ICH occurrence.

Role of Cerebral Infarction in Causing Intracranial Hemorrhage After rt-PA Use in Myocardial Infarction

Cerebral infarction has been suggested as playing a role in the intracranial hemorrhagic complications of anticoagulant therapy [13]. Since clinically apparent cerebral infarction secondary to cardiogenic embolism occurs in about 2.4% of patients with acute MI [12], it is conceivable that either overt or "silent" cerebral embolism may precede ICH in patients acutely treated with intravenous rt-PA and heparin. However, some features of the reported examples of post-rt-PA ICH argue against this being the main mechanism of these hemorrhages: (a) in 9 of the 15 instances (60%) of ICH reported by Kase et al. [10, 11], the MIs were of inferior location, a feature that carries a very low (1.5%) rate of echocardiographically detected left ventricular thrombus formation as a risk factor for systemic embolism, as opposed to a 34% rate for anterior MI [36]; this feature would put the majority of these patients at the lower end of the spectrum of cerebral embolic potential, by virtue of the predominantly inferior type of their MIs; (b) the frequent observation of ICH at sites outside the brain substance, in the subdural or subarachnoid space in 8 of the 28 (28.5%) patients reported by Kase et al. [10, 11] and O'Connor et al. [19], suggests that presumably silent cerebral embolism is not likely to be a common, uniform causative factor of these hemorrhages. Although it is possible that a fraction of these ICHs may be preceded by cerebral embolism, the analysis of these cases suggests that other factors may operate in a significant number of these patients.

Platelet Antiaggregant Effect Due to the rt-PA and/or Antiplatelet Agents

There are data to suggest that rt-PA, by promoting plasmin formation, results in a platelet antiaggregant effect, which is delayed and prolonged, in relationship to the rt-PA infusion [18, 22]. This effect has been recently corroborated by both in vitro assessment of platelet aggregability [25] and documentation of prolonged template bleeding time in patients tested 90 min after rt-PA infusion [7]. The latter authors found that prolongation of the bleeding time correlated with hemorrhagic complications, and suggested that the monitoring of this laboratory value may become an important factor for the identification of patients at increased risk of bleeding complications after rt-PA use. It is thus possible to speculate that plasmin-induced decreased platelet aggregability, which occurs as a late effect after rt-PA infusion, may be implicated in the frequently delayed ICHs that occur after rt-PA use [10]. This effect on platelets may be further enhanced by previous or concomitant use of antiplatelet agents [7], resulting in an increased potential for hemorrhagic complications, including ICH.

Local Cerebral Vascular Pathology,
Not Related to the Acute Myocardial Infarction

The role of local cerebral vascular abnormalities in the production of ICH in the setting of rt-PA treatment of acute MI may be an additional factor to consider. These may include conditions with spontaneous hemorrhagic potential, such as cerebral amyloid angiopathy [35] or occult arteriovenous malformations, the former being more likely in the age groups generally affected by MI. The relative frequency of such conditions in patients with ICH after thrombolysis for MI will only be assessed by much needed systematic pathologic studies of autopsy or surgical biopsy materials. Other local vascular factors, such as those related to prior stroke or recent head trauma, are clinically obvious, and currently constitute appropriate exclusions for thrombolytic treatment.

Conclusions

Intracranial hemorrhage after rt-PA and heparin use for treatment of coronary occlusion occurs at a low frequency of about 0.5%–0.75%. The mechanisms of ICH after rt-PA therapy are unknown, a combination of hematologic and local vascular factors probably being implicated. Further analysis of cases of ICH after rt-PA and heparin therapy should help clarify its mechanisms, and result in increased safety in the use of this highly effective thrombolytic agent.

References

1. Anglo-Scandinavian Study of Early Thrombolysis (ASSET) (1988) Trial of tissue plasminogen activator for mortality reduction in acute myocardial infarction. Lancet 2:525–530
2. Bates ER, Topol EJ (1989) Thrombolytic therapy for acute myocardial infarction. Chest 95 (Suppl):257S–264S
3. Califf RM, Topol EJ, George BS Boswick JM, Abottsmith C, Sigmon KN, Candela R, Masek R, Kereiakes D, O'Neill WW, Stack RS, Stump D and the Thrombolysis and Angioplasty in Myocardial Infarction Study Group (1988) Hemorrhagic complications associated with the use of intravenous tissue plasminogen activator in treatment of acute myocardial infarction. Am J Med 85:353–359
4. Carlson SE, Aldrich MS, Greenberg HS, Topol EJ (1988) Intracerebral hemorrhage complicating intravenous tissue plasminogen activator treatment. Arch Neurol 45:1070–1073
5. Collen D, Topol EJ, Tiefenbrunn AJ, Gold HK, Weisfeldt ML, Sobel BE, Leinbach RC, Brinker JA, Ludbrook PA, Yasuda I, Bulkley BH, Robison AK, Hutter AM, Bell WR, Spadaro JJ, Khaw BA, Grossbard EB (1984) Coronary thrombolysis with recombinant human tissuetype plasminogen activator: a prospective, randomized, placebo-controlled trial. Circulation 70:1012–1017
6. Fennerty AG, Levine MN, Hirsh J (1989) Hemorrhagic complications of thrombolytic therapy in the treatment of myocardial infarction and venous thromboembolism. Chest 95 (Suppl):88S–97S
7. Gimple LW, Gold HK, Leinbach RC, Coller BS, Werner W, Yasuda T, Johns JA, Ziskind AA, Finkelstein D, Collen D (1989) Correlation between template bleeding times and spontaneous bleeding during treatment of acute myocardial infarction with recombinant tissue-type plasminogen activator. Circulation 80:581–588
8. Gore J, Sloan MA, Price TR, Terrin ML, Bovill E, Collen D, Knatterud G, Randall AMY, Sopko G (1990) Intracranial hemorrhage after rt-PA and heparin for acute myocardial infarction – The TIMI II pilot and randomized trial combined experience. J Am Coll Cardiol 15:15A (abstract)
9. Guerci AD, Gerstenblith G, Brinker JA, Chandra NC, Gottlieb SO, Bahr RD, Weiss JL, Shapiro EP, Flaherty JT, Bush DE, Chew PH, Gottlieb SH, Halperin HR, Ouyang P, Walford GD, Bell WR, Fatterpaker AK, Llewellyn M, Topol EJ, Healy B, Siu CO, Becker LC, Weisfeldt ML (1987) A randomized trial of intravenous tissue plasminogen activator for acute myocardial infarction with subsequent randomization to elective coronary angioplasty. N Engl J Med 317:1613–1618
10. Kase CS, O'Neal AM, Fisher M, Girgis GN, Ordia JI (1990a) Intracranial hemorrhage after use of tissue plasminogen activator for coronary thrombolysis. Ann Int Med 112:17–21
11. Kase CS, Pessin MS, Zivin JA, Del Zoppo GJ, Furlan AJ (1990b) Intracranial hemorrhage following coronary thrombolysis with tissue plasminogen activator. Neurology 40 (Suppl 1):191 (abstract)

12. Komrad MS, Coffey CE, Coffey KS, McKinnis R, Massey EW, Califf RM (1984) Myocardial infarction and stroke. Neurology 34:1403–1409
13. Lieberman A, Hass WK, Pinto R, Isom WO, Kupersmith M, Bear G, Chase R (1978) Intracranial hemorrhage and infarction in anticoagulated patients with prosthetic heart valves. Stroke 9:18–24
14. Linnik W, Tintinalli JE, Ramos R (1989) Associated reactions during and immediately after rt-PA infusion. Ann Emerg Med 18:234–239
15. Loscalzo J, Braunwald E (1988) Tissue plasminogen activator. N Engl J Med 319: 925–931
16. Mueller HS, Rao AK, Forman SA, and the TIMI Investigators (1987) Thrombolysis in myocardial infarction (TIMI): comparative studies of coronary reperfusion and systemic fibrinogenolysis with two forms of recombinant tissue-type plasminogen activator. J Am Coll Cardiol 10:479–490
17. National Heart Foundation of Australia Coronary Thrombolysis Group (1988) Coronary thrombolysis and myocardial salvage by tissue plasminogen activators given up to 4 hours after onset of myocardial infarction. Lancet 1:203–208
18. Niewiarowski S, Senyi AF, Gillies P (1973) Plasmin-induced platelet aggregation and platelet release reaction: effects on hemostasis. J Clin Invest 52:1647–1659
19. O'Connor CM, Aldrich H, Massey EW, Uglietta J, Mark DB, Califf RM (1990a) Intracranial hemorrhage after thrombolytic therapy for acute myocardial infarction: clinical characteristics and in-hospital outcome. J Am Coll Cardiol 15:213A (abstract)
20. O'Connor CM, Aldrich H, Uglietta J, Massey EW (1990b) Risk factor profile of patients with intracranial hemorrhage after thrombolytic therapy for acute myocardial infarction. Neurology 40 (Suppl 1):192 (abstract)
21. Rao AK, Pratt C, Berke A, Jaffe A, Ockene I, Schreiber TL, Bell WR, Knatterud G, Robertson TL, Terrin ML for the TIMI investigators (1988) Thrombolysis in myocardial infarction (TIMI) trial-phase I: hemorrhagic manifestations and changes in plasma fibrinogen and the fibrinolytic system in patients treated with recombinant tissue plasminogen activator and streptokinase. J Am Coll Cardiol 11:1–11
22. Schafer AI, Adelman B (1985) Plasmin inhibition of platelet function and of arachidonic acid metabolism. J Clin Invest 75:456–461
23. Simoons ML, Arnold AER, Betrin A (1988) Thrombolysis with tissue plasminogen activator in acute myocardial infarction: no additional benefit from immediate percutaneous coronary angioplasty. Lancet 1:197–203
24. Sloan MA, Price TR, Randall AMY, Solomon RE, Terrin ML (1990) Intracerebral hemorrhage after rt-PA and heparin for acute myocardial infarction: the TIMI II pilot and randomized trial combined experience. Stroke 21:28 (abstract)
25. Terres W, Umnus-Schnelle S, Hamm CW, Bleifeld W (1990) In vitro effects of thrombolytic agents on platelets. J Am Coll Cardiol 15:189A (abstract)
26. The TIMI Study Group (1985) The thrombolysis in myocardial infarction (TIMI) trial: phase I findings. N Engl J Med 312:932–936
27. Topol EJ, Bell WR, Weisfeldt ML (1985) Coronary thrombolysis with recombinant tissue-type plasminogen activator: a hematologic and pharmacologic study. Ann Int Med 103:837–843
28. Topol EJ, Califf RM, George BS (1987a) A randomized trial of immediate versus delayed elective angioplasty after intravenous tissue plasminogen activator in acute myocardial infarction. N Engl J Med 317:581–588
29. Topol EJ, Morris DC, Smalling RW, Schumacher RR, Taylor CR, Nishikawa A, Liberman HA, Collen D, Tufte ME, Grossbard EB, O'Neill WW (1987b) A multicenter, randomized, placebo-controlled trial of a new form of intravenous recombinant tissue-type plasminogen activator (Activase) in acute myocardial infarction. J Am Coll Cardiol 9:1205–1213
30. Topol EJ, George BS, Kereiakes DJ, Candela RJ, Abbottsmith CW, Stump DC, Boswick JM, Stack RS, Califf RM, and the TAMI Study Group (1988) Comparison of two dose regimens of intravenous tissue plasminogen activator for acute myocardial infarction. Am J Cardiol 61:723–728

31. Werf F van de, Arnold AER (1988) Intravenous tissue plasminogen activator and size of infarct, left ventricular function, and survival in acute myocardial infarction. Br Med J 297:2374–2379
32. Verstraete M, Collen D (1986) Thrombolytic therapy in the eighties. Blood 67:1529–1541
33. Verstraete M, Bernard R, Bory M, Brower RW, Collen D, de Bono DP, Erbel R, Huhmann W, Lennane RJ, Lubsen J, Mathey D, Meyer J, Michels HR, Rutsch W, Schartl M, Schmidt W, Uebis R, von Essen R (1985) Randomised trial of intravenous recombinant tissue-type plasminogen activator versus intravenous streptokinase in acute myocardial infarction. Lancet 1:842–847
34. Verstraete M, Bleifeld W, Brower RW, Charbonnier B, Collen D, de Bono DP, Dunning AJ, Lennane RJ, Lubsen J, Mathey DG, Michel PL, Raynaud Ph, Schofer J, Vahanian A, Vanhaecke J, Kley GA van de, Werf F van de, Von Essen R (1985) Double-blind randomised trial of intravenous tissue-type plasminogen activator versus placebo in acute myocardial infarction. Lancet 2:965–969
35. Vinters HV (1987) Cerebral amyloid angiopathy: a critical review. Stroke 18:311–324
36. Weinreich DJ, Burke JF, Pauletto FJ (1984) Left ventricular mural thrombi complicating acute myocardial infarction. Ann Int Med 100:789–794

Predictive Factors for the Effective Treatment of Acute Stroke with Intravenous Thrombolytic Agents

S.M. WOLPERT

Patients treated with intravenous thrombolytic agents for acute stroke due to atherosclerotic disease are not without risk for bleeding, and a number of studies in which cerebral and extracerebral hemorrhages have occurred as a complication of the therapy have been reported. Ascertaining the correct dose of a drug to obtain recanalization of an occluded intracerebral artery with an acceptably low hemorrhagic risk is therefore an important aim of any study in which the effectiveness of thrombolytic therapy is to be assessed.

Early results of a dose escalation, multicenter trial to evaluate the safety and efficacy of intravenous tissue plasminogen activator (t-PA) in patients presenting with an acute thrombolic or thromboembolic stroke is promising, with recanalization of occluded vessels being seen in many patients. Unfortunately hemorrhagic infarcts or intracerebral hematomas also occurred in some of the patients. It is impossible clinically to predict which patients will respond to the therapy or which patients will have hemorrhagic intracerebral complications.

In order for patients with acute stroke to be entered into the multicenter trial, they need to have an entry CT scan without evidence of hemorrhage and a cerebral arteriogram with an occluded intra- or extracranial artery. In some of the patients early signs of infarct were seen on the entry CT scans. On the angiograms there is considerable variability in the nature of the occlusions; the occlusions may involve the extracranial carotid artery, the intracranial carotid artery, or the intracranial cerebral arteries. Various combinations of occlusions may also occur.

A retrospective study was therefore carried out to attempt to determine whether the pretherapy CT scans or the pretherapy cerebral angiograms defined any pattern of abnormalities which could correlate with recanalization of the occluded arteries or determine those patients in whom intracerebral hemorrhagic transformations would occur. Also the size of the infarcts that occurred, as determined by a 24-h scan after the initiation of therapy, was examined to examine any relationship between infarct size, angiographic outcome, and hemorrhagic transformation.

Department of Radiology, Division of Neuroradiology, New England Medical Center Hospitals, 750 Washington Street, Boston, MA 02111, USA.

Hacke et al. (Eds)
Thrombolytic Therapy in Acute Ischemic Stroke
© Springer-Verlag Berlin Heidelberg 1991

Results

A number of conclusions were derived from this preliminary study.

1. Recanalizations occurred more frequently with isolated intracranial occlusions than with occlusions involving the internal carotial artery alone, or the internal carotid artery together with the intracranial arteries.
2. Recanalizations were more common with smaller infarcts as seen on the 24-h scan than with larger infarcts.
3. There appeared to be no relationship between the presence of a recently visible infarct and recanalization.
4. Hemorrhagic infarcts or hematomas occurred more frequently when treatment commenced after 6 h than before 6 h from the onset of stroke.
5. The presence of early infarction probably does not predispose to either hemorrhagic infarcts or intracerebral hematomas.
6. Intracerebral hematomas occurred in patients with middle cerebral artery occlusions distal to the lenticulostriate arteries or in patients with complete occlusions of the internal carotid artery and middle cerebral arteries. Hematomas did not occur in patients with internal cerebral artery occlusions alone, with distal middle cerebral artery occlusions (except in one patient in whom the hematoma occurred in the cerebellum), or with proximal middle cerebral artery occlusions involving the lenticulostriate arteries.
7. There appeared to be no relationship between the size of the infarct seen on the 24-h scan and the development of a hemorrhagic infarct.

Discussion

Before determining the efficacy of any form of treatment for patients with acute stroke, the natural history of the disease must be considered. Emboli causing occluded intracranial arteries may lyse spontaneously. Also the lysis may result in hemorrhagic transformation with resultant hemorrhagic infarction or hematoma.

Occluded vessels recanalize more commonly in embolic than in thrombotic stroke. Yamaguchi et al. [8] demonstrated the disappearance of occlusions on repeat angiograms in 28 of 42 patients with occluded arteries. The shortest interval between the initial and repeat angiograms was 4 days. When migration of emboli to distal branches was included, at least partial reestablishment of circulation to ischemic regions occurred in 38 of the 42 cases. Okada et al. [6] showed reopening of the initial occluded arteries in 56 of 59 patients with cerebral emboli studied a median of 20 (range, 3–47) days after the initial ictus. Irino et al. [3] demonstrated by angiography a case in which a follow-up angiogram on day 2 after an occlusion showed partial recanalization of the occluded artery with full recanalization on day 5. Possibly in some of these reported cases the emboli lysed within hours of the initial embolic event, but this was not documented. The goal of anticoagulant therapy is to promote reopening of occluded vessels within hours of the initial occlusion in order to overcome the deleterious effects of sustained cerebral ischemia. Experience with late thrombolytic therapy (beyond 24 h) for completed stroke has shown little benefit for return of neurological function [2].

The present study is based on the angiographic visualization of the effects of therapy within a time frame in which benefit from lysis of emboli is expected to occur. The study suggests that the site of the occlusion may be a significant factor in the reopening of occluded vessels. Peripheral occlusions at the level of the divisions or branches of the middle cerebral artery appear to be more likely to respond to therapy than more proximal occlusions. Intraarterial thrombolytic therapy delivered through a microcatheter may be the method of choice for the treatment of this latter group of patients, with intravenous thrombolytic therapy being the preferred treatment for patients with more peripheral occlusions.

The size of the infarct may also be a significant factor for recanalization. In the setting of an acute stroke, analysis of lesion size as measured by CT has received little attention although correlation between lesion volume and neurological function has been demonstrated [1, 5]. Our results show that recanalization appears more frequently after small than after large infarcts, indicating that the extent of the vascular compromise and resultant cerebral ischemia may also be significant factors in the recanalization of occluded intracranial arteries.

Hemorrhagic transformation, both hemorrhagic infarcts and hematomas, has been found by computed tomogruphy (CT) in 6% of embolic patients in the first 4 days after the onset of the stroke, and in 40% of the patients in the 1st month in one study [6]. Autopsy studies have shown that hemorrhagic events occur in up to 70% of embolic strokes [4]. This incidence of hemorrhagic complications in the natural course of the disease needs to be weighed against the reports of hemorrhagic events (both hemorrhagic infarctions and hematomas) seen in patients with acute stroke treated with fibrinolytic agents [7, 9]. The present study indicates that hemorrhagic events occur less frequently when intravenous treatment commences sooner rather than later after vascular occlusion. Presumably ischemic alteration of the endothelium of the occluded arteries is aggravated by prolonged occlusion of the vessels.

References

1. Brott T, Marler JR, Olinger CP Adams HP, Tomsick T, Barsan WG, Biller J, Eberle R, Hertzberg V, Walker M (1989) Measurements of acute cerebral infarction: lesion size by computed tomography. Stroke 20:871–875

2. Fletcher AP, Alkjaersig N, Lewis M Tulevski V, Davies A, Brooks JE, Hardin WB, Landau WM, Raichle ME (1976) A pilot study of urokinase therapy in cerebral infarction. Stroke 7:135–142
3. Irino T, Taneda M, Minami T (1977) Angiographic manifestations in postrecanalized cerebral infarction. Neurology 27:471
4. Jorgensen L, Torvik A (1966) Ischemic cerebrovascular disease in an autopsy series. Part 1. J Neurol Sci 3:490–509
5. Kertesz A, Harlock W, Coates R (1979) Computer tomographic localization, lesion size, and prognosis in aphasia and non-verbal impairment. Brain Lang 1:34–50
6. Okada Y, Yamaguchi T, Minematsu K, Miyashita T, Sawada T, Sadoshima S, Fujishima M, Omae T (1989) Hemorrhagic transformation in cerebral embolism. Stroke 20:598–603
7. Theron J, Courtheoux P, Casasco A, Alachkar F, Notari F, Ganem F, Malza D (1989) Local intraarterial fibrinolysis in the carotid territory. AJNR 10:753–765
8. Yamaguchi T, Minematsu K, Choki J Sawada T, Jkeda M (1984) Clinical and neuroradiological analysis of thrombotic and embolic cerebral infarction. Jpn Circ J 48:50–58
9. Zeumer H (1985) Vascular recanalizing techniques in interventional neuroradiology. J Neurol 231:287–294

Invasive Imaging Techniques in the Evaluation of Patient Selection and Cerebrovascular Recanalization

H. ZEUMER, G. SIEPMANN, M. MÜLLER-JENSEN, and H. GOOSSENS-MERKT

Introduction

Digital subtraction angiography (DSA), isoosmotic dye, and microcatheters have significantly improved the technical approach to local intraarterial fibrinolysis (LIF). These methods also have much potential for providing information about the stroke-related thrombembolic process in the cerebral vessels [6].

Methods

The technique of choice for cerebral angiography is intraarterial selective digital subtraction angiography (IADSA). We use iopromide containing 150 mg iodine/ml, which is a dye isoosmotic with blood. After a 5-French sheath set has been placed in the groin, diagnostic angiography is performed using a 5-French Softip catheter (Schneider). A 45° oblique or postero-anterior projection of the vertebrobasilar territory after an injection at the orifice of the vertebral arteries is usually sufficient to demonstrate the major angiological findings, e.g., bilateral intracranial vertebral or basilar artery occlusion. While the fibrinolytic drugs are prepared for infusion, we make an injection into the right and left carotid arteries to demonstrate possible collaterals via the communicating posterior cerebral arteries.

In patients with carotid territory stroke, the first injection is made on the side of the hemiplegia. This enables us to study the collateral crossflow and is particularly helpful if carotid occlusion is the underlying pathogenetic mechanism of stroke. Secondary emboli into the middle cerebral artery (MCA) can easily be detected by this technique. The second injection is made on the side of the suspected vascular occlusion, and a long series is exposed in order to visualize the leptomeningeal collateralization as an important prognostic sign [2, 7].

University Hospital Eppendorf, Department of Neuroradiology, Martinistr. 52, W-2000 Hamburg 20, FRG.

Hacke et al. (Eds)
Thrombolytic Therapy in Acute Ischemic Stroke
© Springer-Verlag Berlin Heidelberg 1991

A steerable microcatheter, Tracker 18 (Target Therapeutics), is easily guided through the 5-French catheter with continuous coaxial flushing so that it is usually possible to place the catheter into the intracranial vessels. The microwire is bent at its tip into a "J" shape and protrudes about 2.5 cm beyond the catheter tip.

Clinical Appearance of Different Types of Stroke

The treatment of stroke by means of fibrinolysis has to be performed before vascular lesions are visible on CT. In order to satisfy the correct indications for diagnostic angiography, it is necessary to recognize and differentiate the different types of stroke using clinical signs, symptoms and patient history.

In some cases it can be difficult to differentiate clinically basilar from carotid territory stroke in the very beginning. In both vascular territories, lesions may only cause hemiparesis as the initial sign. If, however, a basilar occlusion is the underlying lesion, clinical progression is usually seen, with the appearance of tetraparesis, ataxia, or cranial nerve lesions. In contrast lacunar strokes in the basilar area or strokes due to arteriosclerotic occlusion of the circumferential arteries usually do not show such clinical progress but an acute clinical syndrome which can be localized at a definite place in the brain stem.

Chronic arteriosclerotic occlusion without additional thrombosis may be tolerated with only intermittent or minimal persistent clinical signs.

In contrast to the basilar territory, clinical signs and symptoms of carotid embolic strokes usually occur very rapidly. The natural course is extremely variable. Emboli into the M1 segment of the MCA usually more or less occlude the lenticulostriate arteries, which are terminal branches without any collateralization. Thus the involvement of the internal capsule usually leads to complete loss of motor function very early. Nevertheless morphological deterioration in the dependent vascular territories may proceed but this is not demonstrable by means of clinical tests or imaging techniques in the first 6 h after stroke. None of the clinical signs, however, is reliable enough to indicate fibrinolytic treatment, particularly if a longer period of observation cannot be performed.

Thus, angiography is necessary to make the correct indication for LIF. The causal relationship between clinical signs and symptoms and the thrombembolic pathogenesis of stroke has to be proven in advance of a potentially risky treatment. Moreover, the superselective angiography may also enable a prognosis to be made.

Superselective Angiography of Cerebral Vessels

It is well known that a small embolic occlusion in the M1 segment of the MCA may undergo early spontaneous dissolution and recanalization due to intrinsic

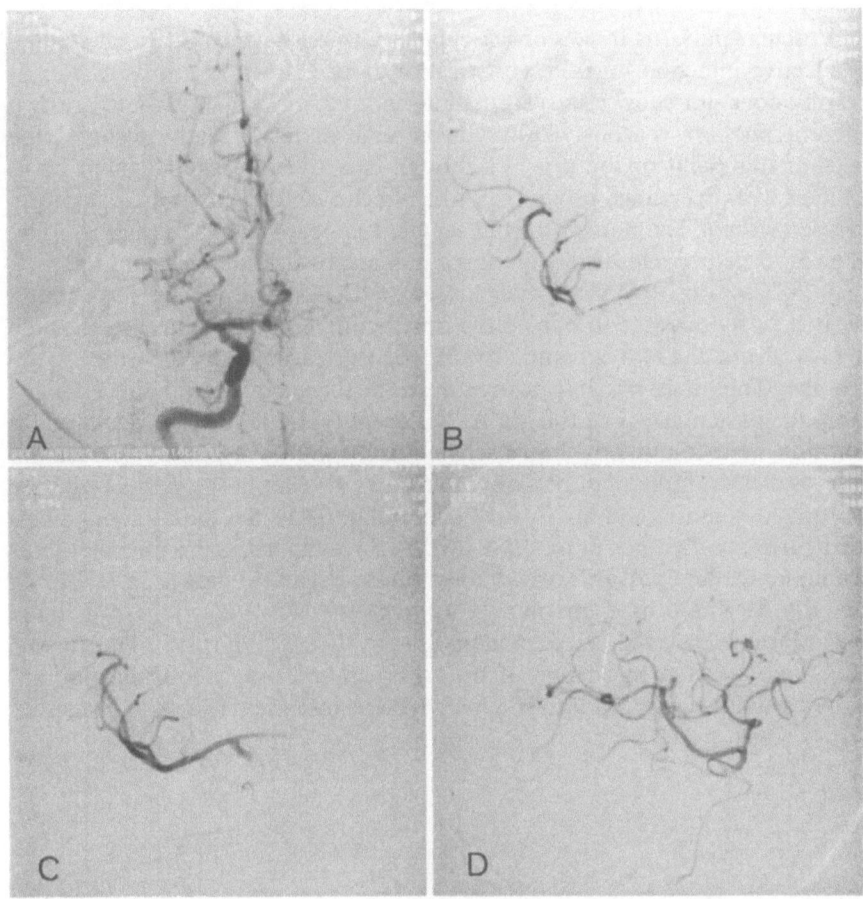

Fig. 1A–D. Acute hemiplegia due to: **A** MCA occlusion; **B** type II MCA occlusion; **C** frontal view and **D** lateral view after MCA recanalization – complete clinical improvement

fibrinolytic activity [1, 4, 5]. Under the protection of a good collateral flow only a minor infarction in the lentiform nucleus and excellent clinical recovery may occur spontaneously. But such a course is not the rule in either the MCA or the basilar artery, because of the lack of intrinsic fibrinolysis or due to widespread embolism into the peripheral vascular bed. Similarly LIF is more successful if only a short segment of a vessel is to be recanalized, while the peripheral vessels are free of thrombotic material (Fig. 1). With regard to stroke progression, the lack of sufficient intrinsic fibrinolytic activity or missing collaterals are not the only causes for clinical and morphological deterioration [2]. Obviously secondary thrombi are often built on the embolus. New thrombotic material gradually increases the size of a primarily floating embolus filling the gaps between the embolus and the vessel wall. In some cases the originally formed embolus become visible only after the secondary thrombi have been lysed.

Vascular patterns in cerebrovascular occlusion have so far been studied by selective injection into the vertebral or carotid artery. However, if angiography does not show contrast medium in a vessel segment, there are two different possible reasons: Either thrombotic material really occludes the vessel at this point or there is not enough flow to submerge stagnant pools of blood with dye, since proximally to an occlusion there is usually a poorly perfused stump. The noncontrasted segment appears larger on angiography, which is to be expected from the large amount of thrombotic material.

In all cases of embolic basilar artery or MCA occlusion we have found that it is easily possible to bypass the obstructing embolus with the steerable guidewire and then to advance the tip of the catheter to the side of the embolus. Thus it is possible to demonstrate the extension of the embolus within the basilar artery or the MCA. Different types of acute vertebrobasilar occlusion were found, which are schematically shown in Fig. 2. Performing these studies we found that basilar emboli are adherent to the vessel wall only in a small circumscribed area usually contralateral to the initial hemiparesis (for figures see Zeumer et al. 1989 [8]). LIF results using the microcatheter technique in comparison with earlier treatments are shown in Table 1. Similarly we found that embolic occlusion of the MCA has quite a variable appearance when superselective angiography is used (Fig. 3). The tips of MCA emboli often reach one of the trifurcational branches while the end of the embolus protrudes into the M1 segment to a greater or lesser degree.

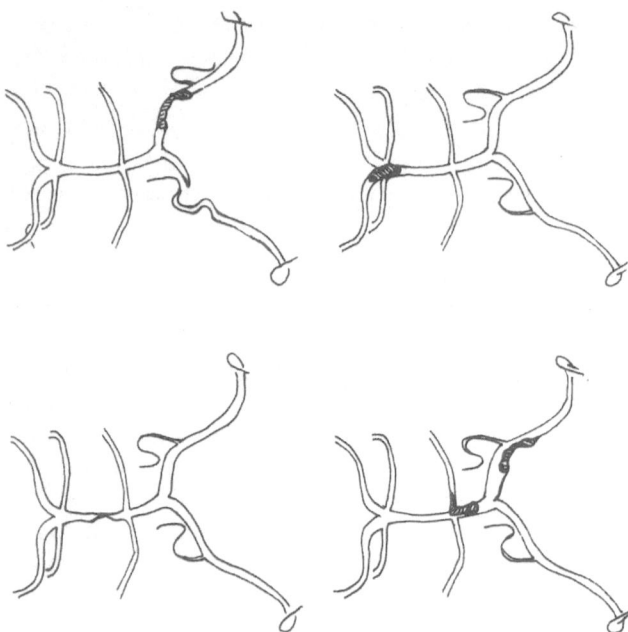

Fig. 2. Types of vertebrobasilar occlusion

Table 1. Acute vertebrobasilar occlusion treatment results

	1972–1979[a] Heparin, systemically	1980–1986[a] Urokinase selective administration	1987–1989[b] Urokinase, microcatheter administration
N	22 (100%)	44 (100%)	16 (100%)
Deaths	20 (91%)	29 (65%)	6 (37%)
Survivals	2 (9%)	15 (35%)	10 (63%)
Deficits			
Severe		1 (2.5%)	2 (12%)
Moderate	1 (4.5%)	13 (29%)	3 (19%)
Mild	1 (4.5%)	1 (2.5%)	5 (31%)

[a] RWTH Aachen.
[b] UK Eppendorf, AK Barmbek, Hamburg.

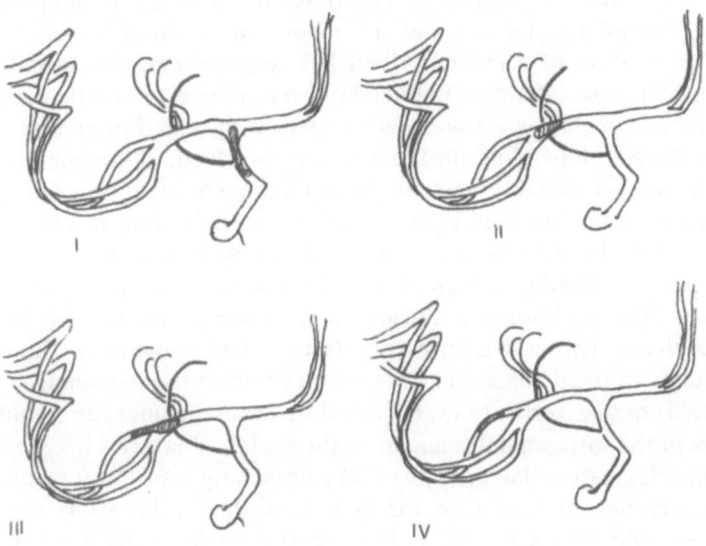

Fig. 5. Types of MCA occlusion: I–IV

After we found that it is possible to bypass the embolus for LIF we now place the tip of the catheter into the small gap between the vessel wall and the embolus. With this technique a much higher concentration of fibrinolytic agents can be delivered to the thrombus than is possible by administration of the drug into the proximal stump of the vessel. In addition superselective angiograms provide another advantage: When the catheter tip is placed distal to the embolus, the subsequent superselective angiography demonstrates either the patency of the distal vessels or the lack of flow due to other throm-

Table 2. Local intraarterial fibrinolysis for carotid territory stroke

Outcome with neurological deficits	No.	Type of occlusion				Recanalization		
		I	II	III	M	Complete	Incomplete	None
Mild	5	1	4			5		
Moderate	2			1	1		2	
Severe	1			1			1	
Death	3				3		1	2

boembolic particles downstream. This is probably of particular importance in the MCA territory as the prognosis turned out better in cases with free downstream vessels than in cases with large or fragmented emboli lodging in the peripheral MCA branches. Table 2 shows the results of LIF using the superselective microcatheter technique. The outcome in these preliminary cases seems to depend on the site and the extension of thromboembolic material. The dissolution of a circumscribed M1 segment embolus usually leads to lentiform nucleus infarction only and often to minor clinical deficits. An additional branch occlusion is usually accompanied by a territorial infarction leading to deficits depending on the territory involved. If fragmented emboli occlude several distal branches, hemispheric softening, swelling, and herniation are to be expected since complete recanalization in time is obviously impossible. In the case of basilar embolic occlusion, the downstream territories are usually visualized via the communicating posterior cerebral arteries. The additional occlusion of peripheral branches as for example the posterior cerebral arteries points to a bad prognosis. These patients are usually in deep coma and are tetraplegic from the beginning.

In the vertebrobasilar territory [3, 8], arteriosclerotic plaques are found most frequently in the intracranial segment of the vertebral arteries between the posterior inferior cerebellar artery (PICA) branching and the junction of the vertebral arteries. However, major stenosis of the basilar artery may also occur in the midbasilar segment. Using selective angiography it is very difficult to describe the true extent of such an occlusion. With the aid of microcatheters the site of the occlusion is demonstrable in more detail. Nevertheless even with the aid of microcatheters it is very difficult to differentiate pure arteriosclerotic occlusion from an occlusion which is caused by a minor atherosclerotic plaque with a major adherent thrombus. In cases with atherothrombotic occlusion of the basilar artery, the bypassing of the occlusion site has never been possible. Thus the tip of the catheter has to be placed to the outmost tip of the occluded vessel. Only if the mechanism of occlusion is predominantly thrombotic may recanalization occur. If however, the occlusion is predominantly due to arteriosclerosis leaving only a minimal residual lumen, no or only transient recanalization can be achieved.

During recent years we have learned to handle urokinase as a safe fibrinolytic drug, which influences the intrinsic hemostatic system only mildly if used with a "high-dose, short-term" strategy: 500 000 IU in the 1st h and 250 000 IU in the 2nd h. However, in the past we have repeatedly observed patients whose thrombotic material did not respond to urokinase at any rate. Furthermore we observed that it usually takes 90–120 min to achieve complete recanalization by using urokinase. Recent publications show that tissue plasminogen activator (t-PA) may be used in very low doses locally in order to recanalize peripheral vessels. Since its mechanism of action is known to be more specifically thrombolytic than urokinase or streptokinase, we try to speed up the recanalization time by applying 20 mg t-PA over 2 h. The results, however, in the ten cases examined so far have been disappointing despite high expenditure.

References

1. Adams HP, Damasio HC, Putman SF, Damasio AR (1983) Middle cerebral artery occlusion as a cause of isolated subcortical infarction. Stroke 14:948–951
2. Bozzao L, Fantozzi LM, Bastianello S, Bozzao A, Fieschi C (1989) Early collateral blood supply and late parenchymal brain damage in patients with middle cerebral artery occlusion. Stroke 20:735–740
3. Brückmann H, Ferbert A, del Zoppo GJ, Hacke W, Zeumer H (1986) Acute vertebrobasilar thrombosis. Angiological – clinical comparison and therapeutic implications. Acta Radiol (Suppl) 369:38–42
4. Saito I, Serugawa H, Shiokawa S, Tsutsumi K (1987) Middle cerebral artery occlusion: correlation of computed tomography and angiography with clinical outcome. Stroke 18:863–868
5. Taneda M, Shimada N, Tsuchiya T (1985) Transient neurological deficits due to embolic occlusion and reopening of the cerebral arteries. Stroke 16:522–524
6. Zeumer H (1989) Stellung der zerebralen Angiographie in der neuroradiologischen Diagnostik. Der Bay Int 9:2–8
7. Zeumer H, Hündgen R, Ferbert A, Ringelstein EB (1984) Local intraarterial fibrinolytic therapy in inaccessible internal carotid occlusion. Neuroradiology 26:315–317
8. Zeumer H, Grzyska U, Freitag HJ, Neunzig HP (1989) Local intraarterial fibrinolysis in acute vertebrobasilar occlusion. Recent results and technical developments. Neuroradiology 31:336–340

The Role of Noninvasive Imaging Techniques in Cerebrovascular Recanalization

S.M. Otis

Extracranial Vascular Disease

Although contrast angiography is still considered by some the best choice for evaluation of the intra- and extracranial vascular system, it has significant risks, costs, and discomfort [4]. These considerations have led to a search for a safe, easily repeatable, and accurate noninvasive method for evaluating these arteries.

The combination of high-resolution B-mode imaging with Doppler flow analysis is a significant advancement in noninvasive vascular carotid evaluation [2, 5]. The duplex system, which combines real-time B-mode ultrasonography and range-gaited pulse Doppler, provides simultaneous image and flow information. With the pulse-echo technique, the range-gaited sample volume may be placed at any site chosen within the visualized vessel, allowing the accumulation of Doppler information that is then analyzed employing fast Fourier transformation techniques.

The duplex system uses the physiologic information derived from Doppler to evaluate blood flow velocities and the two-dimensional image to visualize the walls of the vessels and evaluate plaque deposits. The image, which gives anatomical information, acts as a guide to the areas of flow disturbance which are then interrogated carefully. Blood vessels are identified by their characteristic B-mode image allowing systematic study of the common carotid, internal carotid, and external carotid arteries (longitudinally and transversely). Typical abnormalities of flow are found in areas of stenosis. Laminar flow is seen in normal vessels and in the prestenotic area, whereas in areas of stenosis, velocities are increased. As the stenotic jet reaches the post-stenotic area, the flow stream spreads out, rapidly producing disturbed flow patterns with turbulence. Usually, this turbulence subsides 1–2 cm beyond the stenosis. However, some spectral broadening may continue. Laminar flow usually is reestablished within 3 cm of the stenosis, although this is quite variable. As the arterial lumen is reduced, flow velocity must increase with the same volume of blood to traverse the narrowed segment. Peak systolic

Division of Neurology and Vascular Laboratories, Scripps Clinic and Research Foundation, 10666 North Torrey Pines Road, La Jolla, CA 92037, USA.

Hacke et al (Eds)
Thrombolytic Therapy in Acute Ischemic Stroke
© Springer-Verlag Berlin Heidelberg 1991

velocities occur with a lumen of 1–1.5 mm in diameter and, as stenosis progresses beyond this point, velocity falls off. A 50% reduction in diameter corresponds to a cross-sectional reduction in area of 75%, with blood flow remaining stable until the reduction in diameter approaches 60%. Beyond this level of obstruction, flow decreases precipitously [17, 20]. As useful as Doppler techniques are alone, they may not be good for detecting non-stenotic carotid disease that does not reduce flow. However, coupling with B-mode imaging permits the evaluation of the nonstenotic plaque and other wall changes [8, 10, 11, 15].

In cerebral vascular recanalization studies we are, of course, concerned with the recognition of thrombotic occlusions. Absence of detectable Doppler shift signal is an indication of arterial occlusion. However, a Doppler shift signal may not be detected in very severe stenosis (with only a trickle of residual flow) as mentioned above, leading to misdiagnosis of occlusion. Errors in diagnosis of occlusion with duplex examination (false positive or false negative) can be a significant problem, in that subocclusion might be remediable by surgery and occlusion by possible thrombolytic agents. Color Doppler helps to alleviate some of these difficulties by presenting flow information across the entire field of view superimposed upon the gray scale imaging. Color flow has helped in following the course of the carotid branches and in demonstrating smaller branches from the external carotid artery, which aids in vessel identification and helps lessen errors. The misdiagnosis of occlusion, however, remains a fairly constant problem even for the experienced technologist [9, 19]. Nevertheless, color Doppler imaging has increased the accuracy of noninvasive diagnosis of carotid occlusion, in that the systems are quite sensitive to very low flow states, and are clearly superior to conventional duplex systems for the particular problem of occlusion [9, 12, 19].

Intracranial Vascular Disease

In the past, noninvasive ultrasound techniques for detection of cerebrovascular disease in adults have been limited to extracranial circulation because of problems with bone penetration. However, with the development of improved instrumentation using 2-MHz pulse-wave Doppler ultrasound, we can now detect blood flow in all major arteries at the base of the brain [1, 13, 14]. As Doppler ultrasound has been widely accepted as an accurate noninvasive method for diagnosis of carotid extracranial disease, transcranial Doppler (TCD) is an extension of the use of these techniques to the intracranial arteries. The most obvious clinical advantage of TCD is its ability to rapidly screen the acute stroke patient for intracranial high-grade stenosis or complete occlusion, which could have considerable clinical impact. As in extracranial disease, mild stenosis of the basal intracranial arteries increases peak velocity with little change in the rest of the Doppler pattern, whereas moderate or severe stenosis leads to greater increase in peak velocity with spectral broadening, increased diastolic velocity and turbulent flow. A poststenotic drop in peak velocity is usually seen as well.

Occlusion of the intracerebral basal cerebral arteries can be assessed by the lack of the expected arterial signal in spite of the presence of echoes from the surrounding section of the circle of Willis. For instance, the absence of signals from the middle cerebral artery in its expected location, combined with good signals from the anterior and posterior cerebral arteries, indicates an intact temporal access window but occlusion of the middle cerebral artery. However, dislocation or congenital absence of these arteries must be excluded by other means, because they may mimic occlusion. TCD also allows the determination of the relative hemodynamic significance of tandem lesions; for instance, when stenosis occurs both at the cervical origin of the internal carotid artery coexisting with intracranial stenosis, thus influencing clinical decisions [6, 7].

Noninvasive demonstration of intracranial arterial stenosis is an extremely valuable clinical tool but there are a number of typical errors: misinterpretation of hyperdynamic collateral channels as stenosis, displacement of arteries because of a space occupying lesions, misinterpretation of physiologic variables in the circle of Willis, misdiagnosis of vasospasm as stenosis, and misinterpretation of reactive hyperemia as stenosis [16, 18]. However, with time and improved instrumentation these errors should significantly lessen.

Identification of intracranial stenosis can assist in monitoring patients during medical or surgical treatment and clearly, when perfected, will be the method of choice for monitoring medical treatments. Because this technique is relatively new, little information is available about the sensitivity and specificity of TCD in the detection of intracranial occlusions. Thus, for the present, initial angiographic studies should be performed with follow-up TCD studies.

References

1. Aaslid R (ed) (1986) Transcranial Doppler Sonography. Springer, Berlin Heidelberg New York
2. Breslau P (1981) Current status of ultrasonic techniques. In: Heerlen H (ed) Ultrasonic duplex scanning in the classification of carotid artery disease. Schrijen-Lippertz, Voerendaal, The Netherlands
3. Chikos PM, Fisher LD, Hirsch JH, Harley JD, Thiele BL, Strandness DE (1983) Observer variability in evaluating extracranial carotid stenosis. Stroke 14(6):885–892
4. Clark WM, Hatten HP Jr (1981) Noninvasive screening of extracranial carotid disease: Duplex sonography with angiographic correlation. AJNR 2:443–444
5. Comerota AJ, Cranley JJ, Katz ML, Cook SE, Sippel BJ, Hayden WG, Fogarty, TJ, Tyson RR (1990) Real-time B-mode carotid imaging: a three-year multicenter experience. J Vasc Surg (in press)

6. DeWitt LD, Wechsler H (1988) Transcranial Doppler. Stroke 19:915–921
7. Hennerici M, Rautenberg W, Schwartz A (1987) Transcranial ultrasound for the assessment of intracranial arterial flow velocity-part II. Surg Neurol 27:523–532
8. Imparato AM, Riles TS, Mintzer R, Baumann FG (1983) The importance of hemorrhage in the relationship between gross morphologic characteristics and cerebral symptoms in 376 carotid artery plaques. Ann Surg 197:195–203
9. Jacobs NM, Grant EG, Schellinger D, Byrd MC, Richardson JD, Cohan SL (1985) Duplex carotid sonography: criteria for stenosis, accuracy, and pitfalls. Radiology 154:385–391
10. Johnson JM, Ansel AL, Morgan S, Decesare D (1982) Ultrasonographic screening for evaluation and follow-up of carotid artery ulceration. Am J Surg 144:614–618
11. Lusby RJ, Ferrell LD, Ehrenfeld WK, Stoney RJ, Wylie EJ (1982) Carotid plaque hemorrhage: its role in production of cerebral ischemia. Arch Surg 117:1479–1488
12. O'Leary DH (1985) Vascular ultrasonography. Radiol Clin North Am 23(1):39–56
13. Otis S, Ringelstein EB (1990) Transcranial Doppler sonography. In: Bernstein CV (ed) Noninvasive diagnostic techniques in vascular disease. Mosby, St. Louis, p 59
14. Padayachee TS, Kirkham FJ, Lewis RR, Gillard J, Hutchinson MCE, Gosling RG (1986) Transcranial measurement of blood velocities in the basal cerebral arteries using pulsed Doppler ultrasound: a method of assessing the circle of Willis. Ultrasound Med Biol 12(1):5–14
15. Reilly LM, Lusby RJ, Hughes L, Ferrell LD, Stoney RJ, Ehrenfeld WK (1983) Carotid plaque histology using real-time ultrasonography: clinical and therapeutic implications. Am J Surg 146:188–193
16. Ringelstein EB, Ley-Pozo J (1990) Noninvasive detection of occlusive disease of the carotid siphon and middle cerebralartery. Ann Neurol 28:758–765
17. Spencer MP, Reid JM (1979) Quantitation of carotid stenosis with continuous-wave Doppler ultrasound. Stroke 10:326–330
18. Spencer MP (1983) Intracranial carotid artery diagnosis with transorbital pulsed wave (PW) and continuous wave (CW) Doppler ultrasound. J Ultrasound Med 2 [Suppl]:61
19. Taylor DC, Strandness DE Jr (1987) Carotid artery duplex scanning. J Clin Ultrasound 15:635–644
20. Zwiebel WJ, Zagzebski JA, Crummy AB, Hirschner M (1982) Correlation of peak Doppler frequency with lumen narrowing in carotid stenosis. Stroke 13:386–391

II. Thrombolysis and Stroke Models

Thrombolytic Therapy in Ischemic Stroke: Relevance and Limitations of Animal Models

G.F. MOLINARI

We have recently asked the question: "why model stroke?" [29] in reaction to still further proliferation of new devices and techniques for inducing infarction. Currently the combinations of methodologies and various animal species have produced options as variable as the natural history of stroke itself. Indeed we may select the model that gives us the results we want. Unfortunately it is the enthusiasm generated by such planned optional results that places patients at risk in premature clinical trials [7, 12, 23].

Exercising the alternative to animal modeling, using arteriographic etiological diagnoses and images of outcome lesions, an impressive collection of anecdotal cases and small uncontrolled series suggests quantitative if not absolute efficacy for local intraarterial fibrinolysis (LIF) in man in both the vertebrobasilar [5, 19, 32, 43, 44, 47] and carotid artery territories [19, 43, 45].

Unfortunately the known spontaneous conversions of a relatively larger (10%) subsample of primary middle cerebral artery (MCA) infarctions into secondary hemorrhages [2, 22] and the persistent risk of brain hemorrhage in the absence of infarction using streptokinase [36] and in cardiac patients receiving tissue plasminogen activators (t-PA) [2] still require careful assessment of the risk-benefit ratio in the application of this important therapeutic option to large numbers of acute strokes in humans. Prospective protocols currently in use call for intravenous injection of t-PA within a brief interval after stroke, less than 90 min to a maximum of 3 h, which does not enable the "proper angiographic diagnosis" previously required for LIF to be made [44, 46].

Although technical feasibility and at least partial efficacy have been established by clinicopathoradiological studies, before large-scale statistical studies are undertaken scientifically to establish efficacy of fibrinolytic therapy in acute stroke, it is entirely appropriate and ethical first to establish safety as well as efficacy in animal models.

By its nature the study of fibrinolytic agents requires that the arterial occlusion be caused by clotted blood, thus narrowing the scope of the available experimental models considerably.

Department of Neurology, George Washington University, 2150 Pennsylvania Avenue, NW, Washington, DC 20037, USA.

Hacke et al (Eds)
Thrombolytic Therapy in Acute Ischemic Stroke
© Springer-Verlag Berlin Heidelberg 1991

Qualitatively the biological model should resemble the condition to be treated in man. The usual standard for that resemblance is pathological validation of the model in a subsample of animals surviving long enough into the natural history of the disease to permit documentation of infarction at the light microscopic histopathological level, permitting time-dependent events and complications to run their natural unmodified course. Specifically, a subset of animals must survive long enough to permit evolution of spontaneous hemorrhagic complications.

While thrombosis at the site of a pathologically narrowed or distorted arterial lumen is the most common cause of ischemic stroke in man, no animal model precisely duplicates that combination of mechanisms. Embolism on the other hand is much more common as a proximate cause of arterial occlusion than had been thought at one time [24] and that event lends itself readily to modeling using homologous and even autologous blood clots.

Focusing on this one major mechanism in man, cerebral embolism is known often to cause hemorrhagic infarction [1, 6, 37] and therefore while the possibility of hemorrhagic transformation should be preserved, a spontaneous rate in the animal model control should not be greater than that observed in untreated man (10% or 5%–30%) [2, 30]. Empirically, three variables seem to contribute to the frequency and intensity of hemorrhagic infarction [28]:

1. The species of animal, cats and dogs having greater propensity toward hemorrhagic infarctions than monkeys [11]. Cats are eliminated from modeling of embolism because of the retention of a rete mirabile [17] and because static occlusive lesions produce hemorrhagic infarcts [18]. Relatively reproducible models of blood clot occlusion have been published involving dogs [14], monkeys [27, 42], rats [16, 20], and rabbits [48]. Resurgence of interest in homologous and autologous blood clot embolism occurred after the costs involved in procurement and maintenance of large species became prohibitive.

While undoubtedly credit for development of the homologous clot embolism model belongs to Hill et al. [14] at the Mayo Clinic, this early work in dogs established that the method produces primarily hemorrhagic infarction. Furthermore, success or failure in producing infarction at all depended upon yet another major variable:

2. The amount and age (or age-dependent physical properties) of clot used. Early work by Swank and Hain [39] established the importance of different-sized emboli in animal modeling. The Mayo Group observed that despite dose of clot emboli, freshly clotted (venous) blood injected into the internal carotid artery of barbiturate-anesthetized dogs rarely if ever caused infarction. Older retracted clots formed in a test tube over 24–48 h after venipuncture, found floating in their own serum, when chopped into small fragments, then injected into the internal carotid caused hemorrhagic multifocal hemispheral infarctions approximately 80% of the time. The Mayo

Group demonstrated in subsequent experiments that anticoagulant therapy makes these hemorrhagic infarctions bloodier still [41].

Our own studies suggested that relatively large amounts of freshly clotted venous blood could pass through the brains of lightly anesthetized rhesus monkeys with transient clinical signs but without pathological damage, while older retracted clots (48 h) produced infarction in the deep lenticulostriate arterial territory blocked at the origin by the segmental clot in the parent artery. Similar deep lesions are described in man caused by cerebral embolism [31].

3. The amount of available collateral circulation along with the integrity of the circulatory structures in the penumbra and perfused parenchyma influence the amount and distribution of hemorrhage into experimental ischemic lesions caused by mobile lysable blood clot emboli, stationary clips, and foreign body emboli.

Experimental Embolism

Embolic infarctions are relatively easy to produce in multiple animal species, using homologous, autologous, or heterologous blood clots, and, as in man, often produce hemorrhagic infarctions. Based on observations in larger laboratory animal models and man, the following facts must be considered in selecting models for use in evaluation of thrombolytic agents.

1. Hemorrhagic transformation is a complication, a secondary event, and may be delayed or evolve over days after the primary vascular occlusion [21, 25, 26].
2. While secondary distal embolic migration is the classically cited mechanism of hemorrhagic complication due to reperfusion [6], in animal models hemorrhagic diathesis may occur by way of collaterals and distal to fixed occlusions [9, 21].
3. Spontaneous hemorrhagic extravasation is more likely to occur in surface (arterial) lesions where collaterals are more abundant, but deep gangliar hemorrhages require reperfusion of previously occluded or otherwise damaged penetrating arterioles [26].
4. After initial embolic occlusion, the collateral vascular beds are dysautoregulatory, and therefore hemorrhagic complications and reperfusion may be both quantitatively and qualitatively adversely affected by systemic blood pressure.
5. Hemorrhagic infarction may be clinically indistinguishable from bland infarctions by neurological evaluations of surviving animals. In animal models as in man, hemorrhagic infarction may be progressing while the subject is clinically improving. Only hematomas (under arterial pressure) produce catastrophic clinical deterioration [2, 21, 26, 33].

6. Hematomas must be caused by collapse of preresistance arterioles (probably multiple) in order to generate the tissue destruction and massive acute intracranial pressure gradients and herniations characteristic of a rapidly expanding intracranial mass. While neurological deficits are dependent upon the almost instantaneous loss of metabolites by neurons, hemorrhagic complications occur when the blood vessels become necrotic, which may be somewhat later, particularly when ischemia is incomplete, as in the penumbra.

7. Probably related to the patterns of collateralization, some animal species are more susceptible than others to hemorrhagic complication.

8. The age and physical properties of the embolized clot. From the very beginning of experimentation using homologous blood clot embolism, both the age and age-dependent physical properties of the clots used were known to be important variables in producing brain infarction in dogs [14]. In both dogs and monkeys, relatively large volumes, up to 0.5 ml of freshly clotted venous blood, may pass through the cerebral arterial tree without causing infarction [25, 26]. When venous blood clots are allowed to stand for 24–48 h, the solid elements retract in their containers, becoming compact, more dense, tougher, and eventually float in the serum which had been intrinsically incorporated into the much larger original clot. When those solid elements are extracted from their own serum, shaped and sized by molding or dissection, then injected intracranially, infarctions regularly occur.

The clots used in most homologous, autologous, and even heterologous embolic models is the ropy, deep-purple stuff found in our unwashed "control" Lee-White clotting tubes 2 days after we started our patients on heparin. But is that the stuff that forms in arteries on arteriosclerotic plaques and in ventricular aneurysms? The clotting process in arteries and in the left ventricle operates at mean arterial pressure despite continuous pulse pressure waves and a solid fluid interface of irregular geometry. My surgical colleagues tell me such clots are white, composed of mainly platelets and fibrin [35]. Not only may there be differences in the kinetics of venous (stagnant) and arterial (dynamic) thrombosis [13], but the pressures under which clots are formed could considerably mold, modify the surface hemodynamics, and specific gravity as well as morphology and color of the thrombus.

One recent model, reported by Rigamonti and coworkers [35], takes some of these variables into account. By scratching the endothelium of the auricular artery in rabbits with a specially modified needle and stylet, intra-arterial thrombosis is induced. Seventy-two hours later white platelet thrombin clots are harvested and reinjected into the internal carotid system to induce cerebral infarction using 1-mm-long segments of clot. Furthermore, the method showed induction of secondary propagation of longer intraarterial clots than attributable to the injected particle. In testing fibrinolytic agents it will be advisable to compare and contrast the effects of t-PA on arterial clots as well as venous clots. In man, a clinicopathoradiological study should examine the fate of supraventricular (large-volume, low-density, oxygenated stagnant clots formed at low pressure) compared with ventricular clots from mural thrombi and ventricular aneurysms (formed from oxygenated blood under high pressure). In the absence of a clinical study in man, appropriate animal studies could provide facts about the natural history of clots from different sources and of different quality. Compact daughter clots propagate, then break away from older, organized, subacute, and chronic lesions following myocardial infarction. Arterial emboli formed at upstream intraluminal sites of injured endothelium and denuded collagen start out in a high-pressure elastic cylinder but embolic tails propagate downstream on the low-pressure side of the luminal narrowing created by the older parts of the clot. Physical properties of such embolic clots may well be transitional between the large fresh supraventricular clots formed in an unstable atrium and those formed as part of the healing of an adynamic ventricular segment. The natural history of infarctions from all three may differ with variable contributions by distal migration, spontaneous fibrinolysis, and hemorrhagic complication; all of these variables should be known before attempting to interpret the modification of these natural histories by exogenous fibrinolysins.

In summary, (a) the older and larger the ischemic zone, the more severe the neurological outcome, but, more important to the issue at hand, the older and larger the vascular lesion, the greater the pathophysiological risk of hemorrhage. (b) Small amounts of blood extravasated into a matrix of viable glia, vascular structures, and injured, nonfunctional neurons may not adversely affect neurological outcome. (c) Clots from different sources may produce different clinical and pathological ischemic and infarction patterns. Doses and modes of administration of fibrinolysins may vary between ventricular arterial embolisms and clots of supraventricular origin.

Experimental Thrombosis

While the serendipitous postembolic propagation of injected arterial clots observed by Rigamonti et al. [35] may be a quasi model of thrombosis in situ, the creation of a true model of nonembolic cerebral thrombosis remains a challenge to laboratory investigators. Nonetheless, several models require specific comment on their utility in fibrinolytic experiments.

Del Zoppo and the group at Scripps [3, 4] have more than adequately demonstrated the validity of their model of thrombosis in the lenticulostriate arteries of the baboon. After transorbital placement of an inflatable compressive device around the proximal MCA, inflation of the silicone cuff produces closure of the MCA, which is reversed after 3 h. Patency of the MCA after decompression was confirmed arteriographically, while permanent platelet thrombin occlusions of the ipsilateral lenticulostriate arteries was established by deposition of preocclusion-administered [111]indium-labeled platelets into these arteries, by emission scintigraphy, autoradiography, and fluorescent and light microscopy. Clotting was always associated with a deep gangliar ischemic infarct. Infusion of intraarterial urokinase reduced infarction size, improved neurological outcomes, and did not cause hemorrhagic transformation when given in adequate doses, while lower doses did not change clinical or pathological outcomes over controls.

Given the same hemodynamic consideration as discussed with embolism, the thrombosis in the lenticulostriate vessels in this model is most likely stagnant (low-pressure) thrombosis but surely this is a model of a common, even frequent clinical pathogenesis in man and deserves further use in testing t-PA. The author understands that the clotting system of the baboon is remarkably similar to man.

The expense and ethical debate over use of higher species are the major limiting factors to the utility of the Scripps modification of the Spetzler [38] chronic reversible ischemia model.

Somewhat more recently, Hirschberg and Hofferberth [15] have described a new method of induction of intraarterial thrombosis in situ at the trifurcation of the MCA in dogs. Tiny copper coils are delivered embolically and, because of the differential sizes of the lumina of the MCA and rostral cerebral artery, 14 of 15 trials resulted in selective embolization of the coils into the MCA. Thrombosis at the site of the coils occurred within 5–15 min of injection. The clots within the coil were described microscopically to be composed of mainly platelets, fibrin, and erythrocytes "in the form of platelet-fibrin thrombus," while propagated clot accumulated within the ascending and descending parts of the vessels could be distinguished by a relatively higher erythrocyte content.

Infarctions were produced in all cases but surviving animals were killed at 12 h so that it is not known whether hemorrhagic transformation may have occurred after that time. This indeed should provide a useful model for testing fibrinolysins and anticoagulants and especially for examining the maximal latency after thrombosis that administration of exogenous fibrinolysins may be effective.

Finally, for all of the reasons cited by Ginsberg and Busto [8] in their comprehensive review of rodent models of cerebral ischemia, particularly the lower costs of animals and materials, and both ecological and ethical acceptability, rats should and will continue to be dominant in cerebral vascular research.

Two models deserve specific comment as being useful in fibrinolytic experiments, one embolic, one "thrombotic." While there have been several published reports of homologous clot emboli in rats and in rabbits [48], a recent method reported by Papadopoulos et al. [34] uses heterologous human blood clots injected into rats in order to test the efficacy of human t-PA. Clots used were only 18 h old and were allowed to clot at room temperature (stagnant clot); although not specified, this was presumably venous blood. The response to t-PA was favorable.

In a remarkably neat, reproducible, and simple method, Watson et al. [40] induced in situ thrombosis of selected cortical vessels transcranially in the rat. Intravenous rose Bengal dye is activated by 560-nm light transcranially after mere retraction of the scalp. The light activates dye through generation of singlet oxygen parasitized lipids within the endothelial wall and blood elements, to induce platelet aggregation. While the platelet aggregation which is so prominent early on suggests adaptability of this method to studies of fibrinolysins, progressive endothelial damage and swelling causing microvascular compression at the periphery of the lesion cutting off collateral access may limit the reversibility and even accessibility of the platelet aggregates to exogenous fibrinolysins.

In conclusion, several models exist to test the risk-benefit ratio of fibrinolytic therapy in animals. By far the most rigorously tested and validated is the Scripps model of lenticulostriate thrombosis in baboons. It is also the most expensive and provocative. Many autologous and homologous embolic methods and even one heterologous embolic method have been established in all species. Usually these have involved stagnation-coagulated venous blood injected into arterial systems. Of two new thought-provoking models, one uses intraarterially clotted blood, harvested from the auricular artery and reinjected into the carotid artery of the rabbit and the other involves embolism of a copper coil which then induces thrombosis beginning within the coil but then apparently propagating both proximally and distally. Pathological changes caused by these models should certainly be compared with lesions induced by venous clots, because dose adjustments, administration routes, and duration of fibrinolytic treatment may vary according to the type and origin of the occlusive clot.

Although pretesting for safety of fibrinolytic agents in scale models, i.e., the smaller experimental animals, is still desirable and ethical, the ultimate proof of efficacy may be more expeditiously obtained from full scale man, for whom equipment resources already exist in most modern hospitals that allow direct quantitative measurement of blood flow, blood clotting, lesion size, and clinical outcome.

References

1. Cerebral Embolism Study Group (1984) Immediate anticoagulation of embolic stroke: brain hemorrhage and management options. Stroke 15:779–789
2. Del Zoppo GJ, Zeumer H, Harker LA (1986a) Thrombolytic therapy in stroke: possibilities and hazards. Stroke 17:595–601
3. Del Zoppo GJ, Copeland BR, Waltz TA, et al. (1986b) The beneficial effect of intracarotid urokinase on acute stroke in a baboon model. Stroke 17:638–643
4. Del Zoppo GJ, Copeland BR, Harker LA, et al. (1986c) Experimental acute thrombotic stroke in baboons. Stroke 17:1254–1265

5. Druschky KF, Erbguth F, Kilian KD, Neundorfer B, Huk W, Gmeiner HJ (1986): Erfahrungen mit fibrinolytischer Therapie bei Arteria-basilaris-Thrombose. Akt Neurol 13:III-XII

6. Fisher CM, Adams RD (1951) Observations on brain embolism with special reference to the mechanism of hemorrhagic infarction. J Neuropathol Exp Neurol 10:92-94

7. Fletcher AP, Olkjaersig N, Lewis M, Tulerski V, Davies A, Brooks JE, Hardin WB, Landau WM, Raichle ME (1976) A pilot study of urokinase therapy in cerebral infarction. Stroke 7:135-142

8. Ginsberg MD, Busto R (1989) Rodent models of cerebral ischemia. Stroke 20: 1627-1642

9. Globus JH, Epstein JA (1953) Massive cerebral hemorrhage: spontaneous and experimentally induced. J Neuropathol Exp Neurol 12:107-131

10. Hacke W, Zeumer H, Ferbert A, Brückmann H, Del Zoppo GJ, (1988) Intraarterial fibrinolytic therapy improves outcome in patients with acute vertebrobasilar occlusive disease. Stroke 19:1216-1222

11. Hain RF, Westhaysen PU, Swark RL (1952) Hemorrhagic carotid infarction by arterial occlusion. J Neuropathol Exp Neurol 11:34-43

12. Hanaway J, Terach R, Fletcher AP, Landau WM (1976) Intracranial bleeding associated with urokinase therapy for acute ischemic hemispheral stroke. Stroke 7:143-146

13. Harker LA, Slichter SJ (1974) Arterial and venous thromboembolism. Kinetic characterization and evaluation of therapy. Thromb Diath Haemorrh 131:188-203

14. Hill ND, Millikam CH, Wakin KG, et al. (1955) Studies in cerebrovascular disease: experimental production of cerebral infarction by intracarotid injection of homologous blood clot. Mayo Clin Proc 30:625-633

15. Hirschberg M, Hofferberth B (1988) New model of cerebral thrombosis in dogs. Stroke 19:741-746

16. Kameko D, Nakamura N, Ogawa T (1985) Cerebral infarction in rats using homologous blood emboli. Development of a new experimental model. Stroke 16:75-84

17. Kamijyo Y, Garcia J (1975) Carotid artery supply of feline brain. Stroke 6:361-369

18. Kamijyo Y, Garcia JH, Cooper J (1977) Temporary regional cerebral ischemia in the cat: a model of hemorrhagic and subcortical infarction. J Neuropathol Exp Neurol 36:338-350

19. Karnick R, Slany J, Perneczky G, Ausmerer HP, Brenner H, Leitner N (1988) Regionale Fibrinolyse akuter Verschlüsse intracerebraler Gefäße. Intensivmed 22: 31-34

20. Kudo M, Aoyoma A, Ichimori S, Fukunaga N (1982) Animal model of cerebral infarction homologous blood clot emboli in rats. Stroke 13:505-508

21. Laurent JP, Molinari GF, Oakley ML (1976) Experimental model of cerebral hematoma. J Neuropathol Exp Neurol 35:560-568

22. Lodder L, Krune-Kubat B, Broekman J (1986) Cerebral hemorrhagic infarction at autopsy: cardiac embolic cause and the relationship to the cause of death. Stroke 17:626-629

23. Meyer S, Gilroy J, Barnhart MI, Johnson JP (1963) Therapeutic thrombolysis in cerebral thromboembolism. Neurology 13:927-937

24. Mohr JP, Caplan LR, Melski JW, et al. (1978) The Harvard Cooperative Stroke Registry: a prospective registry of cases hospitalized with stroke. Neurology 28: 754-762

25. Molinari GF (1970) Experimental cerebral infarction II. Clinicopathological aspects of deep cerebral infarction. Stroke 1:222-244

26. Molinari GF (1970) Experimental cerebral infarction I. Selective segmental occlusion of intracranial arteries in the dog. Stroke 1:224-231

27. Molinari GF (1979) Clinical relevance of experimental stroke models in cerebrovascular diseases. In: Price TR, Nelson E (eds) Princeton conference on cerebrovascular disease, 11 March 1978, proceedings. Raven, New York, pp 19-33

28. Molinari GF (1986) Experimental models of ischemic stroke. In: Barnett HJ, et al. (eds) Stroke, pathophysiology, diagnosis and management. Churchill Livingstone, New York, pp 57-73

29. Molinari GF (1988) "Why model strokes?" Stroke 19:1195–1197
30. Molinari GF, Rajoub R, Lightfoote WE (1970) Experimental transient ischemic attacks, neurologically silent infarctions and strokes caused by blood clot embolism. Neurol 28:379 (abstract)
31. Morinkovic SV, Milsavlyevic MM, Koracevic MS, Stevic ZD (1985) Perforating branches of the middle cerebral artery. Stroke 16:1022–1029
32. Nenci GG, Gresele P, Taramelli M, Angelli G, Signorini E (1983) Thrombolytic therapy for thromboembolism of vertebrobasilar artery. Angiology 34:561–571
33. Ott BR, Zamani A, Kleefield J, Funkenstein HH (1986) The clinical spectrum of hemorrhagic infarction. Stroke 17:630–637
34. Papadopoulos SM, Chandler WF, Salamat MS, et al. (1987) Recombinant human tissue type plasminogen activator therapy in acute thromboembolic stroke. J Neurosurg 67:394–398
35. Rigamonti D, Uede T, Johnson PPC, et al. (1989) A new model of cerebral embolic ischemia using autologous arterial thrombus. BNI Quarterly 5:2–7
36. Ropper A (1989) Neurological intensive care. In: Toole RF (ed) Handbook of clinical neurology, vol 11 (54). Vascular diseases, part III. Elsevier Science BV, Amsterdam, pp 203–232
37. Shields RW, Laureno R, Lachman T, Victor M (1984) Anticoagulant related hemorrhage in acute cerebral embolism. Stroke 15:426–437
38. Spetzler RF, Selman WR, Weinstein P, et al. (1980) Chronic reversible ischemia: evaluation of a new baboon model. Neurosurgery 7:257–261
39. Swank RL, Hain RF (1952) The effect of different sized emboli on the vascular system and parenchyma of the brain. J Neuropathol Exp Neurol 11:280–299
40. Watson BD, Prado R, Dietrich WD, et al. (1985) Induction of reproducible brain infarction by photochemically initiated thrombosis. Ann Neurol 17:497–504
41. Whisnant JP (1958) Experimental cerebral vascular disease and dysfunction. In: Wright IS, Millikan CH (eds) Cerebral vascular diseases. Grune and Stratton, New York, pp 53–67
42. Xie Y, Minekata K, Seo K, Hossmann KA (1988) Effect of autologous clot embolism on regional protein biosynthesis of monkey brain. Stroke 19:750–759
43. Zeumer H (1985) Vascular recording techniques in interventional neuroradiology. J Neurology 231:287–294
44. Zeumer H, Hacke W, Ringelstein EB (1983) Local intraarterial thrombolysis in vertebrobasilar thromboembolic disease. Am J Neuroradiol 4:401–404
45. Zeumer H, Hundgen R, Ferbert A, Ringelstein EB (1984) Local intraarterial fibrinolytic therapy in inaccessible internal carotid occlusion. Neuroradiology 26:315–317
46. Zeumer H, Vinuela F, Nadjmi M, Ratzka M (1989): Conventional and interventional angiography. In: Toole RF (ed) Vascular diseases, part II. Elsevier Science BV, Amsterdam, pp 169–194 [Handbook of clinical neurology, vol 10 (54)]
47. Zimmerman R, Heuck CC, Harenburg J, et al. (1981) Fibrinolytische Therapie einer schweren Arteria-basilaris-Thrombose. Dtsch Med Wochenschr 106:464
48. Zivin JA, Fisher M, DiGirolami V, et al. (1985) Tissue plasminogen activator reduces neurological damage after cerebral embolism. Science 230:1289–1292

Update on Animal Model Experience with Recombinant Tissue Plasminogen Activator

M. HIRSCHBERG

Introduction

Animal experiments have demonstrated that release of vessel occlusion with early restoration of blood flow frequently diminishes cerebral infarct size [13]. The recognition of potentially reversible cerebral blood flow thresholds has led to the concept of the ischemic penumbra [1]. The time during which brain tissue can remain in this penumbral state without suffering definitive damage is still a matter of debate ([12, 16], Siesjö, this volume).

These data and the finding that a high proportion (up to 80%) of cerebral infarcts are caused by thromboembolic disease [24, 26] have led to the concept of "limitation of cerebral infarct size" by thrombolytically achieved reperfusion of occluded cerebral vessels to restore cerebral blood flow as early as possible.

Clinical trials of cerebral thrombolysis in the 1960s and 1970s reported a high incidence of cerebral hemorrhages and no benefit after thrombolytic treatment with systemically administered "nonspecific" thrombolytic drugs (e.g., streptokinase, urokinase) ([9, 18, 27], reviews see [6, 23]). With the development of new, so-called relatively fibrin-specific thrombolytic drugs like recombinant tissue plasminogen activator (rt-PA) or single-chain urokinase plasminogen activator (scu-PA), cerebral thrombolysis has received growing interest. It has, therefore, been essential to accurately examine thrombolytic stroke therapy with rt-PA in animal experiments.

Experimental Models

Several methods have been proposed to produce regional cerebral ischemia in experimental animals for the investigation of thrombolysis. The most relevant models are listed in Table 1.

The clot embolus model offers a simple way of producing thrombolytically reversible focal cerebral ischemia without intracranial surgery. The model

Neurologische Universitätsklinik Heidelberg, Im Neuenheimer Feld 400, W-6900 Heidelberg, FRG.

Hacke et al. (Eds)
Thrombolytic Therapy in Acute Ischemic Stroke
© Springer-Verlag Berlin Heidelberg 1991

Table 1. Animal models in studies of thrombolysis

Autologous clot emboli	Zivin et al. 1985, 1987, 1988, 1989
	Phillips et al. 1988, 1989, 1990
	Chehrazi et al. 1987, 1989
	Penar and Greer 1987
	Papadopoulos et al. 1987
Embolus (copper coil)	Hirschberg et al. 1986, 1987, 1988
In situ thrombosis	
MCA compression	del Zoppo et al. 1986, 1990
photochemical	Watson et al. 1985, 1987
Vascular occlusion	Slivka and Pulsinelli 1987

is used by many groups interested in animal research of thrombolysis [14, 19–21, 29]. The autologous blood clots, mostly generated by in vitro clotting of venous blood, are of varying degrees of maturity and size. The clots are injected into the internal carotid artery of small mammals: New Zealand white rabbits or Sprague-Dawley rats. According to the opinions of several investigators, the thromboembolism model comes closest to the pathological situation in human patients. However, a major disadvantage of those models is that blood clots may disaggregate and distribute randomly in the cerebral circulation. Consequently, neither infarct location nor infarct size are reproducible and outcome after therapy cannot be evaluated. In an effort to overcome these difficulties Zivin et al. [29] developed a method of measuring the average weight of clot required to produce neurological deficit or death. In this model the weight of clot increases depending on the therapeutic benefit of the thrombolytic agent.

In the second type of embolization model radiopaque copper coils are introduced into the middle cerebral arteries of dogs by a transfemoral (Seldinger) technique [10]. As in the model mentioned above, no cranial surgery is necessary. Within the copper coil an angiographically well-defined clot is formed that occludes the vessel within minutes. Thrombolytically achieved recanalization can be monitored by angiography. It is a model to test recanalization (efficacy) preferentially. As in all models that use embolization techniques the location of the copper coil embolus cannot be influenced, so infarct extent is variable.

There are also models involving production of in situ thrombosis of small cerebral vessels. This can be achieved by two techniques: (1) reversible compression of the middle cerebral artery of baboons by a surgically implanted balloon, causing local thrombosis in the territory of the lenticulostriate arteries [5]; and (2) photochemical thrombosis of cortical vessels after administration of bengal rose and subsequent illumination of the exposed skull [28]. Both techniques cause well-defined reproducible areas of infarction, but the thrombotic mechanisms and the resulting thrombi are unphysiological and extrapolation to the clinical situation is difficult. Reperfusion studies cannot be performed. The baboon MCA compression model especially demands a skilled neurosurgeon.

The fourth type of stroke model for the investigation of thrombolysis that should be mentioned was presented by Slivka and Pulsinelli [22]. They produced cerebral infarction by permanent unilateral occlusion of the carotid and middle cerebral arteries of rabbits with simultaneous hypotension. Thrombolytic drugs were administered at various times after vessel occlusion. This model only addresses the question of thrombolytically induced hemorrhage into infarcted brain areas. Reperfusion studies are not feasible.

All experimental studies of cerebral thrombolysis have focused on three major questions:

1.   Does rt-PA open up thrombotically occluded cerebral vessels?
2.   Does the treatment with rt-PA cause hemorrhage into infarcted brain areas?
3.   Does the treatment with rt-PA improve neurological outcome (e.g., diminished extent of infarction, improved neurological score)?

Reperfusion

When animal experiments on cerebral thrombolysis are compared it should be remembered that a different spectrum of sensitivities is found for rt-PA in various mammals. Compared with human clots, only 10% dissolution occurs with rat clots in the same period of time, 80% in primates, and 60% in rabbits [15]. Furthermore, the half-life of rt-PA in small animals like rats and rabbits is only one-third of that in humans, making higher doses necessary to achieve comparable rt-PA levels in such species.

In Table 2 the four studies are listed that specifically addressed angiographically controlled reperfusion with rt-PA. They were performed in New Zealand white rabbits and Sprague-Dawley rats. Focal cerebral ischemia was produced by intracarotid injection of autologous blood clots of different volumes (data not shown) and different ages.

Clot age ranged from 2 to 24 h. Although in vitro experiments have not shown any significant difference in the amount of clot lysed if the clot is between 1 and 24 h old, experiments with clots in the venous system of dogs showed that clots older than 24 h needed double the dose of a thrombolytic drug that clots only 2 h old needed [15]. Some authors even doubt that clots less than 24 h old can cause reproducible cerebral vessel occlusion (Molinari, this volume). Whether older clots make higher doses of rt-PA necessary in cerebral ischemia cannot be determined from the experiments performed in the studies discussed here. The studies are too heterogeneous with regard to

Table 2. Reperfusion experiments (angiographically controlled)

Investigator	Species	Thrombus	Clot age (h)	Dosage	Treatment onset	Reperfusion
Zivin et al. 1989	NZWR	Autologous clot	24	3–5 mg/kg Bolus + 30 min	10 min	Controls 1/18 3 mg 5/9 5 mg 6/6
Papadopoulos et al. 1987	SDR	Human clot	18	1.5 mg/kg Over 60 min	120 min	On postmortem, All patent
Phillips et al. 1988	NZWR	Autologous clot	18	1.0 mg/kg Bolus + 30 min	15 min	Controls 0/6 rt-PA 7/8
Chehrazi et al. 1989	NZWR	Autologous clot	2	1.0 mg/kg Over 120 min	30 min, 120 min, 240 min	All patent after 120 min i.v. rt-PA

NZWR, New Zealand white rabbit; *SDR*, Sprague-Dawley rat.

administration of rt-PA and assessment of reperfusion. In only two studies [3, 21] was continous angiography during rt-PA infusion performed until the vessel was recanalized. In the remaining two studies only pre- and post-treatment angiograms were taken. Treatment onset in the four studies varied between 10 min and 4 h postembolization. Regardless of treatment regimen, all studies reported a high proportion of reperfused vessels after rt-PA administration. The dosage of rt-PA in three studies was rather low (1.0–1.5 mg/kg). This is approximately the nominal dosage recommended for humans (1.0–2.0 mg/kg). However, because the effect of human rt-PA is weaker in rabbits, the dosage of rt-PA should be at least one third higher than in humans [15]. Only in the study published by Zivin's group [30] was dosage adjusted for the relatively lower activity of rt-PA in rabbits. They showed a dose-dependent response to rt-PA (recanalization of cerebral vessels): after rt-PA 5 mg/kg the recanalization rate was significantly higher than after treatment with rt-PA 3 mg/kg.

    In conclusion, rt-PA produces lysis of thrombi within the cerebral circulation in different animal models and after different doses of rt-PA. A dose-dependent recanalization rate is reported by one study. Because of species differences in the sensitivity to rt-PA the data are not directly applicable to human patients.

Occurrence of Hemorrhages

The most important safety issue in the use of thrombolytic agents in acute cerebral ischemia is the occurrence of intracerebral hemorrhage. It is feared that the hemorrhagic transformation of a bland cerebral infarction may occur and cause increased mortality and morbidity. A review of clinical experience with intra-arterial thrombolytic agents by del Zoppo et al. [6] suggested an incidence of postreperfusion hemorrhage of about 13%.

    It is well known from the natural course of cerebral ischemia that small cerebral hemorrhages subsequently occur. The mechanism of this kind of hemorrhage is not clear, however. Neuropathological investigations have suggested that collateral flow, clot lysis, and fragmentation of clot may result in hemorrhage following embolic vascular occlusion. Since the vasculature distal to the site of occlusion undergoes ischemic injury, dissolution of the thrombus and restoration of blood flow at systemic arterial pressure may cause rupture of the weakened vessel walls, resulting in intracerebral hemorrhage [8]. So-called reperfusion-hemorrhage has been suggested in several animal species [13]. Additionally, a coagulation defect as may result from a "systemic lytic state" after thrombolytic therapy has been suggested as the cause of bleeding into infarcted cerebral tissues. The interaction of these factors in cerebral infarction may create a spectrum of hemorrhages from microscopic to gross.

There are only three experimental studies that have specifically investigated the incidence of intracerebral hemorrhage following the administration of rt-PA. These studies are listed in Tables 3 and 4. Regarding hemorrhage size, criteria for microscopic and gross cerebral hemorrhages have been developed. For the baboon model, criteria from human neuropathology have been adopted [7]. "Microscopic," "punctate," "small," and "petechial" are the terms describing hemorrhages that have the connotation of not causing adverse effects on neurological outcome. Hemorrhages that are considered to be clinically meaningful are characterized as "gross," "large," or "hematoma with mass effect" (Table 3).

All three studies mentioned in Table 4 show that cerebral infarction is frequently associated with microscopic brain hemorrhage, regardless of treatment regimen, start of thrombolytic therapy, or follow-up time until pathological examination.

Concerning the occurrence of gross cerebral hemorrhages, only the study performed by Slivka and Pulsinelli [22] reported a significantly higher incidence of gross hemorrhages after administration of rt-PA 24 h after insult generation. Controls showed no hemorrhages whereas rt-PA-treated rabbits had gross hemorrhage in 75% of cases. Using a permanent vessel occlusion model they could show that the incidence of intracerebral hemorrhages was not dependent on vessel reperfusion. Rabbits treated with streptokinase within 1 h of vessel occlusion showed no gross hemorrhages (data not shown).

Lyden and coworkers [17], using a rabbit autologous clot model, found no relationship between thrombolysis after different doses of rt-PA and the incidence or size of cerebral hemorrhage, when treatment was started 10 min or 8 h after embolization or even when treatment was delayed up to 24 h. The doses of rt-PA used were sufficient to cause a systemic "lytic" state for the first 30 min after treatment, suggesting that cerebral hemorrhage after treatment was not related to coagulation disorders present at the time of vessel recanalization.

Del Zoppo and coworkers [7] found no increase in gross cerebral hemorrhages after treatment with rt-PA at various doses (up to 10 mg/kg over

Table 3. Definition of hemorrhage size

Slivka and Pulsinelli 1987	Microscopic Gross	(evident to unaided eye)
Lyden et al. 1989	punctate Small Large	(barely visible to unaided eye) <1.0 mm diameter, 1 block face >1.0 mm diameter, >2 block faces
del Zoppo et al. 1990	Petechial Confluent petechial Hematoma Other	0.2–2.0 mm ≤1.0 cm mass effect (e.g., subarachnoid)

Table 4. Occurrence of hemorrhages

Investigator	Treatment onset	tPA dosage (mg/kg)	Follow-up	Hemorrhage Microscopic	Microscopic
Slivka and Pulsinelli 1987	24 h	0.5	30 h	79% control 95% rt-PA	0% 75%
Lyden et al. 1989	10 min	Control 3.0 5.0	24 h	ND	7/18 6/9 3/6
	8 h	Control 3.0 5.0	32 h	1/20 1/5 0/20	4/20 1/5 6/20
	24 h	Control 3.0/5.0	48 h	1/8 3/11	2/8 4/11
del Zoppo et al. 1990	3 h	Control 0.3 1.5 10	14 days	7/12 5/6 4/6 6/6	1/12 1/6 0/6 0/6

60 min i.v.) when treatment was begun 3 h after compression of the middle cerebral artery (MCA) although a dose-dependent increase in the number of extracranial hemorrhages was observed. This disparity between the incidence of peripheral hemorrhages and the absence of significant ischemia-related hemorrhagic transformation was interpreted as a "difference in the response of the respective vascular beds to different vascular injuries in the presence of rt-PA." There was no association between the volume of hemorrhage and the volume of infarction or rt-PA dose.

In summary, infarction-related microscopic hemorrhages often accompany stroke in different animal models, regardless of treatment. This may be interpreted as a sign of progressive endothelial disruption. Early infusion of rt-PA does not increase the incidence of clinically meaningful hemorrhagic transformation, indicating that reperfusion-related hemorrhage is not aggravated by rt-PA, at least within a certain time period. There is apparently no association of hemorrhagic transformation with treatment onset time, rt-PA dosage, infarct size, or coagulation disorders. However, these results should be extrapolated with caution to clinical use of rt-PA in humans. All the animals used were young and healthy, free of preexisting atherosclerotic vascular disease or hypertension.

Evidence for Clinical Improvement?

After having looked at reperfusion (efficacy) and the incidence of hemorrhage (safety), the crucial question remains whether there is any evidence indicating a benefit from rt-PA treatment after stroke in animal experiments. Table 5 lists all the major results of animal studies that have examined improvement of outcome after rt-PA treatment.

Besides positron emission tomography (PET), other functional parameters like cerebral blood flow (hydrogen clearance technique and autoradiography), EEG, neurological scores, and measurement of infarct size have been used to evaluate outcome after treatment with rt-PA in different animal models of focal cerebral ischemia.

A rather pessimistic outlook is given by the study performed by De Ley and coworkers [4]. Because of the importance of this study it is mentioned here, although rt-PA effects were not investigated, but rather recanalization by streptokinase. The investigators looked at improvement of oxygen consumption, oxygen extraction, and tissue perfusion (cerebral blood flow, CBF) with PET. Vessel reperfusion was monitored angiographically. They found a normalization of cerebral blood flow and other parameters only when treatment was started 5 min after onset of ischemia. After a treatment delay of 30 min no salvage of tissue or amelioration of CBF was observed despite clot lysis.

In a photochemical cortical infarction model, Watson and coworkers [28] observed an improvement of cerebral blood flow in the infarcted brain area

Table 5. Assessment of improvement

Investigator	Model	tPA-onset (min)	Method	Outcome (significant results)
Watson et al. 1985	Photochemical	10 240	CBF	Improved CBF, smaller infarct volume No improvement
Papadopoulos et al. 1987	Autologous clot	120	EEG, CBF	CBF within 60 min preembol. value EEG better after 150 min
De Ley et al. 1988	Autologous clot	5 30	PET	CBF normalized No improvement
Zivin et al. 1988	Autologous clot	15 and 45 60	3-point clinical scale	Less severe infarcts No improvement
Chehrazi et al. 1989	Autologous clot	30–240	Infarct size	Infarct size smaller up to 30 min
del Zoppo et al. 1990	MCA compression	180	Infarct size Neurol. score	No reduction No improvement

and smaller infarct volume when rt-PA treatment was started as early as 10 min after cerebral ischemia. There was no improvement when treatment was delayed for 4 h.

Significant improvement of cerebral blood flow and EEG was reported by Papadopoulos and coworkers [19] when treatment was begun 2 h after embolization.

Zivin and coworkers [30] showed that, for a treatment onset interval of up to 45 min after embolization, a significantly larger amount of embolic clot was required to cause neurological damage than in controls treated with saline. This difference was not found in animals treated 60 min after embolization.

Infarct size was only reduced when treatment onset occurred after 30 min in another rabbit clot model. Longer treatment delays showed no significant reduction of infarct size [3].

In a study with 30 baboons that were treated with rt-PA in different doses after 3 h of focal ischemia and were followed up for 14 days, no significant reduction in infarct size was observed. An elaborate neurological score showed no significant improvement in comparison to a control cohort [7].

In summary, the results of different animal studies suggest that it may be possible that at least some function can be salvaged by treatment with rt-PA after severe ischemia of as much as 1 h duration. In the penumbral zone it may even be possible to sustain a more protracted insult before tissue destruction is irreversible [1]. It is probable, however, that beyond a few hours of ischemia infarction is inevitable and reperfusion will provide no benefit. The treatment onset period for useful application of thrombolytic therapy with rt-PA is short. A search for other means of protecting the ischemic brain in animal focal ischemia models to extend the latency time for thrombolytic therapy may be helpful.

References

1. Astrup J, Siesjö B, Symon L (1981) Thresholds in cerebral ischemia—the ischemic penumbra. Stroke 12:723–725
2. Brott T, Haley EC, Levy DE, Barsan WG, Reed RL, Olinger CP, Marler JR (1988) Very early therapy for cerebral infarction with tissue plasminogen activator (tPA) (abstr). Stroke 19:133
3. Chehrazi BB, Seibert JA, Kissel P, Hein L, Brock J (1989) Evaluation of recombinant tissue plasminogen activator in embolic stroke. Neurosurgery 24:355–360
4. De Ley G, Weyne J, Demeester G, Stryckmans K, Goethals P, Van de Velde E, Leusen I (1988) Experimental thromboembolic stroke studied by positron emission tomography: immediate versus delayed reperfusion by fibrinolysis. J Cereb Blood Flow Metab 8:539–545
5. Del Zoppo GJ, Copeland BR, Harker LA, Waltz TA, Zyroff J, Hanson SR, Battenberg E (1986a) Experimental acute thrombotic stroke in baboons. Stroke 17:1254–1265
6. Del Zoppo GJ, Zeumer H, Harker LA (1986b) Thrombolytic therapy in stroke: possibilities and hazards. Stroke 17:595–607

7. Del Zoppo GJ, Copeland BR, Anderchek K, Hacke W, Koziol JA (1990) Hemorrhagic transformation following tissue plasminogen activator in experimental cerebral
   infarction. Stroke 21:596–601
8. Fisher CM, Adams RD (1951) Observations on brain embolism with special reference
   to the mechanism of hemorrhagic infarction. J Neuropathol Exp Neurol 10:92–93
9. Fletcher AP, Alkjaersig N, Lewis M, Tulevski V, Davies A, Brooks JE, Hardin WB,
   Landau WM, Raichle ME (1976) A pilot study of urokinase therapy in cerebral
   infarction. Stroke 7:135–142
10. Hirschberg M, Hofferberth B (1988) New model of cerebral thrombosis in dogs.
    Stroke 19:741–746
11. Hossmann KA, Kleihues P (1973) Reversibility of ischemic brain damage. Arch Neurol
    29:375–382
12. Hossmann KA (1982) Treatment of experimental cerebral ischemia. J Cereb Blood
    Flow Metab 2:275–297
13. Kamijyo Y, Garcia JH, Cooper J (1977) Temporary regional cerebral ischemia in the
    cat. A model of hemorrhagic and subcortical infarction. J Neuropathol Exp Neurol
    36:338–350
14. Kissel P, Cherazi B, Seibert JA, Wagner FC (1987) Digital angiographic quantifica-
    tion of blood flow dynamics in embolic stroke treated with tissue-type plasminogen
    activator. J Neurosurg 67:399–405
15. Korninger C, Collen D (1981) Studies on the specific fibrinolytic effect of human
    extrinsic (tissue-type) plasminogen activator in human blood and in various animal
    species in vitro. Thromb Haemost 46:561–565
16. Lassen N, Vorstrup S (1984) Ischemic penumbra results in incomplete infarction: is the
    sleeping beauty dead? Stroke 15:755
17. Lyden PD, Zivin JA, Clark WA, Madden K, Sasse KC, Mazzarella VA, Terry RD,
    Press GA (1989) Tissue plasminogen activator-mediated thrombolysis of cerebral
    emboli and its effect on hemorrhagic infarction in rabbits. Neurology 39:703–708
18. Meyer JS, Herndon RM, Gotoh F, Tazaki Y, Nelson JN, Johnson JF (1961) Thera-
    peutic thrombolysis. In: Millikan CH, Siekert RG, Whisnant JP (eds) Cerebral vas-
    cular disease. 3rd Princeton Conference. Grune and Stratton, New York, pp 160–177
19. Papadopoulos SM, Chandler WF, Salamat MS, Topol EJ, Sackellares JC (1987)
    Recombinant human tissue-type plasminogen activator therapy in acute throm-
    boembolic stroke. J Neurosurg 67:394–398
20. Penar PL, Greer CA (1987) The effect of intravenous tissue-type plasminogen activator
    in a rat model of embolic cerebral ischemia. Yale J Biol Mec 60:233–243
21. Phillips DA, Fisher M, Smith TW, Davis MA (1988) The safety and angiographic
    efficacy of tissue plasminogen activator in a cerebral embolization model. Ann Neurol
    23:391–394
22. Slivka A, Pulsinelli W (1987) Hemorrhagic complications of thrombolytic therapy in
    experimental stroke. Stroke 18:1148–1156
23. Sloan MA (1987) Thrombolysis and stroke. Past and future. Arch Neurol 44:748–768
24. Solis OJ, Roberson GR, Taveras JM, Mohr JP, Pessin MS (1977) Cerebral angiography
    in acute cerebral infarction. Rev Interam Radiol 2:19–25
25. Spetzler RF, Selman WR, Weinstein P, Townsend J, Mehdoric M, Telks D, Crummine
    RC, Macko R (1980) Chronic reversible cerebral ischemia: Evaluation of a new
    baboon model. J Neurosurg 7:257–261
26. Stillman M, Ronthal M, Kleefield J, O'Reilly G, Wang A, Zamani A, Rumbough
    C (1987) Cerebral infarction: Shortcomings of angiography in the evaluation of intra-
    cranial cerebrovascular disease. Medicine 66:297–308
27. Sussman B, Fitch T, Plainfield N (1958) Thrombolysis with fibrinolysin in cerebral
    arterial occlusion. JAMA 167:1705–1709
28. Watson BD, Prado R, Dietrich WD, Busto R, Scheinberg P, Ginsberg MD (1987)
    Mitigation of evolving cortical infarction in rats by recombinant tissue plasminogen
    activator following photochemically induced thrombosis. In: Raichle ME, Powers WJ
    (eds) Cerebrovascular diseases. Raven, New York, pp 317–330

29. Zivin JA, Fisher M, DeGirolami U, Hemenway CC, Stashak JA (1985) Tissue plasminogen activator reduces neurological damage after cerebral embolism. Science 230:1289–1292
30. Zivin JA, Lyden PD, DeGirolami U, Kochhar A, Mazzarella V, Hemenway CC, Johnston P (1988) Tissue plasminogen activator. Reduction of neurologic damage after experimental embolic stroke. Arch Neurol 45:387–391

III. Clinical Trials

Clinical Trials: Some General Considerations

Trials might be compared to the famous little girl with a curl in the middle of her forehead. You recall that when she was good, she was very, very good, but when she was bad, she was horrid. There is no more useful vehicle in all of clinical medicine than an effective, well-designed, well-analyzed trial. There is also, however, an abundance of very bad trials that waste our resources and time and yield few answers.

The main problem of trials can be captured in the dilemma of numbers versus specificity. The substance of clinical trials is numbers and the gods of trials are statisticians who devour numbers as their major food. In order for a trial to be valid a large enough N is needed for analysis. Unfortunately, in order to get numbers, specificity is often lost. Practicing physicians treat patients with very specific problems. In order for the results of a trial to be useful, it must help physicians deal with the specific problems of their patients. General answers are often not helpful. There are only three ways to get numbers: (a) Have a large enough center that can enroll enough patients with a specific problem. Few centers have this capability and even if they do it may take too long to enroll enough patients. (b) Lump together diverse conditions to acquire enough patients; this sacrifices specificity. (c) Have cooperative studies with enough centers working together to enroll enough patients with a specific problem. The intravenous recombinant tissue-type plasminogen activator (rt PA) in acute thrombotic stroke trial discussed in this volume is an excellent example of the latter strategy.

Trials that study general conditions, e.g., one drug for all patients with transient ischemic attacks or cerebral ischemia, have not been helpful. Trials which study specific problems, e.g., prevention of emboli in patients with atrial fibrillation, or prevention of new posterior circulation ischemic attacks in patients with basilar artery stenosis, are examples of potentially good trials which consider important specific problems. The issues in trials should be: easy to define; have clear end points; and be sufficiently common to enable enrollment of sufficient cases!

Considering trials of thrombolysis, the focus of this meeting, there are two different end points: (a) Does the treatment allow recanalization of the

---

Department of Neurology, Tufts University, New England Medical Center Hospitals, 750 Washington Street, Boston, MA 02111, USA.

Hacke et al (Eds)
Thrombolytic Therapy in Acute Ischemic Stroke
© Springer-Verlag Berlin Heidelberg 1991

occluded artery. As far as is known there is no reason to expect improvement in patient function if the artery does not reopen. (b) Does the patient improve or at least not worsen as a result of the treatment. Does thrombolytic treatment do better than no treatment or alternate treatments. This latter end point is more complex than simple recanalization. Ischemic stroke is heterogeneous. It is difficult to compare deficits from a middle cerebral artery (MCA) stroke with a vertebrobasilar lesion. It is even difficult to compare an aphasic deficit from left MCA disease with visual neglect and anosognosia of right cerebral, right MCA disease. Recovery from a given incident of ischemia depends on factors that relate to the anatomy of the lesion, factors that relate to the disease process and extent, factors that relate to the specific function studied, and factors that relate to the individual patient. In my opinion, in thrombolytic trials we must first study recanalization by documentation of the intraarterial lesion, and then turn to the issue of clinically significant improvement.

Intraarterial Urokinase Plasminogen Activator and Streptokinase in Carotid and Vertebrobasilar Territory Stroke: Clinical Outcome

W. HACKE

Introduction

Recent experience with a limited number of patients at several institutions using local infusion of fibrinolytic agents suggests that early use of intra-arterial urokinase-type plasminogen activator (u-PA) and streptokinase may effect clinical improvement without unacceptable intracerebral hemorrhagic complications. This report summarizes the results of two recently published studies on intraarterial thrombolytic therapy in acute carotid territory and in acute vertebrobasilar stroke.

Patients fulfilling the inclusion criteria and not meeting exclusion criteria (Table 1) detailed in the original publications were treated following the protocol as follows:

1. Clinical assessment
   (including Doppler ultrasound, if possible)
2. Cranial CT
3. Angiography
4. Intraarterial infusion of streptokinase or urokinase at various dosages
5. Repeat angiography
6. Heparin
7. Neurologic intensive care unit

They were transferred to the neuroradiologic facility to receive the fibrinolytic agent by intraarterial infusion via the angiographic system as routinely employed for the initial diagnostic study. Repeat selective angiograms were performed immediately following completion of the intraarterial infusion. The patients were then returned to the neurologic intensive care unit for observation and follow-up care. The method of local intraarterial fibrinolytic therapy has been detailed elsewhere [4].

Neurologische Universitätsklinik, Im Neuenheimer Feld 400, W-6900 Heidelberg, FRG.

Hacke et al (Eds)
Thrombolytic Therapy in Acute Ischemic Stroke
© Springer-Verlag Berlin Heidelberg 1991

Table 1. Inclusion and exclusion criteria

Inclusion

1. Recent (<8 h) severe stroke in the carotid or VB territory
2. Angiographically demonstrated corresponding arterial occlusion
3. Age 20–75 years
4. Cranial CT: no hemorrhage; no hypodense lesion
5. Informed consent

Exclusion

1. Usual exclusion criteria for thrombolytic therapy such as:
   a) Malignant hypertension
   b) Recent surgery
   c) Intracranial hemorrhage

Vertebrobasilar Occlusive Disease

In a retrospective analysis the treatment experience in 43 consecutive patients with clinical signs of severe brain stem ischemia with angiographically demonstrated vertebrobasilar (VB) artery thrombotic occlusions who received local intraarterial fibrinolytic therapy with either urokinase or streptokinase has been reported [3]. The data were analyzed with respect to cerebral artery occlusion patterns, posttreatment arterial recanalization, and clinical outcome (survival/death and favorable/unfavorable outcome). In subgroup analyses, recanalization correlated significantly with favorable clinical outcome. In 19 of 43 patients recanalization following thrombolytic therapy was demonstrated angiographically, while in 24 patients the occlusion persisted. All patients without reperfusion died. In contrast, 14 out of 19 patients who showed recanalization survived ($p = 0.000007$), 10 of them having a favorable clinical outcome.

In comparison, 22 patients with VB artery occlusive disease who were given alternative antiplatelet/anticoagulation treatment were reviewed. Only three survived, each with a moderate clinical deficit. When these groups were compared, highly significant differences in both outcome quality ($p = 0.017$) and survival ($p = 0.0005$) were found to depend on establishing reperfusion. Patient characteristics, methods, subgroup analysis, definition of clinical outcome events as well as angiologic data and clinical findings have been detailed in three recent publications [1, 3, 5].

Since the outcome events of arterial recanalization and of clinical improvement are theoretically partly interdependent, a favorable clinical outcome is attributable to the fibrinolytic therapy only if arterial recanalization has been demonstrated.

The improvement in clinical outcome and survival rate in the patients achieving successful arterial reperfusion after fibrinolytic therapy was statistically highly significant compared with those patients not displaying recanalization, and with the retrospective group of conventionally treated VB patients (Table 2).

The clinical features of some VB artery occlusions may make it very difficult to identify the time of symptom onset in order to assess the time limits for reestablishment of flow. Fluctuating symptoms and progressive stroke leading to sudden deterioration with coma and tetraparesis is not uncommon.

Clinical status on admission proved to be a valuable prognostic factor. When coma and/or tetraparesis was present for several hours, no differential benefit of recanalization on survival was noted. Therefore, it seems most important to begin treatment as soon as possible.

To determine prognostically significant angiographic or clinical findings, a number of combinations of admission status and occlusion patterns were tested. Of interest, 11 of 23 patients (47.8%) with an extremely poor admission status had extended VB artery occlusion patterns, consistent with multiterritorial VB syndromes. The number of survivors presenting with the combination of an extremely poor clinical admission status plus a mid-basilar occlusion or an extended multilevel occlusion pattern (2 of 16) was significantly lower ($p = 0.04$) than the number of survivors with the combination of a top of basilar artery (TOP) or caudal vertebobasilar (CVB) occlusion pattern without a poor clinical admission status (10 of 22). The question arises whether this significant result may be attributed to a more favorable natural history of TOP and CVB patients. This does not seem to be the case, as only 2 of 11 patients in groups A and B_2 who presented with the same clinical severity survived without recanalization compared with 8 survivors of 11 patients in group B_1. All other patients died after several days, showing continuous deterioration of their symptoms leading to coma, or the "locked-in" syndrome.

The incidence of hemorrhagic transformation among patients receiving fibrinolytic agents was 4 out of 43 (9.6%). This fits within the range reported for hemorrhage associated with infarction in the carotid territory.

Table 2. Clinical outcome among treatment (sub)groups and paired group comparisons in acute basilar thrombosis

Group		N	Clinical outcome categories			
			Favorable	Unfavorable	Survival	Death
A		22	3	19	3	19
B_1		19	10	9	13	6
B_2		24	0	24	0	24
			Paired group comparisons			
A	B_1		0.017			0.0005
B_1	B_2		0.00005			0.000007
A	B_2		0.10			0.10

A, patients receiving systemic antiplatelet/anticoagulant agents; $B_1 + B_2$, patients receiving intraarterial fibrinolytic agents; B_1, arterial recanalization; B_2, no arterial recanalization.

Interestingly, two patients exhibited hemorrhagic infarction in the absence of recanalization. There was no laboratory test indicative of the impending hemorrhage.

Despite the limitations of retrospective analyses of open studies, and the limited information about the natural history of acute severe brain stem strokes due to VB artery occlusions, this study presents preliminary evidence that early recanalization of VB occlusion may be accompanied by a significant improvement in clinical outcome. Local intraarterial delivery of fibrinolytic agents in patients suffering from acute VB occlusion provides the following useful new insights: (a) recanalization of acute occluded cerebral vessels is possible, (b) recanalization can be achieved without an increased risk of intracerebral hemorrhage, and (c) recanalization is accompanied by a significant improvement in survival and clinical outcome.

Thrombolytic Therapy in Acute Carotid Territory Stroke

A prospective angiography-based pilot study of acute carotid territory stroke patients was undertaken at two centers. The study was designed to look at arterial recanalization as the primary outcome event, while secondary hemorrhage and clinical outcome were assessed separately. Patient characteristics, exclusion criteria, treatment regimen, data review, and statistics were described in the original publication [2].

Recanalization of the previously occluded carotid territory brain-supplying artery was judged by the neuroradiologist as: (a) no reperfusion, (b) partial perfusion, or (c) complete return of perfusion following infusion of the thrombolytic agent. Partial perfusion consisted of residual occlusion of the principal artery or perfusion of only some of the previously occluded major branches.

The appearance of an intracerebral hemorrhage detected by computed tomography (CT) scan was classified as hemorrhagic infarction (without clinical deterioration), secondary cerebral hematoma, or parenchymatous hemorrhage with mass effect and clinical deterioration. Clinical outcome was judged by the clinical status on hospital discharge compared with the neurologic deficits on admission.

Complete recanalization was documented by angiography in 15 patients within 24 h of the baseline study. Ten of the 15 patients demonstrated partial to near-complete resolution of the neurologic (motor) deficits, whereas the two patientys who did not demonstrate recanalization showed no clinical improvement. Partial recanalization (residual stenosis or recanalization of some branches) occurred in three patients (Table 3).

Four patients suffered CT-detectable intracerebral hemorrhagic transformations within 24 h after intraarterial infusion; however, no clinical deterioration or death could be attributed to the intracerebral hemorrhage.

Table 3. Intraarterial thrombolytic therapy in acute carotid stroke: arterial recanalization and intracerebral hemorrhage

Recanalization	n	Complete/ near-complete	Partial	Unchanged	Deterioration/ death
Complete	15 (4)	6 (2)	4 (1)	4 (1)	1 (10)
Partial	3		2		1
Nil	2			1	1

Numbers in *parentheses* are cases of intracerebral hemorrhage.

All four hemorrhagic events occurred in the 15 patients who demonstrated complete arterial recanalization. The hemorrhagic transformations were consistent with hemorrhagic infarctions by CT appearance and absence of clinical worsening; each hemorrhage resolved during hospitalization. Three of the four patients demonstrated clinical improvement despite the hemorrhage. The patients who hemorrhaged had been given concomitant heparin with hydroxyethyl starch in the immediate postinfusion period. All hemorrhagic infarctions occurred in the affected lenticulostriate artery (LSA) territory; no CT-detectable hemorrhagic event occurred in two patients with large hemispheric infarctions, who finally died from transtentorial herniation. A complete recanalization rate of 75% was achieved in our study, a rate similar to that observed for local thrombolytic therapy in acute myocardial infarction patients. The relevance of this recanalization rate compared with the spontaneous recanalization rate in acute carotid territory stroke cannot be determined from currently available data.

This study presents preliminary evidence that recanalization of carotid territory occlusions may be achieved with conventional fibrinolytic agents delivered by interventional techniques.

Conclusions

The recent clinical studies emphasize a number of poorly defined complex factors surrounding the issue of efficacy and safety. Although electrophysiologic studies have suggested that ischemic injury to cerebral tissue may be tolerated for longer periods than previously thought, thrombolytic therapy may only preserve tissue within the ischemic penumbra. In a given individual this is related to the variability of collateral flow. The precise time limits for initiation of thrombolytic therapy in acute stroke relative to the onset of symptoms have not yet been defined. Furthermore, the distinction between a parenchymatous hemorrhage with associated clinical deterioration and the more clinically benign, but evident on CT scan, hemorrhagic infarction will be critical in safety assessments. Other important practical considerations include: (a) the necessity to demonstrate thrombotic occlusion of a cerebral arterial supply appropriate for the symptoms, (b) the distinction between fluctuating or reversible neurologic deficits and those which are fixed and stable, (c) the natural histories of arterial occlusion in the carotid and VB territories and their individual subgroups, and (d) the necessity to exclude alternative diagnoses in the early minutes to hours of the event. A prospective controlled study will be necessary to resolve the question of whether early thrombolytic therapy can salvage function without significant risk.

The conclusions that might be drawn from these two studies are summarized as follows:

1. Recanalization can be achieved in both VB and intracranial carotid/ middle cerebral occlusive disease
2. Clinical outcome is improved significantly in vertebrobasilar occlusion
3. Treatment is safe
4. Hemorrhagic transformation is rare and is not followed by clinical deterioration in hemispheric infarction
5. Brain edema occurs with and without recanalization
6. It seems feasible to extend the treatment to patients with less severe hemispheric stroke
7. In VBO, our pilot study helped to identify a subgroup of patients who would most likely benefit from the treatment

The open studies reported and the lack of any proven therapy of acute ischemic stroke both emphasize the need for further evaluation of this possibly helpful therapeutic approach. Both local intraarterial infusion and systemic use of fibrinolytic agents will have to be studied in the future to ascertain the most promising treatment approach.

References

1. Brückmann H, Ferbert A, Del Zoppo GJ, Hacke W, Zeumer H (1986) Acute vertebral-basilar thrombosis. Acta Radiol 369 (Suppl):38–42
2. Del Zoppo GJ, Ferbert A, Otis S, Brückmann H, Hacke W, Zyroff J, Harker LA, Zeumer H (1988) Local intra-arterial fibrinolytic therapy in acute carotid territory stroke. Stroke 19:307–313
3. Hacke W, Zeumer H, Ferbert A, Brückmann H, Del Zoppo GJ (1988) Intraarterial fibrinolytic therapy improves outcome in patients with acute vertebrobasilar occlusive disease. Stroke 19:1216–1222
4. Zeumer H (1985) Survey of progress: vascular recanalizing techniques in interventional neuroradiology. J Neurol 231:287–294
5. Ferbert A, Buchner H, Brückmann H, Zeumer H, Hacke W (1988) Evoked potentials in basilar artery thrombosis: correlation with clinical and angiographic findings. Electroencephalogr Clin Neurophysiol 69:136–147

Fibrinolytic Recanalization Therapy in Acute Cerebrovascular Thromboembolism

E. Mori

Introduction

Favorable results in the recent trials of streptokinase and urokinase [6, 7, 9, 12, 15, 16] and the development of recombinant tissue-type plasminogen activator (rt-PA) [2, 3, 5, 8, 13] have renewed interest in thrombolytic therapy in ischemic stroke. I describe here my latest findings on fibrinolytic recanalization therapy in acute stroke. The first section describes local intraarterial urokinase plasminogen activator (u-PA) infusion with acute stroke, and the second section outlines the progress which has been made in our ongoing systemic recombinant tissue-type plasminogen activator (rt-PA) trial in acute carotid territory stroke. Basic issues we must resolve with our clinical trials are first whether early recanalization is followed by clinical improvement and second whether fibrinolytic agents can adequately and safely recanalize occluded arteries.

Intraarterial u-PA Trial

Subjects and Methods

The u-PA study group consisted of 44 patients with acute thromboembolic occlusion of the major cerebral artery who were treated with intraarterial u-PA between 1983 and 1990. They included 23 men and 21 women, with a mean age of 61.4 ± 10.3 (SD) years (range, 40–77 years). They included 8 with internal carotid artery (ICA) occlusion, 31 with middle cerebral artery (MCA) occlusion, and 5 with basilar artery (BA) occlusion. Of the 31 patients with MCA occlusion, 4 had multiple cerebral artery occlusions. Criteria for thrombolysis included appropriate clinical signs of ischemia, usually an interval from onset to infusion of less than 6 h or of less than 12 h

Neurology Service, Hyogo Brain and Heart Center at Himeji, 520, Saisho-Ko, Himeji, 670, Japan.

Hacke et al (Eds)
Thrombolytic Therapy in Acute Ischemic Stroke
© Springer-Verlag Berlin Heidelberg 1991

when symptoms were still evolving; age under 80 years; absence of apparent computed tomography (CT) hypodensity related to the ischemic events; and no contraindication for urokinase such as history of gastrointestinal bleeding. The etiology of the arterial occlusions was supposed to be embolic in 28 patients because of an abrupt completion of symptoms and the presence of cardiac diseases as a potential source of emboli.

After obtaining a brief medical history, physical and neurological examinations, blood for routine laboratory work, and brain CT, and after obtaining informed consent for the procedure from accompanying relatives, patients underwent emergency cerebral angiography. The right or left femoral artery was penetrated with a 7-F side-arm valved sheath. A 7-F catheter was used for selective angiography. After advancing the catheter to the internal carotid or vertebral artery, urokinase was continuously infused through the catheter. Angiography was repeated to watch for thrombus dissolution. Once reperfusion was established, the infusion was discontinued. If reperfusion was not established by 30 min, infusion was stopped. Thus, the duration of infusion ranged from 10 to 30 min.

Recanalization

The mean urokinase dosage given was 0.88 ± 0.25 mega units. The interval from onset of symptoms to infusion was from 45 min to 12 h, an average of 236 ± 162 min. Recanalization was achieved in 16 of 44 patients. The recanalization rate for each artery is shown in Fig. 1. The recanalization rate of the MCA and BA was nearly 50%. By contrast, ICA occlusion was opened in only one patient, and multiple arterial occlusions failed to be recanalized. The interval from onset of symptoms to start of treatment of recanalized patients tended to be longer than that of nonrecanalized patients, but the difference was not significant. There was no difference in the dosages given between recanalized and nonrecanalized patients.

Effects of Recanalization: Analysis of MCA Cases

In order to simplify the analysis of effect of recanalization, we studied the outcome of patients with MCA occlusion. The acute MCA ischemic syndromes consisted of sensorimotor deficits, neuropsychological deficits, visual field defects, and conjugate ocular deviation to the ipsilateral side. According to the combination and severity of these symptoms, patients' initial neurological states were divided into four categories as follows: "stuporous," "severe," "moderate," and "mild," and the outcome at the end of the 3rd month after onset was divided into five categories as follows: "excellent," "good," "fair," "poor," and "dead." More details of these categorizations were previously reported (Mori et al. 1988). Prognosis was correlated with

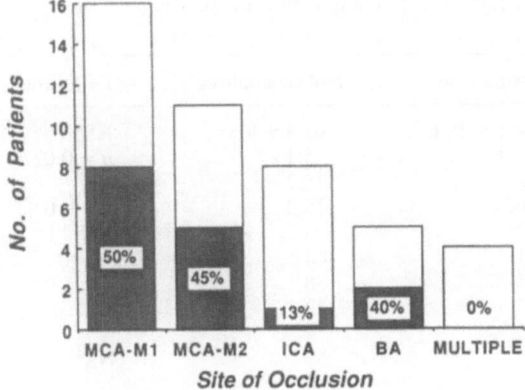

Fig. 1. Recanalization rate of each artery. □, not recanalized; ■, recanalized

Outcome / Initial	Excellent	Good	Fair	Poor	Dead	Total
Mild	⊙⊙⊙ ●●	●●				7
Moderate	⊙⊙	⊙⊙⊙ ●	●			7
Severe		⊙⊙	△●● ●	△●● ●●●		12
Stuporous		⊙		●	●●●	5
Total	7	9	5	7	3	31

Fig. 2. Initial neurological state, recanalization, and outcome of MCA occlusion. ⊙, complete recanalization; ○, partial but effective recanalization; △, recanalization with severe stenosis; ●, no recanalization

the degree of restoration of blood flow ($r_s = 0.633$, $p < 0.001$, Spearman rank correlation test), and with initial severity ($r_s = 0.811$, $p < 0.001$) (Fig. 2). There was no correlation between initial severity and degree of recanalization.

The outcome of the recanalized patient group was significantly better than that of the nonrecanalized group although clinical characteristics at entry, such as age, affected side, initial neurological state, and site of arterial occlusion, did not differ significantly between groups (Table 1). Furthermore, as compared with those treated conventionally and surgically, prognosis of the recanalized group was favorable (Fig. 3). The outcome of the non-recanalized group was approximately the same as those in the literature.

Table 1. Middle cerebral artery characteristics: comparison of recanalized and not recanalized group

	Recanalized	Not recanalized	Difference
Age (years)	54.1 ± 18.6	65.4 ± 9.5	NS[a]
Sex (male:female)	9:4	5:13	$p = 0.027$[b]
Side (left:right)	12:1	15:3	NS[b]
Cause (cardiac:others)	6:7	15:3	$p = 0.036$[b]
Initial neurological state			NS[c]
Stuporous	1	4	
Severe	4	8	
Moderate	5	2	
Mild	3	4	
Site of occlusion			NS[d]
M1 + ACA/PCA	0	4	
Proximal M1	6	6	
Distal M1	2	2	
Proximal M2	5	6	
Interval (h)	242 ± 180	212 ± 140	NS[a]
Dose of urokinase (MU)	0.81 ± 0.35	0.90 ± 0.27	NS[a]
Outcome			$p<0.01$[c]
Dead	0	3	
Poor	1	6	
Fair	1	4	
Good	6	3	
Excellent	5	2	
Volume of infarction (ml)	29 ± 46	173 ± 107	$p<0.01$[a]

[a] Student's t test (one-tailed).
[b] Fischer's exact probability test (one-tailed).
[c] Mann-Whitney U test (one-tailed).
[d] Chi-square test (one-tailed).

In addition, the total volume of the hypodense lesions (or when the lesions contained hemorrhages, total volume of the both hypodense and hyperdense lesions), which was measured by CT obtained 3 days postonset with a personal computer and graphics tablet, was smaller in the recanalized group than in the nonrecanalized group, the difference being statistically significant ($p < 0.01$, Student's t test, Fig. 4). The hypodensity volume was reduced in proportion to the degree of recanalization ($r_s = 0.926, p < 0.001$).

Side Effects: Hemorrhagic Transformation and Systemic Bleeding

Hemorrhagic transformation occurred in ten patients. Some characteristics of those with hemorrhagic transformation are listed in Table 2. All hemorrhages were observed on CT 24 h after treatment. Four of them belonged to the recanalization group. Hemorrhage was petechial in four patients and clinically so insignificant that intracerebral hematoma (ICH) only in the remaining six patients was considered. The start of therapy tended to be later in patients

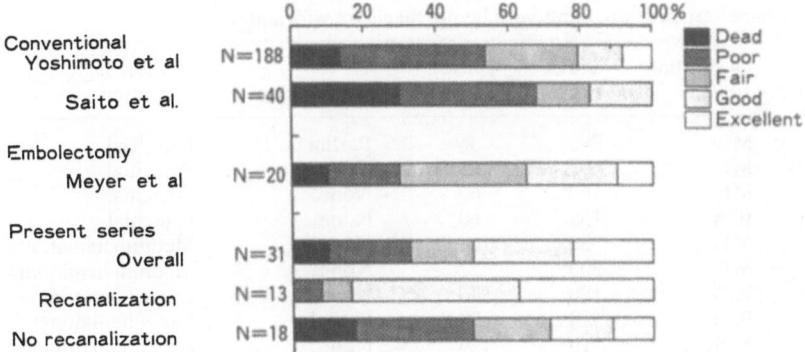

Fig. 3. Prognosis of MCA occlusion: comparison of thrombolytic, conventional, and surgical therapy. For reference see [12]

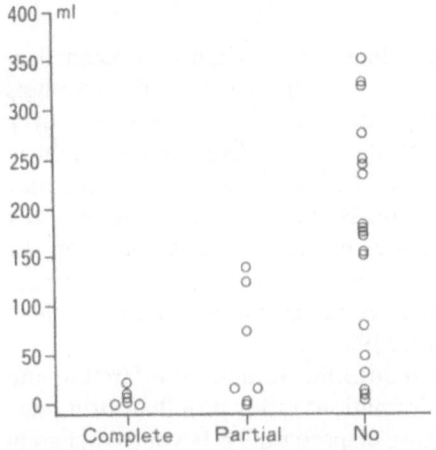

Fig. 4. Relationship between degree of recanalization and size of hypodensity on CTs 3 days after onset

with ICH. It is noteworthy that the elapsed time from onset to initiation of therapy was longer in patients with ICH ($p < 0.05$, Student's t test), in two more than 6 h. Occurrence of ICH was not related to dosage at all. In addition, ICH was apt to occur in unconscious patients ($p = 0.007$, Fisher's exact probability test), although such patients were primarily critical. The incidence of ICH was slightly higher in the recanalized group, but the difference was not statistically significant ($p = 0.216$, Fisher's exact probability test).

Significant systemic bleeding complications for which blood transfusion was required occurred in two patients. A transient systemic lytic state was observed in almost all patients. It was marked when more than 1 million units were given.

Table 2. Characteristics of patients with hemorrhagic transformation

Patient	Occlusion site	Time (min)	Dose (units)	Reperfusion	Hemorrhagic infarction
1	M1	280	36	Partial	Petechial
2	M1	93	90	Complete	Petechial
3	M1	160	60	None	Petechial
4	ICA	155	60	None	Petechial
5	M1	50	108	None	Medium hematoma
6	M1	300	72	None	Medium hematoma
7	ICA	180	90	None	Large hematoma
8	ICA	720	90	Partial	Large hematoma
9	Multiple	210	120	None	Large hematoma
10	BA	600	96	Complete	Large hematoma

Comments

In summary, intraarterial u-PA appears to increase the chance of recanalization rapidly occurring. Although the process of spontaneous thrombolysis might be involved, recanalization during infusion strongly suggests a drug effect. The recanalization rate varies with the artery. As thrombi caught in the ICA are usually larger than those in the MCA or BA, clot volume may explain the difference in recanalization rate. Blood flow conveying the drug may also be a recanalization factor. As ICA has few branches between the origin and the siphon, blood containing the drug is stagnant when the vessel is blocked at the siphon. It is certain that the interventional neuroradiology technique improves the recanalization rate [9, 16].

Immediate recanalization seems to reduce the volume of infarction and neurological deficit. Hemorrhagic transformation, rarely of lethal form, may occur. This tends to occur in patients whose elapsed time is beyond 6 h, and in patients with coma. Systemic lytic state is common, and, occasionally, there may be systemic bleeding.

Systemic rt-PA Trial

Study Design

Based on our experience of the u-PA trial, the trial of rt-PA in acute stroke was designed. It was started in August 1988, and is now in progress. Besides our institute, two neurological departments, Matsudo City Hospital (Matsudo, Chiba Prefecture, Japan), and Kasai Municipal Hospital (Kasai, Hyogo Pref., Japan), are participating in this trial. The study design is a placebo-controlled double-blind trial. In order to simplify the comparison of neurological deficits, subjects are limited to those with carotid artery territory stroke. Angiographic confirmation of acute occlusion of the ICA or its main branches is a necessary condition for inclusion. Inclusion/exclusion criteria are similar to those of the u-PA study. Timing for treatment is limited to 6 h after onset, and comatose patients are excluded. We are planning to enroll about 30 patients in this study.

The treatment consists of a 60-min intravenous infusion of placebo or rt-PA of either 20 or 30 mega units (Duteplase, Sumitomo Pharmaceuticals Co., Tokyo, Japan). These dosages of rt-PA correspond to those used in the trials for myocardial infarction in Japan. After angiography demonstrating occlusion, administration of the drug or placebo is initiated, and angiographic examination is repeated at 30 and 60 min to determine whether reperfusion has occurred. A standardized neurological examination with the Hemispheric Stroke Score (HSS) [1] and CT is repeated during a 1-month follow-up period; that is, patients are examined before treatment, immediately after treatment, and 24 h, 48 h, 1 week, 2 weeks, and 1 month after treatment. The HSS, developed by Adams and others, has been validated and used in a controlled trial of hemodilution [14]. We are using a translated and slightly modified version. Blood is regularly drawn and stored for several coagulation testings.

Progress of rt-PA Trial: Interim Analyses

The trial is under way, and so far 23 patients have been enrolled. We have treated 5 ICA occlusions, 10 M_1 occlusions, 4 M_2 occlusions, and 4 multiple artery occlusions. The cause of occlusion has been cardiogenic embolism in most cases. Mean elapsed time is approximately 3.5 h.

Recanalization to varying degrees has been achieved in 9 of 23 patients. Supposing recanalization occurred only associated with rt-PA, the recanalization rate could be estimated at a little over 50%, which corresponds to that of our intraarterial u-PA trial. Complete recanalization seems to occur less frequently in this trial than in the u-PA trial. As in the u-PA trial, the MCA is more frequently recanalized than ICA occlusion. Severe systemic complications relevant to the treatment have never developed.

As we cannot, at present, specify whether drug or placebo was given because of it being an ongoing double-blind trial, we compared the nature of the two distinctive groups, i.e., the recanalized group and the nonrecanalized group. Figure 5 illustrates the changes in HSS between the groups. Apparently, the recanalized group shows a better recovery of HSS than the nonrecanalized group. The difference in δ-HSS between the two groups reaches a statistically significant level at 24 h, 48 h, 2 week, and 1 month after onset ($p < 0.05$, Mann-Whitney U test).

Hemorrhagic transformation has occurred in 12 of 23 patients. Most of the hemorrhages were petechial and clinically quite insignificant. Relatively

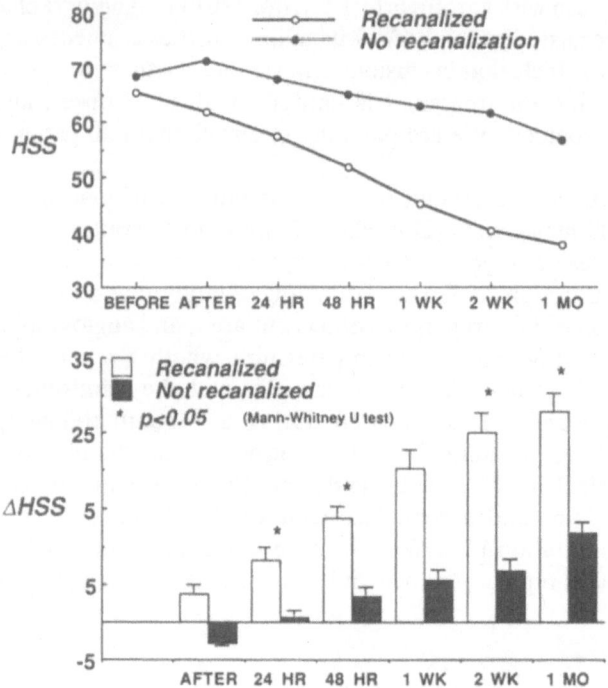

Fig. 5. Changes in hemispheric stroke score. The *line graph* indicates comparison of mean HSS. The more a patient's neurological deficits improves, the more the HSS declines. The *bar graph* indicates comparison of δ-HSS, i.e., changes from baseline value. Thus, δ-HSS reflects the degree of patient recovery

large hemorrhages occurred in two patients of the recanalized group. No one had intracranial hemorrhage appearing outside the infarcted area. It is impressive that all hemorrhages in the recanalized group occurred within 48 h after treatment.

Comments

What we have learned so far from interim analysis of this trial is as follows: In the recanalized group, recovery is apparently favorable. However, hemorrhagic transformation may occur more often, earlier, and sometimes more severely, even if it might not have clinical significance as a whole. Intracranial hemorrhage related to coagulopathy did not occur in the present dosages, but may have occurred with higher dosages of t-PA in nonstroke patients [4, 10]. Although acceleration of edema formation has been suggested to occur as a result of reperfusion [11], we find no evidence of it. Definitive conclusions and comparisons between drug and placebo cannot be made until the completion of this trial.

Conclusion

I believe, based on the evidence derived from both studies, that I can answer at least the first issue mentioned at the beginning of this paper. I would like to stress that early recanalization works for the patient's recovery from ischemia, with the frequency of intracranial bleeding seeming to be within an acceptable limit. However, at present, I cannot conclude that the recanalization has been drug mediated. Although I cannot yet exactly answer the second issue, I think fibrinolytic recanalization therapy is a feasible intervention in acute stroke.

Acknowledgements. I would like to express great thanks to Yukihiro Yoneda, MD, Shingo Ohkawa, MD, Takashi Yoshida, MD, Yukio Ohosumi, MD Masayasu Tabuchi, MD, Asushi Yamadori, MD, Neurology Service, Hyogo Brain and Heart Center at Himeji, Himeji, Kiyomi Minamigumo, MD, Yutaka Shimoe, MD, Takayuki Komatsu, MD, Kunitaka Kitano, MD, Neurology Service, Matudo City Hospital, Matsudo, Kimiko Inoue, MD, and Akira Tsutsumi, MD, Neurology Service, Kasai Municipal Hospital, Kasai, for their generous assistance. This study is much indebted to their hard work.

References

1. Adams RJ, Meador KJ, Sethi KD, Grotta JC, Thomson DS (1987) Graded neurological scale for use in acute hemispheric stroke treatment protocols. Stroke 18:665–669
2. Brott T, Haley EC, Levy DE, Barsan W, Reed RL, Olinger CP, Marler JR (1988) The investigational use of t-PA for stroke. Ann Emerg Med 17:1202–1205
3. Buteux G, Jubault V, Suisse A (1988) Local recombinant tissue plasminogen activator to clear cerebral artery thrombosis developing soon after surgery. Lancet 1:1143–1144
4. Carlson SE, Aldrich MS, Greenberg MS, Topol EJ (1988) Intracerebral hemorrhage complicating intravenous tissue plasminogen activator treatment. Arch Neurol 45:1070–1073
5. Del Zoppo GJ (1988) Investigational use of tPA in acute stroke. Ann Emerg Med 17:1196–1201
6. Del Zoppo GJ, Ferbert A, Otis S, Bruckmann H, Hacke W, Zyroff J, Harker LA, Zeumer H (1988) Local intra-arterial fibrinolytic therapy in acute carotid territory stroke. Stroke 19:307–313
7. Hacke W, Zeumer H, Ferbert A, Bruckmann H, Del Zoppo GJ (1988) Intra-arterial thrombolytic therapy improves outcome in patients with acute vertebrobasilar occlusive disease. Stroke 19:1216–1222
8. Henze TH, Boeer A, Tebbe U, Romatowski J (1987) Lysis of basilar artery occlusion with tissue plasminogen activator. Lancet 1:1391
9. Jungreis CA, Wechsler LR, Horton JA (1989) Intracranial thrombolysis via a catheter embedded in the clot. Stroke 20:1578–1580
10. Kase CS, O'Neal AM, Fisher M, Girgis GN, Ordia JI (1990) Intracranial hemorrhage after use of tissue plasminogen activator for coronary thrombolysis. Ann Intern Med 112:17–21
11. Koudstaal PJ, Stibbe J, Vermeulen M (1988) Fatal ischaemic brain oedema after early thrombolysis with tissue plasminogen activator in acute stroke. Br Med J 297:1571–1574
12. Mori E, Tabuchi M, Yoshida T, Yamadori A (1988) Intracarotid urokinase with thromboembolic occlusion of the middle cerebral artery. Stroke 19:802–812

13. Mori E, Tabuchi M, Yamadori A (1989) Thrombolytic therapy in acute stroke: intra-arterial urokinase and systemic r-tPA. In: Tokyo Satellite Symposia of 12th Congress of the International Society on Thrombosis and Hemostasis, August 26, 1989, Tokyo
14. The Hemodilution in Stroke Study Group (1989) Hypervolemic hemodilution treatment of acute stroke. Stroke 20:317–323
15. Theron J, Courtheoux P, Casasco A, Alachkar F, Notari F, Ganem F, Maiza D (1989) Local intraarterial fibrinolysis in the carotid territory. AJNR 10:753–765
16. Zeumer H, Freitag HJ, Grzyska U, Neunzig HP (1989) Local intraarterial fibrinolysis in acute vertebrobasilar occlusion: technical developments and results. Neuroradiology 31:336–340

Intravenous Recombinant Tissue Plasminogen Activator in Acute Thrombotic Stroke: Study Design, Recanalization, and Clinical Outcome

G.J. del Zoppo[1] and A. Ferbert[2]

Introduction

The study of the efficacy of thrombolytic agents in the treatment of acute stroke derives from the observation that stroke is typically an athero-thrombotic or thromboembolic process [1, 6]. Careful intraarterial infusion of the thrombolytic agents urokinase (u-PA) and streptokinase may lead to thrombus dissolution and clinical improvement in selected patients presenting with acute thrombotic or thromboembolic stroke [1, 2–4, 7]. This experience has provided the practical background for the evaluation of the relatively fibrin specific agent recombinant tissue plasminogen activator (rt-PA), delivered by intravenous infusion. A predominantly two-chain rt-PA preparation (duteplase, Burroughs Wellcome, Beckenham, UK) has been employed in a prospective open multicenter dose-rate safety and efficacy study of thrombolysis in acute thrombotic and thromboembolic stroke.

Study Protocol

This study was designed as a prospective open CT scan/angiography-based dose-range study of recanalization of a documented symptomatic cerebral arterial occlusion (TIMI grade 0) following a 60-min intravenous infusion of rt-PA in patients suffering carotid or vertebrobasilar territory ischemia. In this study, the primary positive outcome event is angiographically demonstrated reperfusion of the documented cerebral artery occlusion (efficacy), while the primary negative outcome event is CNS hemorrhage with neurological deterioration within 24 h of rt-PA infusion (safety). The study protocol is summarized in Table 1.

[1] Department of Molecular and Experimental Medicine and Division of Hematology/ Medical Oncology, Scripps Clinic and Research Foundation, 10666 North Torrey Pines Road, La Jolla, CA 92037, USA.
[2] Abteilung Neurologie, Rheinisch-Westfälische Technische Hochschule Aachen, Pauwelsstr., W-5100 Aachen, FRG.

Hacke et al (Eds)
Thrombolytic Therapy in Acute Ischemic Stroke
© Springer-Verlag Berlin Heidelberg 1991

Table 1. Protocol

Entry
  Clinical assessment
  Informed consent
  Inclusion/exclusion criteria
  (clinical, historical)

CT (cerebral) scan
Angiography (preinfusion)
Intravenous infusion of *rt-PA* (60 min)

Angiography (postinfusion)

CT (cerebral) scan(s) (24 h)

Clinical management (NICU, clinical ward)
  Neurologic assessments
  CT (cerebral) scans
  Noninvasive vascular studies
  Other

NICU = neurological intensive care unit

Strict inclusion and exclusion criteria have been observed for patient entry into the study. Clinical and angiographic inclusion criteria require that patients be 21–80 years of age, have no significant impairment of neurological function prior to the presenting event, which has been acute, occurring no later than 8 h from the expected time of initiating the rt-PA infusion. An unequivocal extracranial or intracranial artery occlusion of the appropriate carotid or vertebral/basilar arteries consistent with the patient's clinical presentation must be demonstrated by angiography. Clinical exclusion criteria include major neurologic deficit(s) implying a large territorial infarction of the carotid or vertebrobasilar territory, or minimal neurologic deficits indicating small, minor, or transient tissue injury; malignant hypertension or an uncompensated systolic blood pressure greater than 200 mmHg; history of neurologic deficit(s) consistent with completed stroke within 6 weeks prior to the presenting event; a previous intracranial hemorrhage; presumed septic embolism; any condition associated with an increased risk of hemorrhage after thrombolytic agents; known sensitivity to contrast agents; or other serious advanced illness with a reduced life expectancy.

After clinical examination, and completion of informed consent requirements, a noncontrast CT cerebral scan is performed to exclude any high-attenuation lesion consistent with hemorrhage of any degree, evidence of mass effect or midline shift, or of an intracranial tumor, arteriovenous malformation, or aneurysm.

Cerebral angiography is performed on patients not excluded by the screening CT scan study. Perfusion of the suspected symptomatic artery (arterial stenosis with or without luminal defect as the sole lesion), suspected arterial dissection, the presence of a nonatherosclerotic arteriopathy (e.g., vasculitis), or a coexistent aneurysm or arteriovenous malformation exclude patients from this study (who are followed separately). Patients with TIMI grade 0 perfusion receive a single preassigned dose of intravenous rt-PA for 60 min. Following completion of the intravenous infusion, the status of the occluded cerebral artery is determined by repeat angiography. The noncontrast CT scan is repeated 24 h and 14 days after rt-PA infusion or, if symptomatic deterioration occurs within this interval, to evaluate the presence/development of new intracerebral hemorrhage. Heparin or other anticoagulants are not used within the first 24 h after symptom onset, but may be instituted at the investigator's discretion thereafter.

Serial neurologic evaluations have been tabulated serially for each patient on extensive data collection instruments, and in short form on the abbreviated Canadian Stroke Scale. For this study, clinical outcome was not formally evaluated in a prospective manner.

Prospective Guidelines and Statistical Analysis

Prospective guidelines for dose escalation/reduction and study termination at each dose rate were derived from expected hemorrhagic infarction and (symptomatic) parenchymatous hemorrhagic or hematoma rates and from arterial recanalization rates suggested from literature sources. Superimposed upon the study are a (a) Primary Safety Rule, which defines a dose-escalation scale based upon "failure to achieve recanalization" versus "hemorrhagic transformation with associated clinical deterioration ($p = 0.05$ of type 1 error)," and a (b) Secondary Safety Rule, for which the study would cease if greater than a predetermined number of treated patients in a dose-rate cohort developed neurologic and clinical deterioration associated with a relevant hemorrhagic transformation. All neuroradiologic and clinical data of patients demonstrating hemorrhagic transformation are reviewed and categorized by the Safety Committee.

Prospective analysis of the neuroradiologic data has been performed at the Neuroradiologic Core facility in the Department of Radiology, Tufts-New England Medical Center (Boston) under the direction of S. Wolpert, MD.

Clinical Centers

Patients have been acquired from 16 major institutional centers in North America and the Federal Republic of Germany, who are participants in the rt-PA/Acute Stroke Study Group.

Outcome

Recanalization and Hemorrhagic Transformation

To date, 71 patients with symptoms of acute cerebrovascular ischemia and angiographically demonstrated TIMI grade 0 perfusion in an appropriate cerebral artery have received rt-PA by intravenous infusion in seven dose-rate groups [5]. The mean time from symptom onset to initiation to rt-PA infusion was 5.4 h. At least partial arterial recanalization occurred in all dose-rate groups. However, at this time the incidence of recanalization has not been optimized.

Hemorrhagic transformation was a common finding in this study, occurring at all dose-rates: (a) hemorrhagic infarction, occurring within 24 h of treatment, was not associated with clinical deterioration. In fact, clinical improvement occurred in approximately one-half of the patients demonstrating early hemorrhagic infarction; (b) parenchymatous hemorrhage or symptomatic hematoma formation was observed in a small number of patients. The incidence of such events remained within the study's prospective safety guidelines. At this time, the study is proceeding with higher dose rates to optimize recanalization efficacy and safety events.

Clinical Consequences

As this is not a randomized or double-blind study, definite conclusions concerning the clinical benefit of rt-PA cannot be drawn. However, the study design does allow comparison of some clinical consequences relative to angiological response. Preliminary analysis for the first 65 treated patients shows that angiographic responders fared better than nonresponders with regard to hand paresis and language function. This limited improvement was correlated with the interval between onset of stroke and recanalization, being more pronounced the earlier the recanalization occurred. There was no difference in survival between the two angiographic responses.

The drawback of this kind of analysis is that some of the patients classified as angiographic nonresponders after the 1 h rt-PA infusion may, in fact, be responders at a later time. This could occur within the 1st hour after the repeat angiography and would only occasionally be documented angiographically.

Some patients with angiographic response showed significant improvement within minutes after recanalization. These preliminary results are in favor of a clinical benefit of recanalization at an early stage in acute thrombotic stroke. Finally, as no untoward clinical consequences of rt-PA infusion or of angiography per se have been noted, the study is proceeding with caution at higher dose rates.

Appendix

Clinical Centers. Scripps Clinic and Research Foundation. (G.J. del Zoppo, S.M. Otis), La Jolla, CA, and the Rheinische Westphalische Technische Hochschule (RWTH) Aachen (A. Ferbert, K. Poeck), Aachen, FRG; Tufts–New England Medical Center (M.S. Pessin), Boston University (C. Kase), Massachusetts General Hospital (D. Grass), Boston, MA; The Cleveland Clinic (A. Furlan), Cleveland, OH; The Neurological Institute (J.P. Mohr), New York, NY; University of California San Diego (J. Zivin), San Diego, CA; Yale University (L. Brass), New Haven, CT; Rhode Island Hospital (E. Feldmann), Providence, RI; University of Pittsburgh (L. Wechsler), Pittsburgh, PA; Klinikum I. Minden (O. Busse), Minden, FRG; Duke University (M. Alberts), Durham, NC; University of Texas, Southwestern Medical Center (R. Greenlee, Jr.), Dallas, TX; University of Iowa (J. Biller), Iowa City, IA; and Karl Ruprechts Universitat-Heidelberg (W. Hacke), Heidelberg, FRG.

Core Neuroradiology Facility. Department of Radiology, Tufts-New England Medical Center (S. Wolpert), Boston, MA.

References

1. Del Zoppo GJ, Zeumer H, Harker LA (1986) Thrombolytic therapy in acute stroke: possibilities and hazards. Stroke 17: 595–607
2. Del Zoppo GJ, Ferbert A, Otis S, Bruckmann H, Hacke W, Zyroff J, Harker LA, Zeumer H (1988) Local intra-arterial fibrinolytic therapy in acute carotid territory stroke: a pilot study. Stroke 19:307–313
3. Hacke W, Zeumer H, Ferbert A, Bruckmann H, Del Zoppo GJ (1988) Intraarterial thrombolytic therapy improves outcome in patients with acute vertebrobasilar occlusive disease. Stroke 19:1216–1222
4. Mori E, Tabuchi M, Yoshida T, Yamadori A (1988) Intracarotid urokinase with thromboembolic occlusion of the middle cerebral artery. Stroke 19:802–812
5. rt-PA Acute Stroke Study Group (1990) An open multicenter study of the safety and efficacy of various doses of t-PA in patients with acute stroke: A progress report. Stroke 21:181
6. Solis OJ, Roberson GR, Taveras JM, Mohr J, Pessin MS (1977) Cerebral angiography in acute cerebral infarction. Rev Interam Radiol 2:19–25
7. Zeumer H (1985) Survey of progress: vascular recanalizing techniques in interventional neuroradiology. J Neurol 231:287–294

Evaluation of Tissue Plasminogen Activator Early in the Course of Acute Ischemic Stroke

J.R. MARLER[1], T. BROTT, E.C. HALEY, and D. LEVY

Introduction

The National Institute of Neurological Disorders and Stroke (NINDS) has initiated a series of studies to evaluate tissue plasminogen activator (t-PA) as a treatment for acute ischemic stroke [1]. To date, an initial pilot dose determination safety study has been completed and, based on the results of the pilot study, an intermediate randomized controlled trial is about to begin. This report will discuss the design considerations for these trials, the details of the study design of the recently completed pilot study, and some special features of the intermediate-sized controlled clinical trial that will soon begin.

Design Considerations: Early Treatment

The NINDS pilot dose determination safety study was intended to form the basis for one or more subsequent clinical trials. For this reason, the pilot study was designed to have inclusion and exclusion criteria as well as outcome variables that would be useful in future trials. For a clinical trial to establish that t-PA is an effective treatment for ischemic stroke, the primary outcome must be long-term death and disability measured on a functional outcome scale. Rather than attempt to carry out an explanatory or mechanistic investigation, the plan from the beginning has been for the NINDS to focus on the long-term practical benefit of treatment to a patient and to attempt the difficult comparison of benefit to risk.

Of many different agents being considered for treatment of ischemic stroke, t-PA is one of the most promising. For this reason, it was decided to give this promising therapy the greatest possible chance to show some benefit. Therefore, serious consideration was given to the large volume of laboratory research which has been performed in the investigation of different models of

[1] National Institute of Neurological Disorders and Stroke. Division of Stroke and Trauma, Federal Building, Room 800, 7550 Wisconsin Avenue, Bethesda, MD 20892, USA.

Hacke et al (Eds)
Thrombolytic Therapy in Acute Ischemic Stroke
© Springer-Verlag Berlin Heidelberg 1991

ischemic stroke. An inescapable fact apparent in almost all of the laboratory models of ischemic stroke is that the extent of infarction increases in proportion to the duration of ischemia. In general, most models would seem to predict that there is little chance of reducing the extent of infarction by increasing perfusion after 6 or 8 h of ischemia; in fact, many laboratory models would predict that the latest possible time for intervention was closer to 30 min. One research model using t-PA in acute ischemic stroke demonstrated no evidence of efficacy after 45 min of ischemia [4]. For this reason, the design of the NINDS pilot study and subsequent clinical trials established and maintains a focus on achieving the earliest possible treatment in order that a new and promising therapeutic agent will have the maximum possibility to demonstrate its efficacy.

In addition to providing an increased opportunity for thrombolytic therapy to reduce the extent of infarction,there is the possibility that early treatment will also reduce the risk of intracerebral hematoma. Previous attempts to use thrombolytic agents such as streptokinase in the treatment of acute ischemic stroke have been made and have shown an unacceptable risk of intracerebral hemorrhage [2]. This was compatible with previous clinical observations that brain tissue injured by ischemia may be a likely site for the initiation of intracerebral hemorrhage. A secondary benefit of early treatment may therefore be a reduced incidence of intracerebral hematoma.

In summary, in order for a treatment of acute ischemic stroke to be effective, it may be most beneficial if given at a time before irreversible neuronal damage occurs. It is conceivable that an agent which would be effective at 60 min or 2 h after the onset of stroke symptoms would be entirely ineffective if given after 8 or 12 h. There is also the possibility that early treatment will reduce the number and extent of intracerebral hemorrhages.

The goal of this emphasis on early intervention following the onset of stroke symptoms is to break the difficult circular cycle that has in the past discouraged the development of new treatments for acute stroke. Stroke is not generally afforded consideration as a serious medical emergency requiring immediate transportation, rapid diagnosis, and early intervention. If the only patients that are treated in a stroke intervention study are those that arrive after the process of infarction is already well on its way to completion, then there is little or no opportunity for a therapeutic agent to show any benefit. Without proven treatment, there is little motivation to make the extra effort required to treat patients early.

The relationship of time from onset of ischemia to the extent of infarction and the incidence of hemorrhage is complex. Based on experience with coronary occlusion reported in the cardiological literature, an optimistic estimate of the rate of reperfusion of brain in response to treatment with t-PA would be 40%–60% [3]. However, the effect on the restoration of function following reperfusion is going to diminish as the duration of ischemia increases. A hypothetical curve, "Response to Therapy," is shown in Fig. 1. The curve, shown only for the purpose of discussion, is probably quite

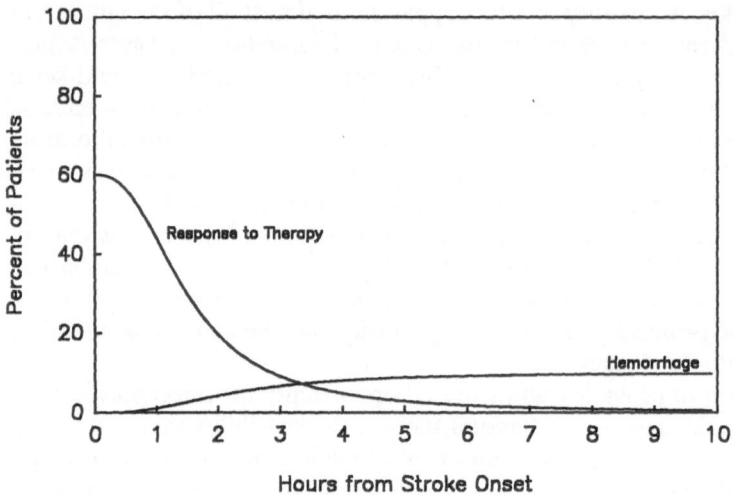

Fig. 1. Comparison of risk of hemorrhage with response to t-PA: change with time from onset

optimistic. It is assumed that few stroke patients would show a significant improvement due to reperfusion after more than 8 h of ischemia.

In addition to the decline in the response to therapeutic treatment, there may also be an increase in the risk of intracerebral hemorrhage as time progresses. Again, there are little or no data on which to base an estimate. We do have human studies that indicate that thrombolytic therapy combined with heparin is associated with intracerebral hemorrhage [2]. This presumably is related to reperfusion of a vasculature that has itself suffered injury as a result of ischemia. Ischemic vascular injury may also increase with the duration of ischemia. The curve in Fig. 1 is based on the assumption that eventually the risk of hemorrhage following reperfusion of infarcted brain will reach a rate of 10%.

If these two curves are overlaid (Fig. 2), it can be seen that very early following the onset of symptoms the number of patients predicted to have serious intracerebral hemorrhage would exceed the number of patients that would show significant benefit from therapy. Another way to look at this is to subtract the expected number of patients that would respond from the number that would have an intracerebral hemorrhage. As can be seen, it is possible that, at some point in time, the benefit from treatment with t-PA may be lost and, in fact, not only would there be no benefit but there would be an actual risk exceeding any possible benefit. This possibility has had a major impact in the design of the NINDS pilot studies and clinical trials to evaluate t-PA in the treatment of acute ischemic stroke and is the primary reason for the 90-min time limit to begin the infusion.

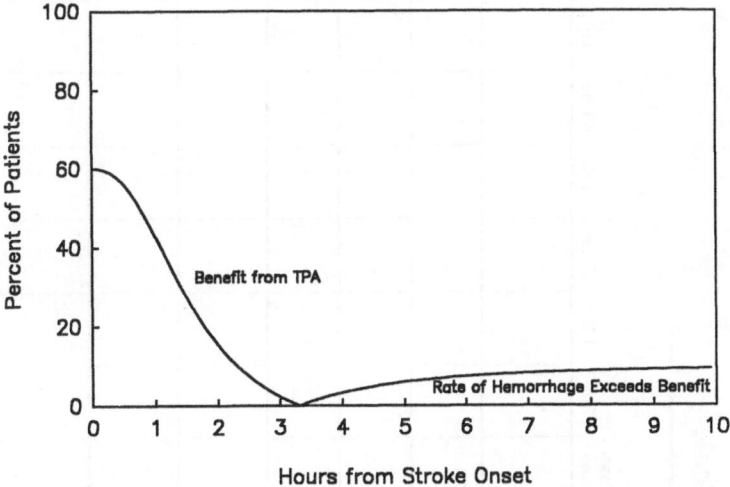

Fig. 2. Benefit and risk from treatment of stroke with t-PA. This depends on the time from onset of stroke

Pilot Study: Methods

In the NINDS pilot study for the evaluation of t-PA early in the course of acute ischemic stroke, the first patient was treated on 11 March 1987. By the end of the study there were over 70 patients in whom an infusion of t-PA could be begun within 90 min of the onset of their symptoms. The objectives of that study were first to estimate a potentially safe dose that could be used in a future trial and, second, to estimate any potential efficacy in order that a larger trial could be designed. The study was coordinated by the NINDS, and was performed at three clinical centers: the University of Cincinnati, the University of Virginia, and Cornell University Medical Center. All patients were treated at the clinical center. The principal investigators at each center were Drs. Brott, Haley, and Levy, respectively. They not only treated the patients but also developed the protocol and data collection forms. The basic study design required very early intervention, the use of no concomitant heparin, frequent evaluation according to a standardized neurological scale, a safety CT scan at 24 h in all patients, and functional outcome and CT scan volume measurements as well as a neurological scale at 3 months. The inclusion criteria were that there be a clinical diagnosis of ischemic stroke, that there be a measurable, significant, deficit on the standardized stroke scale, that the patient be within the age range 18–80 years, and that t-PA infusion could begin within 90 min from the well-defined time of onset of stroke symptoms. Informed consent was obtained for all patients. Prior to the beginning of t-PA infusion, an entry evaluation was carried out and completed within the 90 min from the onset of stroke symptoms. Before

Stroke Scale

		Base-Line	30'	1 Hr	2 Hr	24 Hr	48 Hr	7-10 Days
1.a. Level of Consciousness	Alert 0 Drowsy 1 Stuporous 2 Coma 3							
1.b. LOC Questions	Answers both correctly 0 Answers one correctly 1 Incorrect 2							
1.c. LOC Commands	Obeys both correctly 0 Obeys one correctly 1 Incorrect 2							
2. Best Gaze	Normal 0 Partial gaze palsy 1 Forced deviation 2							
3. Best Visual	No visual loss 0 Partial hemianopia 1 Complete hemianopia 2 Bilateral hemianopia 3							
4. Facial Palsy	Normal 0 Minor 1 Partial 2 Complete 3							
5. Best Motor Arm	No drift 0 Drift 1 Can't resist gravity 2 No effort against gravity 3 No movement 4							
6. Other Arm	For brainstem stroke (Use same scale as above) 0-4							

Item	Description	Score
7. Best Motor Leg	No drift / Drift / Can't resist gravity / No effort against gravity / No movement	0 / 1 / 2 / 3 / 4
8. Other Leg	For brainstem stroke (Use same scale as above)	0-4
9. Limb Ataxia	Absent / Present in upper or lower / Present in both	0 / 1 / 2
10. Sensory	Normal / Partial loss / Dense loss	0 / 1 / 2
11. Neglect	No neglect / Partial neglect / Complete neglect	0 / 1 / 2
12. Dysarthria	Normal articulation / Mild to moderate dysarthria / Near unintelligible or worse	0 / 1 / 2
13. Best Language	No aphasia / Mild to moderate aphasia / Severe aphasia / Mute	0 / 1 / 2 / 3
14. Change from Previous Exam	Same / Better / Worse	S / B / W
15. Change from Baseline	Same / Better / Worse	S / B / W

Fig. 1

treatment the patients were given a neurological examination and a medical examination, and the investigators were made aware of the results of the complete blood count (CBC), prothrombin time (PT), partial prothrombin time (PTT), glucose level, blood urea nitrogen (BUN) level, ECG, and CT scan without contrast. Angiography was not performed prior to treatment in order to avoid delay of treatment. Blood was drawn that was later used to determine baseline fibrinogen and fibrinogen degradation products at a centralized laboratory. To complete this evaluation, it was required in most instances that the patient be in the emergency room within 45 min of the onset of stroke symptoms.

Exclusion criteria excluded patients who already had hemorrhages or had recently had hemorrhages and those who had high blood pressure or other factors thought to increase the risk of hemorrhage unacceptably.

The t-PA was administered as a continuous intravenous infusion. Initial doses were quite low, with escalation of the dose after a review of the clinical course of each of the treated patients at a given tier was completed and a presentation made to a monitoring committee. Any potential clinical response was compared with the incidence of any serious complications by the independent monitoring committee before proceeding to the next higher dose. At tier 1, 0.35 mg/kg was given over 1 h, no bolus was used, and there was a maximum limit of 25 mg/patients. At tier 2 the dose was 0.6 mg/kg over 1 h, no bolus was used, and the maximum dose was 40 mg. At tier 3 the dose was 0.85 mg/kg for 1 h with no bolus and a 60-mg maximum. At tier 4 the method of computing the dosage was changed to be based on body surface area. For tier 4 a 10% bolus was given and the maximum dose was increased from 60 to 90 mg. In most patients, 32 mg/m^2 is very close to the tier 3 dose of 0.85 mg/kg. Tier 4 is essentially the addition of a bolus to tier 3. At tier 5 the dose increased to 37.6 mg/m^2 over 1 h with a 10% bolus and a 90-mg maximum dose. This dose is equivalent to approximately 1 mg/kg so that a 70-kg average adult would receive 70 mg t-PA in the 1st h, 10% given as a bolus infusion. Tier 4 extended is an increase in dose in tier 4, not in the 1st h but in the 30 min following the 1st h. The total dose in tier 4 extended and tier 5 are essentially the same. Only one patient was treated at tier 6.

Prior to and during administration of the t-PA and at scheduled times after administration, a standardized stroke scale was performed by the neurologist investigator who was present when the patient was treated (Fig. 1). The neurological scale was performed at baseline, before treatment, then at 30 min, 1 h, and 2 h after treatment had started, then again at 1 day, 2 days, 7–10 days, and 3 months. In addition, during the first 2 h following the start of treatment, the major sign of the patient's neurological deficit was reexamined every 15 min for 2 h.

Four CT scans were obtained, one at baseline before treatment, one at 18–30 h after treatment, one at 7–10 days, and one at 3 months. The outcome variables which were obtained included symptomatic intracranial hemorrhage in the first 24 h, intracranial hemorrhage on the 24-h CT scan, fibrinogen at

2 h, a clinically significant two-point improvement in neurological scale at 2 h, lesion volume on CT scan at 3 months, a four-point improvement in neurological scale at 24 h, lesion volume on CT scan at 3 months, and a functional outcome scale performed at 3 months. This was an open-label study. The t-PA was provided by Genentech, Inc.

Controlled Trial: Design

Plans for a controlled trial have been made as a result of a recommendation by the monitoring committee. This intermediate-sized trial will have many of the same features as the pilot study with some exceptions. The inclusion and exclusion criteria will be essentially unchanged from the pilot study as will the outcome measures. A more formal assessment of functional outcome will be performed at 3 months.

If the treatment of patients within 90 min is shown to be effective, then the question will remain whether later treatment would not also offer some benefit. Since the 90-min limit is very restrictive, it would be useful to have some information on the relative benefit of early and late treatment. For this reason, two different simultaneous trials are planned. In one, 140 patients who can begin treatment within 90 min will be randomized to t-PA or identical placebo. In another, 140 patients who can begin treatment between 90 and 180 min will be randomized to t-PA or placebo. While the patients in the two time groups will not be strictly comparable, useful information should be gained from the comparison of the two groups.

The pilot study has raised many questions about the early events in ischemic stroke. Since there were no control patients in the pilot study, it is impossible to know that the improvement seen in the treated patients might not have occurred without treatment. The relationship of treatment to eventual outcome at 3 months is even more difficult to define because of greater interpatient variability in functional assessment. For this reason, a primary outcome was chosen that is less variable and better defined; namely, early improvement in neurological scale. The sample size calculations were based on being able to detect a difference in the proportion of patients with a significant early improvement of 20 percentage points. If initial estimates are accurate, there should be ample power to answer the question. It is hoped that there is a close relationship between early improvement and improved function at 3 months. If this is so, it may be possible to establish effectiveness of t-PA for the treatment of ischemic stroke.

Secondary outcomes will include functional assessment scales such as the Barthel index, the measurement of CT scan lesion volume, and a comparison of the standardized neurological scale. As before, no concomitant heparin will be administered and a CT scan will be required in all patients before and after treatment.

Conclusion

A pilot study to estimate the safety of t-PA at different dose levels has been completed. A randomized, controlled clinical trial to evaluate the relative risk and benefit of early treatment with t-PA will begin soon. Both studies emphasize the importance of earliest possible treatment.

References

1. Marler JR, Walker MD (1989) Clinical research on stroke: The NINCDS strategy. Ginsberg MD, Dalton Dietrich W, (eds) Cerebrovascular diseases. Raven Press, New York, pp 17–20
2. Meyer JS, Gilroy J, Barnhart ME (1965) Therapeutic thrombolysis in cerebral thromboembolism: randomized evaluation of intravenous streptokinase. In: Siekert RG, Whisnant JP (eds) Cerebral vascular diseases. Grune & Stratton, New York, pp 200–213
3. The TIMI Study Group (1985) The thrombolysis in myocardial infarction (TIMI) trial: phase I findings. N Engl J Med 312:932–936
4. Zivin JA, Lyden PD, DeGirolami U, Kochhar A, Mazzarella V, Hemenway CC, Johnston P (1988) Tissue plasminogen activator: reduction of neurologic damage after experimental embolic stroke. Arch Neurol, 45:(no. 4) 387–391

Intravenous Recombinant Tissue Plasminogen Activator in Acute Stroke

R. von KUMMER[1], M. FORSTING[1], K. SARTOR[1] and W. HACKE[2]

Introduction

Severe focal ischemia leads to neuronal death within minutes. Due to the cerebral collateral network, in most instances occlusion of a major intracranial artery causes variable degrees of ischemia and oxygen supply within different parts of the vessel's territory. The ability of brain tissue to survive under ischemic conditions is time-dependent [4]. Restoring cerebral blood flow by recanalization of the occluded artery may help to decrease the extent of ischemic necrosis. Recently, new thrombus-selective thrombolytic agents such as recombinant tissue plasminogen activator (rt-PA) and single-chain urokinase plasminogen activator (scu-PA) have become available and are being successfully used in the treatment of ischemic heart disease. Encouraged by reports of successful arterial recanalization associated with favorable clinical outcome following intra-arterial infusion of streptokinase or urokinase [2, 3, 8–10], we studied the efficacy and safety of intravenous rt-PA in patients with acute thromboembolic vertebrobasilar and middle cerebral artery stroke. The purpose of this study was to find the dosage of alteplase (rt-PA) which is safe with respect to intracranial hemorrhage and effective with respect to thrombolysis and clinical outcome in preparation for a controlled study.

Subjects and Methods

In an open, prospective, and nonrandomized trial, a total of 27 consecutive patients (13 women, 14 men) were treated with intravenous infusion of 70 mg ($n = 12$) or 100 mg ($n = 15$) alteplase (Actilyse) over 90 min. Treatment was finished within 6 h of the onset of symptoms. Inclusion criteria were: (1) clinical diagnosis of acute stroke; (2) lack of hemorrhage, local brain swelling, or significant hypodensity due to early infarction as documented by computed

[1] Departments of Neuroradiology and [2] Neurology, University of Heidelberg, Im Neuenheimer Feld 400, W-6900 Heidelberg, FRG.

Hacke et al (Eds)
Thrombolytic Therapy in Acute Ischemic Stroke
© Springer-Verlag Berlin Heidelberg 1991

tomography (CT); (3) angiographic demonstration of corresponding occlusion of large intracranial artery or arteries; (4) age of patient between 20 and 70 years; and (5) informed consent given by patient or relatives. Angiography was repeated immediately after 90 min of rt-PA infusion. Reperfusion was graded in (1) no reperfusion or penetration with minimal reperfusion, (2) partial reperfusion, and (3) complete reperfusion according to angiography. Reperfusion was also assessed 12–24 h after onset of symptoms by a third angiography or transcranial Doppler ultrasound (TCD). TCD assessment of partial or complete reperfusion was done by comparison with the contralateral vessel.

Clinical outcome was defined as good when the patients recovered considerably from their initial deficit and were able to walk without assistance. Outcome was defined as poor when no apparent improvement was seen. Efficacy was likewise assessed by repeated CT or magnetic resonance imaging (MRI), and clinically 2 days, 10 days, and 4 weeks after treatment.

Heparin was given as a bolus of 5000 IU simultaneously with alteplase and continued at 1000 IU/h. All patients remained on the critical care ward for at least 3 days.

Results

Occlusions of Vertebrobasilar Arteries

The five patients with occlusion of the basilar artery ($n = 4$) or both vertebral arteries ($n = 1$) were treated with 70 mg only. In two patients, minor partial reperfusion was achieved within 6 h of onset of symptoms, and in one patient, TCD revealed complete reperfusion after 24 h. Three patients died due to extended ischemic brain stem infarction, and one patient remained "locked-in". One patient recovered well and showed no neurological deficit at discharge despite small brain stem infarctions detected by MRI. Because of this outcome analysis, no further patients with vertebrobasilar occlusions were included in this study but were treated with intra-arterially and locally administered urokinase.

Occlusions Within the Internal Carotid Territory

Internal Carotid Artery (ICA).   Occlusion of the intracranial ICA was present in four patients, in four cases in combination with middle cerebral artery (MCA) occlusion. Two patients additionally showed obliteration of the A1 segment of the ipsilateral anterior cerebral artery (ACA). In these two patients no reperfusion was achieved. They died due to extended ischemic brain edema. The other three patients showed partial ($n = 2$) or complete reperfusion of the ICA within 6h of stroke onset. In one the MCA remained occluded. This patient died from a space-occupying MCA infarction associated with remote parenchymal and intraventricular hemorrhage of the ipsilateral hemisphere. The other patient with partial reperfusion recovered well from severe hemiparesis. The third patient with complete reperfusion and intact collateral flow via ACA and MCA had no neurological deficit at discharge despite small infarcts in the territories of the anterior choroidal artery and the posterior cerebral artery originating from the ICA which were detected by MRI.

Middle Cerebral Artery (MCA) Trunk. Eleven patients had occlusion of the MCA trunk. After rt-PA treatment, five of them showed no reperfusion and five only partial reperfusion. In one patient angiography could not be repeated. The day after stroke, no reperfusion was observed in three patients, partial reperfusion in two, and complete reperfusion in six. With CT or MRI showing ischemia in all patients, brain infarctions were detected in parts of the MCA territories covering the striatum in ten patients. Five patients improved considerably, all showing complete reperfusion within 24 h. Despite partial reperfusion within 6h, one died from space-occupying MCA infarction, while another did not recover from severe hemiparesis. All three patients showing no reperfusion within 24h did not improve.

Branches of the MCA. In six patients, branches of the MCA were occluded at the trifurcation. No reperfusion was observed in two patients and partial reperfusion in four when angiography was repeated immediately after alteplase infusion. The following day, reperfusion was still partial in three patients but complete in the other three. The ischemic infarct was confined to the striatum in three patients and to the insular cortex in one. In one patient, CT revealed a more extended infarction within the MCA territory. One patient was on aspirin because of coronary artery stenosis and developed disseminated parenchymal hemorrhages of both hemispheres from which she died. Four patients recovered well, two of them leaving hospital without any apparent deficit. One patient showed only slight improvement of his severe hemiparesis.

Hemorrhages

Parenchymal hemorrhages occurred in two patients (7%), one with partial reperfusion of an MCA branch and one in whom the MCA remained occluded; both patients had been treated with 100 mg alteplase. In six patients (22%), hemorrhagic transformation of the infarctions was seen. Five of them recovered well. In four patients (15%), severe bleeding from the puncture site occurred 2–4 days after rt-PA treatment without any apparent influence on clinical outcome.

Table 1. Clinical outcome after 70 mg or 100 mg alteplase (intravenous in patients with occlusion within the ICA territory ($n = 22$)

	Dosage	
Outcome	70 mg	100 mg
Good	4	8
Poor	2	3
Died	1	4
Total	7	15

Reperfusion Within ICA Territory and Dosage of rt-PA

Within 6 h of onset of symptoms, at least partial reperfusion was observed in three of six patients treated with 70 mg where repeated angiography was possible and in 9 of 14 patients (64%) treated with 100 mg. After 12–24 h angiography and/or TCD showed the three vessels of the 70 mg group to be still occluded, whereas all vessels except two (86%) were partially or completely recanalized after 100 mg rt-PA.

Outcome in Patients with Occlusions Within ICA Territory

Type of Artery and Outcome. Occlusion of the ICA led to death in three patients; two recovered well. With MCA trunk occlusion, two patients died, four did not improve, and five recovered well. Outcome was best with occlusion of an MCA branch: five of six patients recovered well, and none died.

Table 2. Reperfusion within 6 and 24 h after onset of symptoms and clinical outcome in patients with occlusion within the ICA territory ($n = 22$) after alteplase (intravenous)

	Outcome		
Reperfusion	Good	Poor	Died
6 h[a]			
None	3	4	2
Partial	7	1	3
Complete	1	0	0
24 h			
None	0	3	2
Partial	4	1	2
Complete	8	1	1

[a] In one patient angiography was not performed.

Alteplase Dosage and Outcome. Although reperfusion was more frequent with higher doses, outcome was not different between the two dosage groups (Table 1).

Reperfusion and Outcome. Of the nine patients in whom no reperfusion occurred within 6 h of onset of symptoms, two died, four had a poor outcome, but three improved. On the other hand, 12 patients of the 17 showing complete or partial reperfusion within 24 h improved (Table 2). No reperfusion within 24 h correlated significantly with lack of clinical improvement or death of the patients ($\psi^2 = 5.18$, $p < 0.05$).

Discussion

The main purpose of this study was to find out whether a dosage of alteplase comparable to that used in myocardial infarction is safe with respect to intracranial hemorrhage and to obtain preliminary information about the effect on recanalization of thromboembolic occlusions and clinical outcome. Doses of 70 mg and 100 mg were used in consecutive and nonrandomized groups of patients. No control group existed to compare the effects. The study was open. Results therefore have to be interpreted carefully.

Alteplase treatment was discontinued in patients with vertebrobasilar occlusions because of discouraging results. Thus, the effect of 100 mg alteplase was not observed in this subgroup.

Reperfusion after thromboembolic occlusion can be due to the treatment or to spontaneous recanalization. Spontaneous recanalization was observed in 27%–59% of patients by angiography during the first days after stroke [1, 6, 7]. In our series of 22 patients with carotid circulation occlusions, the recanalization rate was 43% with 70 mg and 64% with 100 mg immediately after alteplase treatment, i.e., within 6 h of onset of symptoms. When reperfusion was assessed later, 24 h after stroke, rates were even higher at 57% and 86% respectively. Reocclusion was not observed. From this it is considered that the reperfusion in our study is mostly alteplase induced.

Reperfusion of the MCA was observed in 56% of patients within 6 h of stroke and in 82% within 24 h. This recanalization rate is high compared to the 45% which was achieved by intra-arterial urokinase infusion [8], but comparable with another study in which streptokinase or urokinase were applied locally within the carotid territory [2].

Immediate assessment after alteplase infusion revealed incomplete recanalization in all patients, with the exception of one short thrombus in the very distal ICA not occluding the A1 and M1-segments. This thrombus could be lysed completely. Assessment the next day, however, showed that late recanalization reduced the number of nonperfused vessels from 11 to 7 and increased the number of completely reperfused arteries from 1 to 10. Obviously, during alteplase infusion the proximal thrombus was lysed, moved, or fragmented first, and thrombolysis continued in distal branches during the subsequent hours. Reperfusion was more frequent with MCA branch occlusion than with occlusion of the MCA trunk or ICA, suggesting that thrombolysis is better the smaller the thrombus. Probably thrombi in larger vessels required higher doses of rt-PA.

Outcome in stroke is influenced by many factors but mainly by the extent and duration of ischemia. Despite reperfusion within 6 h of the insult, infarctions could not be prevented. However, outcome seemed to be better when reperfusion was achieved within 24 h. This suggests that restoration of blood flow could prevent necrosis in parts of the ischemic brain region.

Intracerebral hemorrhagic events were observed in eight patients (30%), two of whom experienced parenchymatous hemorrhages. One of them died showing an extended MCA infarction, which was certainly a cofactor in the fatal outcome. Interestingly, this patient did not exhibit any recanalization. Disseminated bleeding in both hemispheres, including parenchymatous hemorrhage, were observed in one patient who had been pretreated with aspirin, which may be dangerous in combination with rt-PA. Obviously, hemorrhagic transformation of the ischemic infarct did not negatively influence outcome. The rate of all intracerebral bleedings was higher than with intra-arterial urokinase therapy [2, 8], but not higher than expected from the natural course [5].

In conclusion, these preliminary observations show that treatment with 100 mg alteplase is safe and effective in terms of arterial recanalization within the ICA territory. There is the impression that reperfusion, even within 24 h of onset of symptoms, may be beneficial in thromboembolic stroke.

References

1. Bladin PF (1964) A radiologic and pathologic study of embolism of the internal carotid-middle cerebral arterial axis. Radiology 82:615–625
2. Del Zoppo GJ, Ferbert A, Otis S, Brückmann H, Hacke W, Zyroff J, Harker LA, Zeumer H (1988) Local intra-arterial fibrinolytic therapy in acute carotid territory stroke. Stroke 19:307–313
3. Hacke W, Zeumer H, Ferbert A, Brückmann H, Del Zoppo GJ (1988) Intra-arterial thrombolytic therapy improves outcome in patients with acute vertebrobasilar occlusive disease. Stroke 19:1216–1222
4. Heiss WD, Rosner G (1983) Functional recovery of cortical neurons as related to degree and duration of ischemia. Ann Neurol 14:294–301
5. Hornig CR, Dorndorf W, Agnoli AL (1986) Hemorrhagic cerebral infarction: a prospective study. Stroke 17:179–185
6. Irino T, Taneda M, Takaku M (1977) Angiographic manifestations in postrecanalized cerebral infarction. Neurology 27:471–475
7. Mohr JP, Barnett HJM (1978) The Harvard Cooperative Stroke Registry: a prospective registry. Neurology 28:754–762

8. Mori E, Tabuchi M, Yoshida T, Yamadori A (1988) Intracarotid urokinase with thromboembolic occlusion of the middle cerebral artery. Stroke 19:802–812
9. Zimmermann R, Heuck CC, Harenberg J, von Kummer R, Schmidt-Gayk U, Simon B, Wahl P, Mörl H, Weber PG (1981) Fibrinolytische Therapie einer schweren Arteria-basilaris-Thrombose. Dtsch Med Wochenschr 106:464–467
10. Zeumer H, Ringelstein EB, Hassel M, Poeck K (1983) Lokale Fibrinolysetherapie bei subtotaler Stenose der A. cerebri media. Dtsch Med Wochenschr 108:1103–1105

Thrombolytic Therapy in Embolic and Thrombotic Cerebral Infarction: A Cooperative Study

T. Yamaguchi[1], T. Hayakawa[2], H. Kikuchi[3], and T. Abe[4]

Introduction

The application of fibrinolytic therapy to patients in the acute stage of ischemic stroke has been actively discussed since the 1960s [6]. No conclusion concerning its efficacy has been achieved to date, although tissue plasminogen activator (t-PA) with its potent lytic activity and thrombus-specific affinity has become clinically available.

Active thrombolysis with high doses of urokinase (UK) in acute stroke has rarely been applied clinically since a number of fatal intracranial bleedings were reported by Hanaway et al. [3]. However, in a Japanese placebo-controlled double-blind study, in which subjects were restricted to thrombotic cerebral infarction, low-dose UK (60 000 U) was reported to be superior to placebo in its clinical improvement ratio, even though patients were treated up to 5 days after onset [7]. This suggests that the effect of UK may not only be limited to thrombolysis. This notion is supported by the observation that microcirculation in human scleral vessels was markedly improved after intravenous UK infusion [8].

Selecting Dosage According to Cerebral Infarction Subtype

It has long been known that cerebral infarction can be divided according to the mechanism of vascular occlusion into thrombotic and embolic stroke, which are considerably different in pathophysiology and clinical symptomatology. We have previously discussed two possible ways of applying t-PA in acute ischemic stroke (Yamaguchi, at the Satellite Symposium of the 12th Congress of the ISTH, 26 August 1989, Tokyo) and have suggested that, considering thrombolytic therapy in acute stroke patients, it is necessary to

[1] Cerebrovascular Division, National Cardiovascular Center, 5-7-1 Fujishirodai, Suita, Osaka 565, Japan.
[2] Department of Neurosurgery, Osaka University Medical School, Osaka, Japan.
[3] Department of Neurosurgery, Faculty of Medicine, Kyoto University, Kyoto, Japan.
[4] Teikyo University, Tokyo, Japan.

Hacke et al. (Eds.)
Thrombolytic Therapy in Acute Ischemic Stroke
© Springer-Verlag Berlin Heidelberg 1991

choose a dose of drug, timing of application, and a procedure appropriate to the type of stroke.

We have recommended intermittent intravenous administration of low-dose rt-PA for thrombotic stroke and high-dose administration in embolic stroke for the following reasons. Although patients with embolic stroke generally present more profound neurologic symptoms and poorer outcome than those with thrombotic stroke, such serious hemispheric syndrome at onset can improve dramatically within several hours or days. This is probably caused by rapid fragmentation and migration of a large embolus initially lodged in the trunk of the cerebral artery to the peripheral vessels. If rapid clot lysis or fragmentation of the embolus is caused very early after occlusion by administration of t-PA, a dramatic improvement can be expected.

On the other hand, in the case of thrombotic stroke, reasonably good collateral circulation develops, because it takes a fairly long time until the arteries are occluded or highly stenosed by atheroma. In this case, reopening or recanalization by t-PA is hardly expected, and the administration of low-dose t-PA to improve the microcirculation and to prevent further development of the thrombus from the occluded site to the more peripheral site may lead to clinical improvement.

In this paper, (a) preliminary results of high-dose administration for hyperacute embolic stroke, and (b) the final results of a low-dose trial for thrombotic stroke will be introduced briefly. Diagnosis of embolic and thrombotic infarction was made according to our criteria which have been previously reported [9].

Acute Cerebral Embolism Study

Protocol

Inclusion criteria for the study were acute embolic stroke with (a) age not more than 70 years, (b) entry less than 6h after onset, (c) no apparent hypodensity on computed tomography (CT) at entry, and (d) angiographic evidence of occlusion in the carotid axis. Informed consent was obtained from the patient or his/her family in every case. Patients with a history of intracranial hemorrhage, known hemorrhagic diathesis, and severe hepatic disorders were excluded.

Immediately after angiographic confirmation of embolic occlusion of the cerebral artery, 10, 20, or 30 megaunits (MU) of recombinant t-PA (Duteplase) dissolved in 200–250 ml electrolyte solution was given to each patient by drip infusion intravenously over 60 min. After completion of the t-PA infusion, cerebral angiography was again performed to confirm that reopening of the occluded vessels had occurred. CT was repeated at the

24th h, and on the 3rd, 7th, and 28th day after administration of rt-PA. For evaluation of the clinical symptoms and signs, the procedure designed by Mori et al. (presented at the Satellite Symposium of the 12th Congress of the ISTH, 26 August 1989, Tokyo), referring to the Hemispheric Stroke Scale [1] and the Barthel Index [5], was provided to minimize the interobserver variation. Angiographic findings were classified into the following five grades: complete reopening, partial reperfusion $\geq 50\%$, partial reperfusion $<50\%$, slight migration of embolus, and unchanged.

Results and Discussion

Fifty-eight patients with characteristic symptoms of embolic stroke were enrolled in the study (11 patients, 10 MU; 21 patients, 20 MU; 26 patients, 30 MU). Sufficient angiographic responses (complete and partial reperfusion $\geq 50\%$) were obtained mostly at 20–30 MU rt-PA (Table 1). Among 14 patients with sufficient reperfusion, 11 (79%) showed remarkable clinical improvement (judged to be moderately and markedly improved). Particularly, four of eight patients (50%) treated with 20 and 30 MU within 2 h after onset achieved sufficient reperfusion over 50% and remarkable clinical improvement with no hemorrhagic transformation (Fig. 1). This rate appeared to be better than that of delayed (≥ 4 h) treatment (sufficient reperfusion; 5/21, 24%). When the grade of reperfusion was not taken into account, seven of eight patients treated within 2 h showed remarkable improvement, while only 9 of 21 patients treated later than 4 h of onset showed a similar improvement.

Thus, there were a considerable number of patients whose cerebral injury may have been too critical to allow sufficient functional recovery or clinical

Table 1. Angiographic findings of the occluded carotid artery immediately after completion of intravenous rt-PA infusion in patients with hyperacute embolic stroke

Dose (MU)	N	Grade reperfusion						Hemorrhagic transformation
		Compl	$\geq 50\%$	$<50\%$	Migrat	None	?	
10	11	–	1^1 (9)	1 (18)	3^1	6^1	–	3
20	21	2 (10)	3^1 (24)	7^3 (57)	2	5^1	2	5
30	26	2 (8)	6 (31)	3^1 (42)	2	11^3	2	4
Total	58	4 (7)	10 (24)	11 (43)	7	22	4	12

Numbers in the *parenthesis* refer to the cumulative percentage of patients with reperfusion. *Superscript numbers* indicate the number of patients with hemorrhagic transformation.

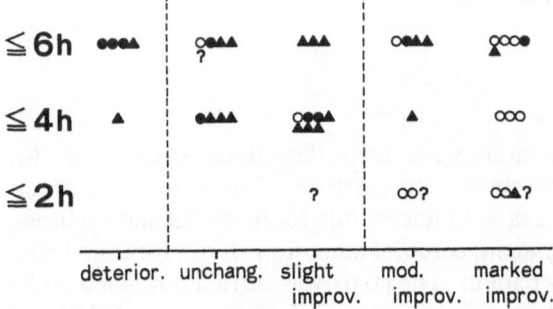

Fig. 1. Improvement rating by the time elapsed and the grade of reperfusion in hyperacute embolic stroke. *Open circle*, complete reopening and reperfusion >50%; *solid circle*, reperfusion <50%; *solid triangle*, minimal reperfusion and no reperfusion

improvement when treated later than 4 h. Therefore, patients for thrombolytic therapy must be selected from the standpoint of the grade of collateral arterial supply and more detailed CT findings, such as an equivocal decrease in attenuation value and the number of cortical sulci on the affected hemisphere, even though the hypodensity is not apparent on CT.

Spontaneous reopening of the previously occluded artery within several hours or days after onset and subsequent hemorrhagic transformation of the infarct are clinically and neuroradiologically important features of embolic stroke, which occasionally cause aggravation of brain edema followed by clinical deterioration. In our experience and from previous reports [2, 4, 9], aggravation was observed in about 80% and clinical deterioration was detected in about 50% of patients with acute embolic stroke following conventional treatment.

Interestingly, hemorrhagic transformation on CT in the present study was seen only in 12 (21%) of 58 patients (3 cases in the 10-MU, 5 in the 20-MU, and 4 in the 30-MU groups), the frequency being lower than in previous reports with conventional treatment. The frequency of hemorrhagic transformation, however, tended to increase with the delay of rt-PA administration (≤2 h, 1/9; 2–4 h, 3/20; 4–6 h, 8/26).

From the results of this study, administration of 20 or 30 MU rt-PA appeared appropriate to achieve major reperfusion in hyperacute embolic stroke. To elucidate the clinical efficacy and therapeutic window in the treatment with t-PA, however, a placebo-controlled randomized study with more detailed analysis is absolutely necessary.

Acute Cerebral Thrombosis Study

Protocol

The inclusion criteria for the study were acute thrombotic stroke with: (a) no clinical evidence of embolic stroke, (b) entry less than 3 days after onset, and (c) age not more than 75 years. Other criteria for inclusion and exclusion were the same as those in the acute cerebral embolism study. Informed consent was obtained from every patient. The study was carried out in a double-blind comparison method between the two doses of rt-PA (1 and 2 MU) and urokinase (6×10^4 U). Patients received intravenous infusion of the test drug (allotted randomly by the controller) once a day for 7 days. Only treatment with 10% glycerol at 400–600 ml was allowed as an additional treatment.

For clinical evaluation, level of consciousness, subjective neurologic and psychiatric symptoms and signs, and activity of daily living (ADL) were compared between three groups before and 7 and 28 days after commencement of the therapy. Clinical improvement (global improvement rating, GIR) was evaluated in five grades; marked, moderate, slightly improved, unchanged, and deteriorated.

Results and Discussion

Two hundred and twenty-two patients (70 patients, 2 MU t-PA; 75 patients, 1 MU t-PA; 77 patients, 6×10^4 U UK) were enrolled in the study. On the 7th day's evaluation, 33 of the 70 patients (47.1%) in the 2-MU and 26 of the 75 patients (38.7%) in the 1-MU rt-PA groups were judged to be more than "moderately improved," while only 15 of 77 patients (21.1%) showed such an improvement. As for chronic recovery, the ratios of patients who more than "moderately improved" increased to 68.6% and 64.0% in the 2- and 1-MU groups on the 28th day's evaluation, respectively, but that of the UK group remained at 44.7%, the differences being statistically significant (Fig. 2).

The baseline characteristics (age, sex ratio, time elapsed after onset, risk factors, past history, site and size of the lesion, etc.) of patients in the three groups were nearly equal, but the only difference obtained was the severity of neurologic symptoms and signs at entry, where the 2-MU rt-PA group consisted of patients with more severe deficits than the UK group.

Hemorrhagic transformation of infarct, which is the most unfavorable side effect in the thrombolytic therapy of cerebral thrombosis, was reported only in the UK group (Table 2). This evidence can be illustrated by the different pattern of fibrinolysis between t-PA and UK. Fibrin degradation products (FDPs) in plasma increased remarkably after rt-PA administration whereas they remained unchanged or slightly increased after UK administration, and

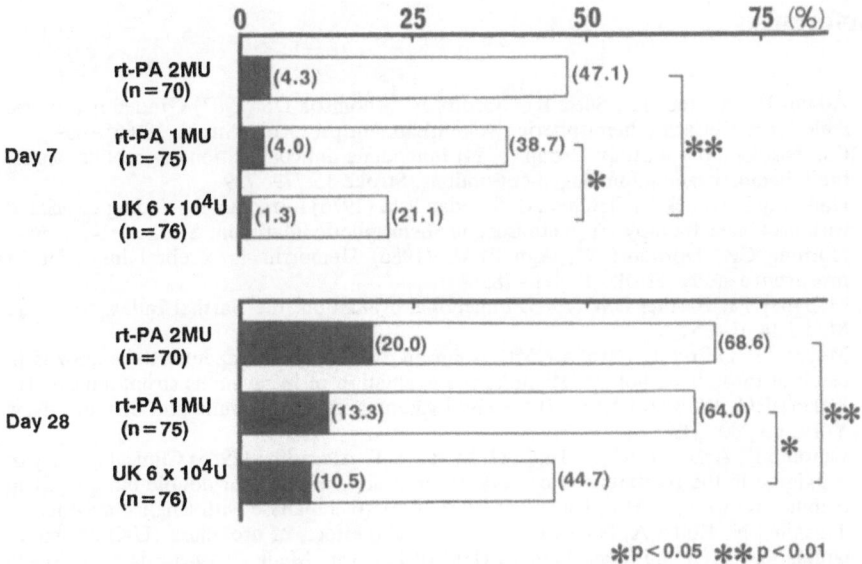

Fig. 2. Global improvement rating of clinical symptoms and signs in three treatment groups with acute thrombotic stroke. *Number in parenthesis*, cumulative percentage of improvement. *dotted column*, marked improvement; *open column*, moderate improvement

Table 2. Side effects of low-dose rt-PA treatment in patients with thrombotic stroke

Item	rt-PA 2 MU ($N = 70$)	rt-PA 1 MU ($N = 75$)	UK 6×10^4 ($N = 77$)
Subcutaneous bleeding	0	1	0
Cerebral bleeding	0	0	1
Hemorrhagic transformation of infarct	0	0	4
Hematuria	0	0	1
Leukopenia	0	2[b]	0
Thrombopenia	1	0	0
Anemia	1[a]	0	0
Miscellaneous[c]	3[a]	4[b]	1
Total	5	7	7

[a,b] Occurred in the same case.
[c] Miscellaneous includes liver dysfunction.

the antiplasmin level was gradually decreased in the prolonged course of treatment with urokinase, rather than with rt-PA.

Thus, the use of low-dose rt-PA for the treatment of acute ischemic stroke was found to be safe and to have considerable efficacy, provided the subjects were restricted to thrombotic cerebral infarction.

References

1. Adams RJ, Meador KJ, Sethi KD, Grotta JC, Thomson DS (1987) Graded neurologic scale for use in acute hemispheric stroke treatment protocols. Stroke 18:665–669
2. Cerebral Embolism Study Group (1984) Immediate anticoagulation of embolic stroke; brain hemorrhage and management options. Stroke 15:779–789
3. Hanaway J, Torack R, Fletcher AP, Landau WM (1976) Intracranial bleeding associated with urokinase therapy for acute ischemic hemispheric infarction. Stroke 7:143–146
4. Horning CR, Dorndorf W, Agnoli AL (1986) Hemorrhagic cerebral infarction: a prospective study. Stroke 17:179–185
5. Mahoney FI, Barthel DW (1965) Functional evaluation: the Barthel Index. Md State Med J 14:61–65
6. Meyer JS, Gilroy J, Barahart ME, Johnson JF (1965) Therapeutic thrombolysis in cerebral thromboembolism. Randomized evaluation of intravenous streptokinase. In: Siekert RG, Whisnant JP (eds) Cerebral vascular diseases. Grune and Stratton, New York, pp 200–213
7. Ohtomo E, Araki G, Ito E, Toghi H, Matsuda T, Atarashi J (1985) Clinical efficacy of urokinase in the treatment of cerebral thrombosis – multicenter double blind study in comparison with placebo. Clin Eval 13:711–751 (in Japanese with English abstract)
8. Tsushima N, Koike A, Nakayama R (1985) The effects of urokinase (UK) on microcirculation (MC) and hemorheology (HMS). Excerpta Medica, Amsterdam, pp 37–45 (Microcirculation Annual 1985)
9. Yamaguchi T, Minematsu K, Choki J, Jkeda M (1984) Clinical and neuroradiological analysis of thrombotic and embolic cerebral infarction. Jpn Circ J 48:50–58

IV. Future Directions

Problems in Formulating Therapeutic Trials

J.P. MOHR

This volume focuses on clinical trials intended to prevent the acute evolution of a brain infarct, and does not concern itself with prevention of stroke in an asymptomatic population or prevention of stroke recurrence. Although many clinical trials share common problems with design, in hyperacute stroke studies, special problems arise with accessing cases of acute stroke, obtaining patient consent, identifying the form of stroke for study, and determining whether the natural history has been altered by the therapy.

Running the Eligibility Gauntlet

The experience at the Neurological Institute during its first 2 years of activity, in which all patients admitted with stroke were surveyed and approached for their willingness to participate in an observational study known as the Stroke Data Bank, demonstrated that only 32% of 1327 patients approached were actually enrolled in this study of acute stroke within the first 7 days from onset. A surprising 51% proved ineligible, as some 22% of all cases diagnosed as stroke on admission were found not to have this diagnosis when studies were complete. Given this high frequency of confounding factors, investigators must be prepared for a huge survey effort for a small yield even in a study with generous entry criteria like the Stroke Data Bank.

Rounding up the Usual Suspects

No studies have been able to enter all patients arriving with stroke, and many constraints on eligibility prove very discouraging. Assuming the study is directed toward brain infarction, not hemorrhage, and there are the usual age criteria, exclusion of cardiac embolism because of its use of heparin, wish for no prior stroke lest the clinical scoring prove difficult, and the patient be

Stroke Service, The Neurological Institute, Columbia-Presbyterian Medical Center, 630 West 168th Street, New York, NY 10032, USA.

Hacke et al. (Eds)
Thrombolytic Therapy in Acute Ischemic Stroke
© Springer-Verlag Berlin Heidelberg 1991

intact enough to be worth the study effort, it is disappointing how few emerge for eligibility. Using the data from the Stroke Data Bank, as a guide, something slightly less than one-third of cases of stroke admitted to the hospital will be eligible for any acute study.

When constraints are imposed, the number screened to those admitted drops drastically. In the nimodipine study, the requirement that the patients agree to the trial, take no other medications, have a motor deficit, and arrive within 48 h resulted in a total of 13 437 patients with acute stroke screened at 53 institutions for a mere 1064 entered into the protocol, of whom 83% of patients completed the trial.

Emergency Ward Arrival Time and First Examination After Infarct

As if the foregoing were not difficult enough, severe constraints on recruitment come from any attempts to limit recruitment based on time. Any attempt to catch patients early requires some form of detection mechanism operative in the emergency ward with rapid transit to a brain imaging facility. The time of arrival from onset of stroke documented below comes directly from the data from the NINCDS Stroke Data Bank project for 413 patients with acute stroke entered at the Neurological Institute, 1 of 4 centers in this project. The figures below are the actual intervals between onset and initial examination by a principal investigator. In the Stroke Data Bank project, there was no specific requirement for hyperacute contact with the patients. Nonetheless, the data indicate speedy contact can be obtained. It also indicates there is a steady flow of patients into the emergency ward and that only a small fraction find their way within the initial hours. For the Data Bank, 3.4% arrived in the 1st h, another 1.5% in the 2nd h, 2.4% in the 3rd h, and by 12 h a total of 18% of the total admissions for stroke had reached the hospital.

A similar disappointing experience was encountered during the nimodipine study, where 144 of the total 1064 patients reached the hospital and received medication within the 12-h period. To implement acute clinical trials, faster arrival times will be needed.

Time to First Brain Image

For patients who have had their first stroke event or a new event while hospitalized, magnetic resonance (MRI) imaging has been carried out in six patients in as short a time as 30 min from documented stroke deficit onset, when the onset has been in the Neurological Institute and the patient rushed immediately to the unit by the physicians. For those transported through our underground tunnel from the emergency room, delays average about 15 min. The data indicate that there is only a slight delay in determining by brain imaging if the patient has had a hemorrhage or an infarct. It is also clear that it is often the case that an alert management team can bring a patient to the imaging setting before a responsible investigator can be called.

By the end of the 1st h, 3.4% were scanned in the Data Bank, by 6 h 17%, and by 12 h 31%. Considering the rate of patient arrival for stroke, these delays force an additional burden on the team trying to start therapy. It would be preferred that a therapy being used would be safe enough that it could be started without regard for the exact diagnosis, as now seems possible for nimodipine.

Deciding Whether and How Much Infarction Has Already Occurred

The decision whether a patient has had a stroke can be made on clinical grounds alone, on clinical grounds buttressed by computed tomography (CT) scan data, or by CT scan data alone. CT scan data alone has the advantage of offering evidence which could be interpreted by an adjudicator blinded to the treatment arm for a given case and unfamiliar with the clinical features which brought the patient to attention. This simple test would be quite desirable should it give a high frequency of positive findings in a cohort of cases deemed clinically to have had acute stroke. However, the results of this survey indicated that insistence on a symptomatic, clinically related, CT-positive infarct as the basis for entry into a trial would probably lower both the proven eligible case rates and the proven recurrence rates too far to permit the recruitment rates sought by the study.

The Stroke Data Bank is a suitable source to test the rates for positive CT scan in the first 30 days after hospitalization for a clinically diagnosed acute stroke. Excluding all forms of hemorrhage, the frequency of positive CT scans for all subtypes of infarction was a mere 63% on the first scan, and 73% for those whose cause was embolism.

Yet these figures refer to any abnormality found on CT scan. When further consideration was given to those lesions on CT which were considered clinically symptomatic and related to the infarct syndrome, the rate of CT-positive lesions was lower at 42%, and the individual frequencies scattered widely over the subtypes from a high of 55% in the large artery stenosis or occlusion group to a low of 31% in the lacunar syndromes.

There may be some ready explanations for the surprisingly low rate of CT-positive infarction in these data; yet these frequencies are holding up rather well in subsequent studies. For the Stroke Data Bank project there was no requirement that the CT scan be positive, only that it be performed.

As a result, for fully 35% of the patients no subsequent scanning was undertaken after the initially negative study, some for reasons that the patient was
too devastated by the stroke to have the information be of management
value, while in other cases management plans were based on the simple
absence of hemorrhage.

When analysis was extended to those who had more than one CT scan,
the frequency of clinically related positive scans rose as might be expected,
but only from a total of 42% to 52% when these observations were limited
to those lesions which were symptomatically related to the syndromes. The
highest rate was 80% for embolism and the lowest 42% for lacunes. Although these rates seem more satisfactory, they still leave at least 31% with
no clinically related CT scan findings despite two CT scans in a patient with
a clinically apparent ischemic stroke. CT scans performed when the initial
scan was negative do not have a sufficiently high positive rate to explain
the initially negative scans.

One explanation for the 31% frequency of negative CT scans for symptomatic stroke might be that the technology of the scanners used for imaging
in the Stroke Data Bank, modern for their time (1983–1986), seems a bit
antiquated compared with those available now. Whatever the explanation,
the data here can be taken to represent the minimum frequency of positive
CT scans in brain infarction. The rates of CT-positive infarcts may prove far
higher than those encountered in the Stroke Data Bank, for reasons outlined
above.

When considering patients within the first few hours of stroke, the frequency of the initially positive CT scans is lower still. Based on our experiences to date with the MR/CT contract, the use of the initial scan as a guide
to developing ischemia may be a bit misplaced and the MR may not be any
more sensitive than is the CT scan for the detection of early lesions.

Assessing Stroke by Brain Areas Injured

In addition to syndromes, a study was made of the brain sites affected by
ischemic stroke to try and create a similar manageable subset for the purposes
of data collection and estimation of stroke severity. The frequency data
demonstrated the expected clustering of vascular sites which were further
refined to a manageable small number of 12 subtypes, here presented in
descending frequency. This clustering also provides a ready means of assessing infarct size, which should help determine any differences between the
initial and the recurrent stroke.

We hoped this list could avoid problems which have arisen in prior studies
which, in attempting to capture all of the relevant data on CT or MRI studies,
have created a data set so unwieldy that the detailed analyses originally

planned are not fully undertaken. For this list to apply, however, there must be a brain image with a detectable abnormality.

Forty-two percent of cases are accounted for by frontoparietal infarction or convexity infarction not involving the frontal lobe. The remaining hemisphere sites are very low in frequency. These findings indicate there is more similarity than there is difference in the distribution of brain lesions on CT scan. Separate studies underway with these data also indicate the clinical correlation with the motor deficit is also somewhat limited and that the homuncular profile expected from focal hemispheral infarction in the Rolandic region is rather uncommon.

Estimating Stroke Severity Using Syndrome Analysis

Because some effects of acute therapy should be to reduce the severity of the syndrome on admission, it seemed worthwhile to try and characterize the frequency of the more easily recognized clinical syndrome using the Stroke Data Bank data to do so. An effort was made to rank the syndromes by frequency, combining those with very low frequencies to arrive at a manageably small group which might be subject to working definitions. The main elements of clinical examination were also surveyed and those elements frequently encountered or necessary for delineation of given syndromes were then included. Study was made of the frequencies with which certain commonly recognized syndromes occurred, in order to narrow down and group the expected syndromes into manageable groups. The result of the effort is reported below, in which combinations were made of syndrome subtypes to include all those represented by at least 1% frequency.

This list is not comprehensive but is designed to permit gross classification of the initial and recurrent strokes to allow some estimate of the relative severity of the entry stroke and any that might occur during the course of a study. The findings indicate the usual syndromes are not so discrete as to permit their easy use as a means of classifying stroke by severity; some other method is necessary. Major hemisphere syndrome occurred in 37.4%, followed by pure motor syndromes in 17.9%, the remaining syndromic types lagging rather far behind.

Determining the Patency of the Vessels

It is this step in an acute protocol where a tissue plasminogen activator (t-PA) study has difficulty recruiting patients. For an angiogram to be performed, a room must be made ready or one in use hastily evacuated, a radiologist and his or her team must be brought to the site, and valuable time is lost while the angiogram is performed. This step alone has blocked us at the Neurological Institute from entering many patients in such a study, as our rooms are usually in use when the emergency patient arrives, forcing delays which have in some cases exceeded the time limit.

In our own institution, the Internal Review Board took the position that angiography is not the standard of care for all cases of acute stroke so we were forced to undertake some additional steps before we could approach a patient for angiography. This step was transcranial Doppler scan, a technique we use regularly. When we were able to find evidence of stenosis or patency of the large vessels, we were compelled to cease any further workup. Only when we had findings that would be consistent with occlusion of an extra- or intracranial major artery could we then proceed with the angiogram. This constraint has kept our participation lower than we would have liked.

Early Discontinuation of Study Medication

In the nimodipine study, we were dismayed to find a high frequency of discontinuation from the study because of what we inferred to be adverse effects. It is of interest that the frequency of such effects in the placebo group were the same as those for the various doses. Despite the irony of presumed placebo effects throughout the whole subset of those who withdrew, the problem created by these withdrawals is reduction in size of the cohort in each of the groups, a reduction that interferes with the power of the calculations for a drug effect. Planning a sample size roughly twice what you need seems prudent.

Efforts to Avoid Concomitant Therapies

In the nimodipine study, it was deemed important to exclude any patient already receiving another calcium antagonist for fear the two agents would confound the interpretation of results from those receiving study drug. This requirement proved to eliminate a large number of patients who would otherwise have been eligible. Future trials must settle this point to minimize patients lost to a study.

We also faced a problem with the use of heparin. Although it would have been ideal to use no ancillary treatment, many centers regularly used intravenous heparin anticoagulation for patients with obvious cardiac atrial fibrillation. A standard throughout the study was made on this drug. Heparin was given for 3–5 days from admission, during which time coumadin was started for those cardiogenic in origin. The exact period depended on the time required for a given case to change his/her coagulation profile in response to the coumadin medication.

Studies Within Studies

Some of the problems created by the goal of comparability of findings across studies can be gleaned by the layering of testing we undertook for the American Nimodipine study. In designing our study, we attempted, where possible, to provide an opportunity to replicate the elements of other studies so as to permit a comparison between our cohort and those previously reported. Within our large cohort is a subset of patients who were treated within 24 h of onset with 120 mg nimodipine and others with placebo. This subset is actually a study within a study whose numbers are larger than those reported by Gelmers et al.

A number of uncertainties tempered these hopes, among them the most useful dose of nimodipine, the importance of time from onset of stroke to treatment, the severity of the ischemic process and its cause, embolic or thrombotic, and the lack of certainty that the measures used for estimating the severity of the stroke would prove adequate. In its more narrow focus, the trial was designed to achieve four definite goals, in descending order of importance. First, the study was to settle the dose and safety issues should the results require a larger study using the results of this dose and safety study. Second, it was to determine if a certain time interval seemed crucial for any benefits as might be seen. Third, it should permit estimates of the type of ischemic stroke likely to show benefit, including such factors as severity of the initial syndrome and its likely cause. Fourth, it was hoped a satisfactory assessment method would emerge to determine the outcomes of interest. Finally, the specific design used was being tested as a prototype for ensuring success in entering patients in a study, in hopes of encouraging high levels of effort among the study participants.

In selecting the scales to be used for evaluation, the Mathews Scale was deemed necessary because it was used in the Gelmers study and a direct comparison between this and the Gelmers study was desired. Since the Mathews scale was unfamiliar to many in the United States, the Toronto Scale was also included so the two scales could be compared. Analysis of these two scales left the investigators somewhat dissatisfied with the precision of the correlation between the motor deficit and the CT scan findings, so many elements of the forms created for the NIH Stroke Data Bank project were added to the protocol. The Barthel Index of Disability was also incorporated to assess the functional deficit separate from that found on the neurological examination.

Randomization was into four groups: nimodipine 60, 120, or 240 mg daily, or placebo. This design permitted a comparison of any nimodipine against placebo, and allowed the most tested dose of 120 mg day to be compared against half and double that dose.

The patients were examined at onset and on days 4, 10, and 21 using six separate neurological scales. These epochs were chosen in hopes they might provide some insight into temporal effects which could not be noted in earlier trials comparing only the onset status with that at 28 days. To detect any obvious changes in clinical status, the patients were also seen daily for a formal but brief neurological examination to detect major changes in the clinical syndrome.

Repeat CT scan was undertaken between day 3 and 5 to seek confirmation of the diagnosis of ischemic stroke, evidence of hemorrhagic transformation, mass effect, or change in lesion site and size. At that time, it was planned to exclude those patients who had been entered erroneously for the wrong diagnosis. Further, those whose course appeared to be complicated by hemorrhagic transformation or massive brain edema could also be dropped from the trial so as to avoid any concerns that the active agent might contribute to further neurological worsening. Accordingly, postrandomization exclusion was made for those whose investigations disclosed the presence of brain tumor, intracranial hemorrhage, or other causes of an acute focal deficit inconsistent with acute ischemic infarction or those for whom it became known after randomization that they suffered a medical condition which precluded their continued participation.

Assessing Outcome

It is easier to document reestablishment of a lumen than it is to show there has been neurological benefit. In the nimodipine study, there was a disappointing lack of prominent benefits in neurological outcome. In both our study and in the Gelmers studies, the mean score on the neurological scales showed the patients suffered obvious neurological disabilities from the effects of the ischemic stroke. A small number of patients had only the minimum of signs while many had a large deficit. As in the Gelmers studies, those minimally affected had little improvement they could show while those heavily affected had little chance to show improvement, leaving the bulk of the changes for those patients with syndromes of intermediate severity. Changes overall in any of the neurological scales were disappointingly small, some 10% compared with baseline no matter what the scale used. These findings indicate that the benefits, where documented, although functionally important, are not the sort that lead to total reversal of a major neurological deficit evident on admission.

Ranking Stroke Events

We suggest something like the following in order to rank cases into categories, beginning with the stroke types least subject to disagreement in adjudication, and continuing to those with the least certainty as to events. Although the data will be ranked in these categories, the primary analysis will be conducted by lumping the data across all five categories. These categories seem necessary because several of the current studies indicate the effects of aspirin and possibly those of ticlopidine are mainly on the reduction of minor stroke events, not the major events, and the same argument may apply to other drugs, including t-PA.

Each category should separate whether a patient has the first or subsequent event, how late after the onset the brain image was obtained, whether the brain image was positive and explained the syndrome, and whether the subsequent course featured worsening or recurrence.

Invasive and Noninvasive Vascular Imaging Techniques and Their Role in Clinical Stroke Trials

W.J. HUK

In the past 1½ decades, technological geniuses have invented new diagnostic tools, computed tomography (CT) and magnetic resonance imaging (MRI), which produce excellent images of the brain sometimes superior to anatomical sections, and which – their latest achievement – are able to visualize vascular structures without the need for contrast medium. With respect to acute cerebrovascular disease and fibrinolytic therapy, these promising techniques evoke the following questions:

- Can we analyze the hemodynamic situation in acute stroke reliably with these noninvasive techniques, or do we still need direct arteriography? How reliable is magnetic resonance angiography (MRA)?
- Can we obtain reliable information on the prognosis of acute stroke, i.e., will it be only a transient attack or will it end up as completed stroke with more or less extensive necrosis of brain tissue?
- Can we decide the indication for thrombolysis on the basis of the results of noninvasive imaging techniques alone or do we need conventional angiography?

Conventional arteriography, either by direct puncture or preferably by the transfemoral approach, bears potential risks, which are increased in severe cerebrovascular disease, when large amounts of contrast medium are used, when repeated injections are administered, when allergic reactions occur, etc; they are reduced when the examination is performed by a skilled and experienced physician. Nevertheless, in the most vulnerable phase of brain tissue in early acute stroke, one wants to avoid any means which could affect the blood flow and oxygen supply to the ischemic territory.

However, since thrombolysis is most effective and associated with the least risk of side effects when performed as soon as possible after the acute event, early diagnosis is mandatory. In order to identify among the large number of cerebrovascular events those with acute thrombotic or embolic vascular occlusions which are accessible for lysis, i.e., more than 30% of the total number, the vascular tree of the brain has to be visualized. When

Neuroradiology Department, Neurosurgical Hospital of Erlangen-Nürnberg, Schwabachanlage 6, W-8520 Erlangen, FRG.

Hacke et al. (Eds)
Thrombolytic Therapy in Acute Ischemic Stroke
© Springer-Verlag Berlin Heidelberg 1991

conventional angiography is employed in all cases, too many patients, for whom no therapeutic benefits result from the examination, undergo unnecessary risks. In this situation CT and MRI can provide valuable and reliable information.

In 1988, Schuierer [7] from our department reported on a small series of four patients, demonstrating that a hyperdense middle cerebral artery (MCA) in the noncontrast CT scan reflects acute cerebral embolism or thrombosis within the first hours of clinical symptoms appearing (Fig. 1). Although basal cerebral arteries especially in older patients are visualized on modern noncontrast CT images, only very few cases of clots in the MCA detected by CT have been reported up to the present time [1, 5, 10]. As clots possess a higher absorption value on CT than moving blood, they appear as hyperdense areas in the course of intracranial arteries. Gacs et al. [1] and Pressman et al. [5] proved the presence of cerebral emboli in three patients who had angiography and evidence of an embolus on CT in their respective studies. Since there usually is a normal contralateral MCA for comparison, a study with intravenous contrast medium, as proposed in basilar artery thrombosis by Vonofakos et al. in 1983 [9], does not seem necessary. Positioning of the patient in the scanner should therefore be as symmetrical as possible even though these patients are often difficult to handle. Reduction of slice thickness to 4 mm or less will also improve the detectability of a clot within the basal cerebral vessels. Discretely hyperdense bilateral MCAs can be seen

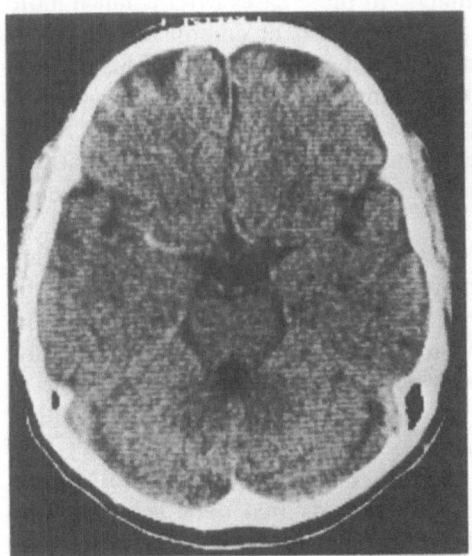

Fig. 1. Hyperdense left MCA in a 40-year-old man about 4 h after acute spontaneous hemiplegia on the right. Angiography verified a complete occlusion of the M1 segment

in aged patients with extensive arteriosclerosis, but the absence of clinical signs of acute ischemia prevents misinterpretation. Calcified emboli showing higher localized densities may also be found.

As already mentioned, more than 30% of cases of cerebral ischemia are, according to the Harvard cooperative stroke registry of 1978 [3], caused by cerebral embolism. Cardiac and cerebrovascular abnormalities are the main source of these emboli, which was also the case in three out of our four patients. Sherman and coworkers in 1984 [8] found a higher incidence of cerebral embolism in patients with atrial fibrillation, and they pointed out that cerebral infarctions in these patients had a poor prognosis, with more than 50% of their patients dying or showing extensive disabilities.

The hyperdense MCA can be considered a reliable early sign of impending cerebral infarction. In our small series in one case it was seen 2 h after the acute event. Theoretically the affected vessel should appear hyperdense as soon as the clot has become located or formed in the vessel lumen. In all four patients of the published series as well as in several others since then, clinical signs and CT monitoring showed complete MCA territory infarction, explaining the unfavorable outcome. A hyperdense MCA might, therefore, also be considered to predict a poor prognosis. This observation could be an important argument for local or systemic thrombolysis in selected cases.

In patients with occlusion of the MCA, CT is superior to MRI in the very acute phase. It provides a longitudinal section of the vessel involved, and the usually uncooperative patients can be managed more easily with CT. The basilar artery is, however, only seen on CT as a small cross-section in an area which is subject to multiple artifacts. In these cases MRI is much more reliable in demonstrating basilar artery thrombosis or embolism (Fig. 2). If an occlusion of the basilar artery is suspected from the clinical history and the neurological findings, MRI is the imaging technique of choice, which in noncooperative patients justifies general anesthesia to achieve good image quality. However, this has to be performed as fast as possible in patients who fullfil the inclusion criteria of local thrombolysis. Otherwise immediate arteriography should be preferred.

With the exception of the hyperdense MCA just mentioned, the demonstration of acute occlusion of proximal portions of cerebral arteries, by either CT or MRI, does not provide reliable information concerning the further course of the disease. Neither technique shows the collateral supply, e.g., via leptomeningeal anastomoses. Theoretically it may be possible to visualize anastomotic channels or collateral supply with MRI modalities, such as MRA or MRI perfusion studies.

In MRA [6], inflow and phase effects of moving protons are utilized with gradient echo sequences and three-dimensional data acquisition to demonstrate intravascular flow without contrast medium. To acquire two-dimensional projections, which are preferred to sequential two-dimensional slices for the evaluation of vascular structures, the MRA series are post-

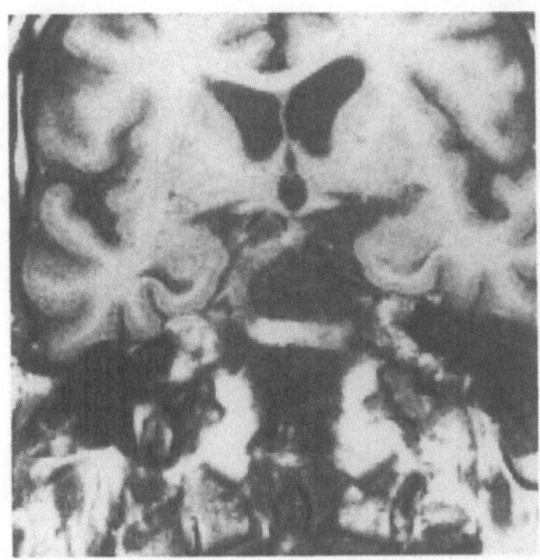

Fig. 2. Acute occlusion of the basilar artery in a 62-year-old man. Angiography did not show the elongated and tortuous artery; the extensive embolus/thrombus can only be evaluated properly on the coronal MR scan (SE = 0.45 s/15 ms, 1.5 *T*)

processed by means of a ray-tracing algorithm incorporating a maximum intensity projection (MIP). This technique visualizes laminar flow of a certain velocity (Fig. 3a); slow flow, such as in narrow arteries or small veins, might not be seen. The present sequences are also prone to artifacts from turbulent flow, which decreases the signal intensity. This turbulence may cause the impression of a narrowing of the vessel lumen, making it difficult to estimate the true degree of stenosis. Stenosis is thus easily overestimated. In the area of flow dividers, such as the carotid bifurcation, turbulence is a normal finding in the arteriogram of healthy carotids; this possible risk of false-positive diagnosis must therefore be kept in mind. Another risk of misinterpretation arises from structures or tissues with high magnetic susceptibility, for example, acute thrombosis, which cause a hyperintense signal similar to intravascular flow (Fig. 3b). In the very acute phase, therefore, T1- or T2-weighted spin echo images might be more reliable in demonstrating vascular occlusion than MRA.

With contrast medium the spatial resolution of MRA can be improved and with optimized sequences it should in the future be possible to demonstrate the retrograde flow of leptomeningeal anastomoses in acute stroke. This, of course, does not answer the question of whether the collateral supply is sufficient for brain function and whether the ischemic brain tissue will survive or not. So far we have had no chance to study this in acute stroke patients.

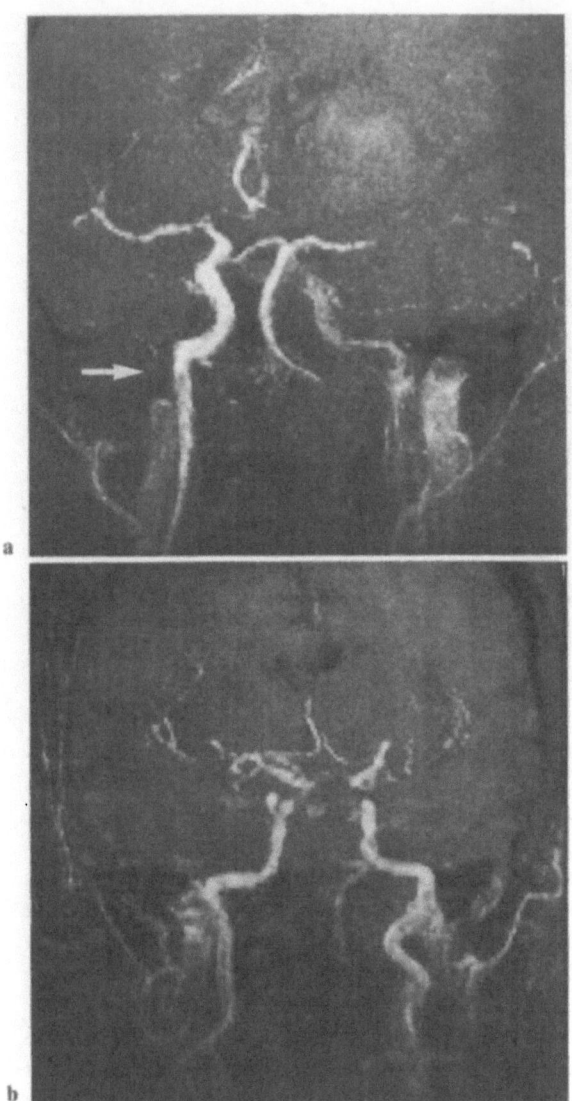

Fig. 3a,b. Coronal MRA of **a** a 65-year-old man with thrombosis of the basilar artery. Only the left vertebral artery (*arrow*) is shown. **b** Coronal MRA of a 40-year-old man with acute occlusion of the left internal carotid artery (ICA) by spontaneous dissection. The fresh thrombus appears less hyperintense than the normal blood flow of the opposite ICA

Magnetic resonance imaging perfusion studies (Deimling M, personal communication, 1990) use very fast sequences, so-called turbo-FLASH, with a 64 or 128 matrix and very short imaging parameters TR and TE which make images possible every 1–2 s for dynamic studies. In this sequence an inversion pulse precedes the data acquisition. When contrast medium is injected as a bolus during the sequence, the inflow of contrast medium into the different anatomical structures can be compared by means of signal intensity curves. The results correlate with those of dynamic CT studies, where fast CT scanners are used to detect the uptake, clearance, or circulation of radio-dense materials, for example, iodinated compounds and nonradioactive xenon. The time course of the absorption values in each pixel is used to calculate cerebral blood flow. As in dynamic CT studies, sequential scans at each brain level are also required by MRI perfusion studies, and exact reproducibility of patient position during the study is necessary, thus limiting the application of this technique to cooperative patients. Theoretically a multislice sequence could be used in cases were a high time resolution is not required. This type of MRI perfusion study is not very time consuming; only about 10 additional minutes are needed for the data acquisition and calculation of 25 images of a single slice.

The initial portion of this curve, which is drawn by the bolus after its first passage through the lungs and the heart, seems to be useful for the evaluation of local tissue perfusion. When compared with the major vessels, the perfusion rate of normal and pathological tissues can be estimated (Fig. 4). This technique, of course, provides only relative data of the amount of blood flow. It could perhaps give some information on the retrograde flow of collateral

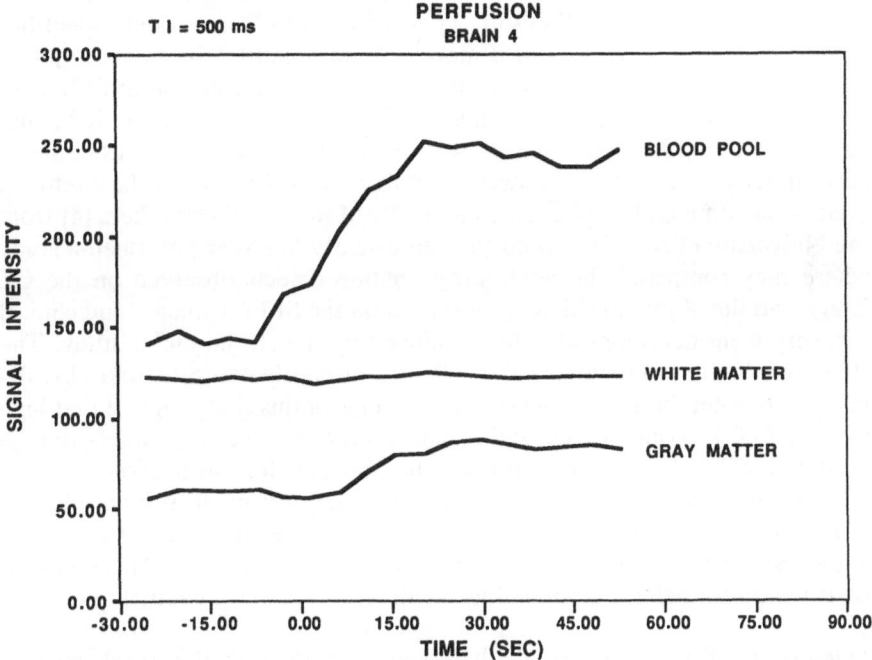

Fig. 4. Perfusion study of gray and white matter compared with major intracranial vessels (blood pool) after bolus injection of 10 ml gadolinium DTPA

channels in acute occlusion of cerebral arteries. The first very preliminary results of our study to evaluate the clinical relevance of this technique show that there is almost no enhancement of the white matter compared with gray matter, reflecting the higher perfusion rate of gray matter. In different kinds of tumors, different signal intensity curves could be correlated with their degree of vascularity. In healthy individuals we have seen no significant difference between the two hemispheres. In elderly patients a more gentle slope of the curve could be observed.

Another imaging technique which provides information on tissue perfusion is single photon emission computed tomography (SPECT). New tracers have been developed, for example, iodine-123 iofetamine and technetium-99m hexamethyl propyleneamine oxime (HMPAO), that cross the blood-brain barrier, distribute within the brain proportional to regional blood flow, and remain fixed within the brain for sufficient time to permit cross-sectional imaging with either rotating gamma cameras or special-purpose ring-type imaging systems.

A most dramatic difference between emission and transmission tomography is described by Holman et al. [2] within the first day or two after an acute cerebral infarction. Images produced by magnetic resonance and X-ray computed tomography, which rely on changes in anatomy and morphology, remain normal for some time after the onset of symptoms, while SPECT documents the changes in blood flow and metabolism that are present at the onset. According to the literature, perfusion SPECT accurately identifies chronic cerebral infarction and is more accurate than CT in the early phase of acute infarction. The extent of the defect is often greater on SPECT than on CT as alteration in perfusion may occur because of diaschisis, ischemia, or neuronal loss. Delayed imaging with iodine-123 spectamine differentiates peri-infarct ischemia from central necrosis and may therefore be useful to predict outcome and to plan treatment (2). Mountz and coworkers [4] from the University of Michigan Medical Center early this year published a study where they compared the anatomical volume defects observed on the CT image and the blood flow defects observed on the SPECT image; and clinical recovery from neurological deficits induced by the stroke under study. The study was limited to patients ($N = 27$) with primarily cortical strokes involving only one cerebral hemisphere. The findings of this study suggest that high SPECT to CT volume defect ratios indicate the presence of viable – though dysfunctional – tissue which retains the capacity for restoration of more normal function, possibly due to subsequent improvement in blood flow to this tissue. On the other hand, where SPECT to CT volume defects are nearly equal, no such capacity for restoration of lost function exists. This seems to be true also for MRI. Summarizing, I will try to answer my initial questions.

Question 1. Can we analyze the hemodynamic situation of acute stroke reliably enough for therapeutic decisions on the basis of the noninvasive imaging techniques just mentioned? At the present time we are able to demonstrate an acute occlusion of major cerebral vessels by an embolus or thrombus with CT and MRI using SE sequences. Minimal remaining flow through the affected vessel and collateral flow via leptomeningeal anastomoses has not yet been shown. This is also true for the present version of MRA. However, it should theoretically be possible to improve the sensitivity and spatial resolution of angiographic sequences, which in addition can be increased with intravenous contrast medium. With this optimized MRI technique it should be possible to demonstrate collateral flow, although without reliable quantitative information. The small lenticulostriate branches of the MCA, which are end vessels, cannot be seen in MRI; chances of their recanalization in cases of MCA occlusion have been poor in our limited number of cases.

In thrombosis of the basilar artery the collateral supply of the brain stem and the basal ganglia will also be beyond the spatial resolution of MRA, as it is of conventional angiography. Many of the small perforating arteries are also end branches of the basilar artery. MR, however, can depict the shape and course of the basilar artery and the extent of the embolus or thrombus better than conventional arteriography (see Fig. 2).

Question 2. Can we obtain reliable information on the outcome of an acute cerebrovascular occlusion from the initial findings of imaging techniques? The answer is yes and no. Yes, because hopefully we will be able to see to some extent a collateral supply, which means a lesser degree of tissue damage. No, because we do not know whether this collateral supply is adequate to meet the minimum requirements of tissue survival in the acute or late phase of stroke. And no, because we get no idea of whether there will be adequate spontaneous thrombolysis and recanalization of the affected vessel before definite damage of brain tissue has occurred. Especially in acute embolic occlusion of the anterior circulation of younger individuals, a high percentage of spontaneous recanalizations is stated by several authors. But to wait for spontaneous lysis means to lose the only chance of effective treatment in cases where it does not happen. Conventional arteriography, of course, is also not able to predict spontaneous recanalization. In the subacute phase, perfusion studies with dynamic CT, MR, and/or SPECT are of certain prognostic value with respect to the final outcome following stroke.

Question 3. Can we decide for or against local or systemic thrombolysis on the basis of CT, MR, or SPECT alone? The answer depends greatly on the time that is available for diagnosis and the availability of the various imaging techniques for acute examinations. If the patient is not a candidate for lysis because of exclusion criteria, noninvasive techniques should be employed. If she or he is a candidate for thrombolysis, then we should differentiate between the anterior and posterior circulation: In acute occlusion of the MCA the initial CT scan, which is performed to differentiate between hemorrhage and ischemia as the cause of stroke and to ascertain whether there are already early signs of hypoxic edema, can be used to look for a hyperdense

MCA. If this sign is present, immediate transfemoral arteriography should be performed to confirm the diagnosis and to advance the microcatheter to the thrombus for local thrombolysis without losing valuable time.

In patients with suspected thrombosis of the basilar artery, the diagnostic modality which should be used initially depends on the patient's clinical history and neurological status. If there was acute onset with severe symptoms indicating a larger embolus, the management should be similar to that for MCA occlusion, i.e., immediate angiography with subsequent lysis. If there is a gradual onset of symptoms pointing to the brain stem, suggesting the buildup of a thrombus, MRI together with MRA should be performed for differential diagnosis. Angiography with lysis should, if indicated, follow thereafter.

As time is a very important factor in the management of acute stroke and the decision for or against thrombolysis has to be made as soon as possible, only examinations of short duration and instant results such as those from CT and angiography, are justified. In this very early phase of stroke the most relevant information we want to verify is whether there is an acute embolic or thrombotic occlusion of the vessel or not. Only when the results of MRI, MRA, MR perfusion studies, and SPECT can be obtained within a few minutes can the use of these techniques be justified in the acute phase; after this it takes additional time to bring the patient to the angiographic unit for local thrombolysis. MRI will hopefully be able to fulfil these requirements in the near future. Until then, MRA, MR perfusion studies, and SPECT can only be used in stroke patients after thrombolysis or in those cases where thrombolysis cannot be performed for other reasons, in order to evaluate the degree of tissue damage for prognostic considerations.

References

1. Gacs G, Fox AJ, Barnett H, Vinuela F (1983) CT visualisation of intracranial arterial thromboembolism. Stroke 14 (5):756–862
2. Holman BL, Tumeh SS (1990) Single-photon emission computed tomography (SPECT). Application and potential. JAMA 263(4):561–564
3. Mohr JP, Caplan LR, Melski JW, Goldstein RJ, Duncan GW, Kistler JP, Pessin MS, Bleich HL (1978) The Harvard cooperative stroke registry: a prospective registry. Neurology 28:754–762
4. Mountz JM, Modell JG, Foster NL, DuPree ES, Ackerman RJ, Petry NA, Bluemlein LE, Kuhl DE (1990) Prognostication of recovery following stroke using a comparison of CT and technetium-99m HMPAO SPECT. J Nucl Med 31(1):61–66
5. Pressman BD, Tourje EJ, Thompson JR (1987) An early sign of ischemic infarction: increased density in a cerebral artery. AJNR 4:525–528
6. Ruggieri PM, Laub E, Masaryk T, Modic M (1989) Intracranial circulation: pulse sequence consideration in 3-dimensional MR angiography. Radiology 171 (3):785–791
7. Schuierer G, Huk W (1988) The unilateral hyperdense middle cerebral artery: an early CT-sign of embolism or thrombosis. Neuroradiology 30:120–122

8. Sherman DG, Goldman L, Whiting RB, Jürgensen K, Kaste M, Easton JD (1984) Thromboembolism in patients with atrial fibrillation. Arch Neurol 41:708–710
9. Vonofakos D, Marcu H, Hacker H (1983) CT diagnosis of basilar artery occlusion. AJNR 4:525–528
10. Yock DH (1981) CT demonstration of cerebral emboli. J Comput Assist Tomogr 5(2):190–196

Strategies for Early Treatment
of Acute Cerebral Infarction

T. Brott[1], E.C. Haley[2], D. Levy[3], W. Barsan[1], J. Broderick[1],
and J.R. Marler[4]

Introduction

For cerebral infarction, potentially effective therapeutic agents include calcium channel antagonists, excitatory amino acid receptor blockers, free
radical scavengers, and agents promoting thrombolysis [7]. To evaluate these
interventions in patients, they must be administered very early after symptom
onset, ideally within several hours. The time threshold in humans for irreversible cellular injury following focal cerebral ischemia has not been established.
No doubt it will vary depending on the degree of ischemia and its location
within the brain. In primates laboratory studies indicate a threshold for
neocortex of 3 h or less [9].

For cerebral infarction therapy trials, such a threshold for irreversible
injury suggests a paradox. The results from a trial including patients treated
beyond the threshold may falsely suggest that the treatment is ineffective,
even though the trial may have included the hundreds of patients estimated
necessary for adequate statistical power. Results from a much smaller trial,
including only patients treated within the threshold, could be more valid
biologically. Such a trial may actually require fewer patients than estimated
for adequate statistical power if many of the patients are treated well within
the threshold.

Unfortunately, early treatment has either not been a feature of stroke
therapy trials or has been very difficult to accomplish. Between 1972 and
1981, only one trial began treatment within 6 h of stroke onset [4]. Recent
trials of prostacyclin [8] and nimodipine [6] allowed patient entry up to

[1] Departments of Neurology and Emergency Medicine, University of Cincinnati Medical
Center, 231 Bethesda Avenue, 4010 Medical Science Building, Cincinnati, OH 45267-0525,
USA.
[2] University of Virginia, Health Sciences Center, Box 394, Charlottesville, VA 22908,
USA.
[3] Department of Neurology (A-569), Cornell University Medical College, 1300 York
Avenue, New York, NY 10021, USA.
[4] National Institute of Neurological Disorders and Stroke, Division of Stroke and
Trauma, Federal Building, Room 800, 7550 Wisconsin Avenue, Bethesda, MD 20892,
USA.

Hacke et al (Eds.)
Thrombolytic Therapy in Acute Ischemic Stroke
© Springer-Verlag Berlin Heidelberg 1991

24–48 h after symptom onset. Treatment within 8 h of symptom onset (and after a cerebral angiogram) has been required in a multicenter dose-escalation trial of intravenous tissue plasminogen activator (t-PA) [14], but fewer than 100 patients could be treated over the first 3 years of patient entry at multiple hospitals. Treatment within 90 min was required in a recent dose-escalation trial of t-PA sponsored by the National Institutes of Health (NIH) [3] in which pretreatment angiography was not performed. Only 74 patients were entered at 13 hospitals over 30 months.

Delays in Treatment and Evaluation

In an observational study of 457 patients with stroke reported by Albert [1], only 42% of patients presented to the hospital within 24 h of symptom onset. Delays were significantly related to stroke type. Patients with cerebral infarction were least likely to present within 24 h (36%), and patients with intracerebral hemorrhage were most likely to present within 24 h (63%). The authors suggested several reasons for delay: (a) patients' lack of knowledge about the symptoms of stroke; (b) delay in deciding to seek medical attention in the hope that the deficit will improve spontaneously; (c) delay because of transportation; (d) delay because of inability of elderly or demented patients to communicate their complaints effectively to medical personnel; and (e) delay because of denial of a deficit.

Timerding [13] identified delays in evaluation after patient arrival to the hospital. The steps required for entry into a trial of ancrod for ischemic stroke were analyzed. Approximately 50% of the patients for whom the therapy team responded were eventually excluded from the trial. There were no consent refusals. Time until treatment was signficantly affected by time of patient hospital arrival, time for completion of bleeding time and fibrinogen assay, time of arrangement of CT until its completion, and site of treatment. Patients were treated more rapidly if therapy was begun in the Emergency Department instead of the Neurology Intensive Care Unit, and patients entered in the later months of the study were evaluated and treated more rapidly than were the initial patients.

Timerding suggested that ischemic stroke patients have historically not been considered to be critically ill, being classified to have moderately low medical acuity. She cited a recent time study in which patients with moderate medical acuity required 123–142 min in the Emergency Department for evaluation and treatment. Patients judged critically ill required an average of only 35 min in the Emergency Department for evaluation and treatment [17]. The conclusion was that medical staff perception of acuity for ischemic stroke patients must be changed if rapid treatment is to be accomplished in future stroke therapy trials.

Shortening Patient Response Time

In the United States approximately 40% of people recently surveyed did not know the warning signs of stroke, and only 1% were aware that stroke is a leading cause of death [1]. Public education has been effective in facilitating early treatment for myocardial infarction [10] and has the potential of greatly facilitating early treatment for stroke.

For television, the story must have visual impact with the stroke investigators' "message" interwoven. For example, ABC News broadcast a story on emergency stroke therapy in the United States, entitled "Brain Attack" (8 June 1990), as part of the network program "20/20". This story was in preparation for many months but was finalized for broadcast when videotaping of helicopter transport and treatment of actual patients could be accomplished. The educational messages were secondary to the dramatic elements but were an integral part of the feature. In Cincinnati, approximately five television stories have run describing recent stroke therapy trials. The producers have been consistently enthusiastic in arranging coverage as long as individual patients were available to be featured. The anecdotal format may actually be ideal for education. The medical importance of stroke, the symptoms of stroke, and the need for early evaluation following stroke may be more memorably conveyed when visually linked to actual patients – particularly when those patients have improved following therapy.

The print media will report results without anecdotes, but the long-term nature of stroke therapy trials keeps the number of such stories very limited. However, national and local print media will run stories on a more frequent basis if they are topical and feature a vivid case history with a positive outcome. Recent stroke therapy stories in the New York Times and the Washington Post began with and emphasized individual patient experiences. The details of stroke symptoms, stroke warning symptoms, and available therapies were conveyed as they related to the patients.

Radio may be particularly underutilized for stroke public education. The "talk show format" has become particularly popular in the United States. With hours of such programming to provide, radio station directors can be persuaded by the enthusiastic and available investigator to run stories on stroke. Few other diseases provide such memorable examples of behavioral dysfunction, and the great majority of patients improve.

For television, print, and radio public education, the multihospital network approach to therapy has important advantages. Reporters are less concerned that a suggested story is actually an advertisement for a particular hospital or investigator. The editors will find a given story of more interest the more citywide medical implications. The public relations departments of the hospitals may cooperate with each other and assist in the preparation of stories and news conferences. Such cooperation in the competitive hospital environment found in the United States is becoming uncommon but is feasible if the hospitals are engaged in a common mission.

The multihospital approach also allows the exposure of individual investigators to be easily shared. Each member of the team may have a turn in the "spotlight," and no single team member need be overexposed, a situation which may become counter-productive by alienating other physicians in community leadership positions.

Enlarging the Referral Base

Evaluation and treatment of acute ischemic stroke patients within 90 min of symptom onset has been accomplished by the Cincinnati stroke team in 60 patients over the previous 4 years. Over the most recent 16 months, 37 patients with spontaneous intracerebral hemorrhage have been studied within 3 h of symptom onset in a prospective observational study requiring early serial neurological examinations and CT scans. Over the same 16-month period, 11 additional acute ischemic stroke patients have been evaluated and treated within 6 h as part of a multicenter randomized trial of ancrod. Of this total of 108 patients, only 24 were recruited at the University of Cincinnati Medical Center. The remaining 84 patients were evaluated and treated at one of ten cooperating community hospitals in Ohio and Kentucky.

The specific techniques for developing a multihospital acute stroke network are beyond the scope of this discussion, particularly as they may have limited application to other metropolitan areas. Our experience with this network has underscored several patterns of medical practice. The sophisticated medical resources once limited to major university medical centers are now frequently available at the local community hospital. Perhaps more important, the local community hospital is usually perceived by the public, the pre-hospital care system, and many physicians to have equipment and resources comparable to those of tertiary centers. The medical resources available to the investigator within a hospital network may be multiplied many times over through active participation of the numerous patient care departments at each of the hospitals. For example, instead of one or two CT scanners, the investigator may have access to 10 or 15.

Enlisting the Pre-Hospital Care System

In major trauma, the mean time from injury to hospital arrival has ranged from 20 to 38 min [5]. We have attempted to duplicate that performance for stroke patients.

The pre-hospital care system varies from metropolitan region to metropolitan region and even varies in its operation from hospital to hospital. Accordingly, the active participation of a physician specializing in emergency medicine may be particularly helpful. Such a physician may easily develop the local knowledge and professional contacts which facilitate emergency referrals. In Cincinnati, William Barsan has helped coordinate the pre-hospital care system for acute stroke investigation. A central telemetry system at our University Medical Center monitors all life squad radio communication. A fail-safe digital paging system with three investigators carrying a pager with the same telephone number assures absolute investigator availability. One of these three experienced investigators arrives on the scene to supervise the evaluation of every patient. Accordingly, life squad members see one of the stroke team investigators on most occasions that they transport a stroke patient to a study hospital. Follow-up letters are sent regarding individual patients, and general update letters are widely distributed through a pre-hospital care mailing list. Study update presentations are given by the investigators at the various life squad group meetings.

The importance of pre-hospital care in the t-PA pilot study is indicated in Tables 1–3. To be evaluated and treated within 90 min usually meant patient arrival had to be within 30–40 min. These patients were more likely to call 911, and the life squad personnel were more likely to be the first persons aware of the study.

Table 1. Time from stroke onset to hospital presentation[a]

Hours	n	%
0–1.5	401	27
1.5–4.0	268	18
4–12	287	19
12–24	160	11
Unknown	394	26

[a] Obtained from a prospective analysis of 1510 stroke patients screened for possible entry into the NIH pilot trial of tPA.

Table 2. First medical contact[a]

	n	%
Pre-hospital care (e.g., 911)	615	41
Hospital ED	600	40
Personal physician	173	11
Other	116	8

[a] Obtained from a prospective analysis of 1504 stroke patients screened within 24 h of symptom onset for possible entry into the NIH pilot trial of tPA.

Table 3. Person first aware of tPA stroke study[a]

	n	%
Pre-hospital care	300	20
Hospital ED	943	63
Personal physician	177	12
Other	89	5

[a] Obtained from a prospective analysis of 1509 stroke patients screened within 24 h of symptom onset for possible entry into the NIH pilot trial of tPA.

Parallel Processing in the Hospital

The NIH pilot t-PA trial was not designed to temporally dissect the in-hospital evaluation and treatment of patients with acute ischemic stroke, and so the precise time requirements of the various evaluations have not been measured. Obvious bottle-necks were delays for completion of laboratory studies, delays in completion of the pre-treatment CT scan, and delays in preparation of the study drug. Nonetheless, the average patient-arrival to patient-treatment time has been 52 min [2]. Cellular telephone communications with parallel processing have played an important role. For example, an investigator would be informed of a potential patient through a page from the Emergency Department and would respond immediately by conventional telephone, or, if hiking or bicycling, etc., could in most instances respond immediately via a transportable cellular telephone. The initial return call could be brief but still activate CT and laboratory evaluation as well as initial preparations in the pharmacy. Subsequent calls could then follow, assuring that each of the necessary steps was being accomplished simultaneously. By the time of the investigator's arrival at the Emergency Department or CT scanner, more time would then be available for neurological examination and discussion of the study with the patient and family.

Additional time-saving has been accomplished by initiating treatment in the CT scanner, before transporting the patient back to the Emergency Department or to the patient's assigned in-hospital unit. Further time-saving could be accomplished if completion of hematological laboratory studies were not required prior to treatment (e.g., prothrombin time, partial thromboplastin time). Completion of these studies is neither required nor recommended prior to thrombolytic therapy for myocardial infarction [11]. In the NIH pilot trial, not a single patient was excluded because of an abnormal hematological laboratory result.

The Discipline of Time

Since 1983 we have recruited patients into emergency stroke therapy protocols with successively more demanding entry deadlines – 48 h, 24 h, 6 h, 3 h, and 90 min – using a trauma style approach. Patient entry has not had a biological pattern, but rather has clustered at the "last minute" as physicians, nurses, and technicians rush to beat the particular entry deadline. For example, in the 90-min study (t-PA), 56 (73%) of the 74 patients were treated between 85 and 90 min from symptom onset. The capacity for exceptional speed on the part of hospital personnel was obvious in that study. In the other studies, patients arriving early to the hospital too often had their evaluations carried out in a nonurgent fashion as the 6 h (or later) entry deadline did not enforce a discipline of time – until the last minutes. We suggest that stroke therapy entry deadlines beyond 3 h may slow the in-hospital evaluation and treatment of patients arriving very early to the hospital (i.e., within 30–60 min).

Conclusions

Ultra-early stroke patient evaluation and treatment has been accomplished but only in small numbers. To improve early recruitment, greater efforts must be made in public education, pre-hospital care, and in-hospital emergency evaluation and treatment. Success in these areas was achieved for the care of acute trauma in the 1980s, and is precedent that real progress can be made for emergency stroke therapy in the 1990s.

References

1. Albert MJ, Bertels C, Dawson DV (1990) An analysis of time of presentation after stroke. JAMA 263:65–68
2. Barsan WG, Brott TG, Olinger CP (1989) Early treatment for acute ischemic stroke. Ann Intern Med 111:449–450
3. Brott TG, Haley EC, Levy D, Barsan W, Sheppard G, Broderick J, Reed R, Marler J (1990) Safety and potential efficacy of tissue plasminogen activator (t-PA) for stroke. Stroke 21:181 (abstract)
4. Capildeo R, Haberman S, Rose FC (1982) Stroke trials: the facts. In: Rose FC (ed) Advances in stroke therapy. Raven, New York
5. Cwinn AA, Pons AT, Moore EE, Mary JA, Honigman B, Dinerman N (1987) Prehospital advanced trauma life support for critical blunt trauma victims. Ann Emerg Med 16:399–402
6. Gelmers HJ, Gorter K, DeWeerdt CJ, Wiezer HJA (1988) A controlled trial of nimodipine in acute ischemic stroke. N Engl J Med 318:203–207
7. Grotta JC (1987) Current medical and surgical therapy for cerebrovascular disease. N Engl J Med 317:1505–1516

8. Hsu CY, Faught RE Jr, Furlan AJ, Coull BM, Huang DC, Hogan EL, Linet OI, Yatsu
   FM (1987) Intravenous prostacyclin in acute nonhemorrhagic stroke: a placebo-
   controlled double-blind trial. Stroke 18:352–358
9. Jones TH, Moraweta RB, Crowell RM, Maccoux FW, Fitzgibbon SJ, DeGirolami V,
   Ojemann RG (1981) Threshholds of focal cerebral ischemia in awake monkeys. J
   Neurosurg 54:773–782
10. O'Rourke MF, Ballantyne K, Thompson PL (1989) Community aspects of coronary
    thrombolysis: public education and cost effectiveness. In: Julian D, Kubler W, Norris
    RM, Swan HJC, Collen D, Verstraete M (eds) Thrombolysis in cardiovascular disease.
    Dekker, New York, pp 309–324
11. Sane DC, Califf RM, Topol EJ, Stump DC, Mark DB, Greenberg CS (1989) Bleeding
    during thrombolytic therapy for acute myocardial infarction: mechanisms and man-
    agement. Ann Intern Med 111:1010–1022
12. Saunders CE (1987) Time study of patient movement through the emergency depart-
    ment: sources of delay in relation to patient acuity. Ann Emerg Med 16:1244–1248
13. Timerding BL, Barsan WG, Hedges JR, Brott TG, Vanligten PJ, Spiluer JA, Olinger
    CP (1989) Stroke patient evaluation in the emergency department before pharma-
    cologic therapy. Am J Emerg Med 7:11–15
14. tPA Acute Stroke Study Group (1990) An open multicenter study of the safety and
    efficacy of various doses of tPA in patients with acute stroke: a progress report. Stroke
    21:181 (abstract)

V. Open Communications

Topical Intraarterial Urokinase Infusion for Acute Stroke

K. Matsumoto and K. Satoh

Cerebrovascular accidents are a common disease and the third leading cause of death in Japan. In 1986 we began topical intraarterial urokinase (UK) infusion therapy for cases of acute major stroke [2–4] and have now administered it to 50 patients, 27 males and 23 females, ranging in age from 44 to 85 years [1–4]. Obstructive lesions were located in the internal carotid artery (ICA) in 19 cases, the middle cerebral artery (MCA) in 20 cases, the posterior cerebral artery (PCA) in 1 case, and the basilar artery (BA) in 10 cases.

Indication and Method

The indication for UK therapy was defined as acute ischemic cerebral stroke within 24 h after onset of symptoms, absence of a low-density area in high-resolution computed tomography (CT), and obstruction of the major or principal cerebral artery demonstrated by diagnostic angiography with the lesion thought to be the cause of clinical symptoms. Subsequent to diagnostic angiography, UK solution (240 000 IU in 20 ml) was infused through the angiographic catheter for 10 min to a site proximal to the obstruction. Infusion of the UK solution was repeated with intermittent angiography according to the patient's condition. The maximal total dose of UK was limited to 1 200 000 IU. Motor symptoms were evaluated with a manual muscle testing scale [1]: normal strength (5/5), movement against resistance with reduced strength (4/5), movement against gravity but not resistance (3/5), joint movement but not against gravity (2/5), visible contraction but no joint motion (1/5), and no visible contraction (0/5). The 2-month outcome was assessed using five grades: complete recovery with no deficit (excellent), satisfactory recovery with minor deficits (good), improvement with major deficits in daily living activity (fair), a vegetative state or confined to bed (poor), and dead.

Department of Neurological Surgery, School of Medicine, University of Tokushima, 2-chome, Kuramoto-Cho, Tokushima 770, Japan.

Hacke et al (Eds)
Thrombolytic Therapy in Acute Ischemic Stroke
© Springer-Verlag Berlin Heidelberg 1991

Table 1. Summary of cases (ICA and MCA occlusion)

Case	Age (years)	Sex	Cons.	Motor symptom	Operation timing (h)	AF (ECG)	Site of occlusion	UK dosis (x10⁴ IU)	Recan.	HI	Outcome (2 months)
1	77	M	C	L 1/5	4.00	+	IC-S	120	+	–	Excellent
2	78	M	C	L 1/5	2.00	+	IC-S	72	+	–	Excellent
3	70	F	A	L 3/5	5.00	–	IC-C	24	+	–	Good
4	59	M	B	L 3/5	8.00	–	IC-S	24	–	–	Good
5	62	M	C	R 1/5	1.50	+	IC-C	96	+	+	Fair
6	62	F	B	R 3/5	4.00	+	IC-P	72	+	+	Fair
7	76	F	C	L 0/5	4.00	–	IC-C	84	+	+	Fair
8	68	F	C	R 1/5	8.00	–	IC-S	48	–	–	Fair
9	57	F	B	R 1/5	4.00	–	IC-C	24	–	–	Fair
10	46	F	C	R 2/5	4.20	+	IC-S	48	–	–	Fair
11	82	F	C	L 0/5	4.00	–	IC-S	24	–	+	Poor
12	85	F	C	L 0/5	8.00	+	IC-C	48	+	–	Poor
13	71	M	C	L 0/5	5.00	+	IC-P	48	+	+	Poor
14	73	F	C	L 0/5	15.00	+	IC-S	96	–	–	Dead
15	61	F	C	R 0/5	15.00	+	IC-S	48	–	–	Dead
16	73	M	C		5.00	–	IC-C	72	+	–	Dead
17	79	M	C		5.00	+	IC-S	72	–	–	Dead
18	70	M	C	R 1/5	10.00	+	IC-S	72	–	++	Dead
19	71	F	C	R 1/5	3.00	+	IC-S	72	+	–	Dead
20	72	F	C	L 1/5	4.00	+	M1-D	72	++	–	Excellent
21	72	M	A	R 3/5	12.00	–	M1-P	48	–	–	Excellent
22	70	M	A	R 3/5	1.00	–	M2	18	++	–	Excellent

No.	Age	Sex	Cons.	Motor			Site				Outcome
23	62	M	A	L 3/5	24.00	−	M1-P	72	++	−	Excellent
24	50	F	B	L 2/5	2.00	+	M1-P	72	++	++[a]	Good
25	66	M	A	R 0/5	13.00	−	M1-P	48	++	−	Fair
26	67	F	C	R 1/5	6.00	+	M1-D	72	−	+	Fair
27	54	M	C	R 0/5	5.00	+	M2	72	++	−	Fair
28	78	F	C	R 0/5	8.00	−	M1-P	48	++	+	Fair
29	58	M	B	L 2/5	8.00	−	M1-P	48	−	−	Fair
30	73	M	B	R 1/5	4.00	−	M1-P	84	−	−	Fair
31	65	F	C	L 1/5	6.00	−	M1-P	36	++	++	Fair
32	70	M	C	L 3/5	0.00	+	M1-P	72	++	+	Poor
33	80	F	C	R 1/5	3.00	−	M1-P	84	+	−	Poor
34	72	M	B	R 1/5	9.00	−	M1-D	72	++	−	Poor
35	69	M	C	L 1/5	10.00	++	M1-D	24	++	++[a]	Poor
36	76	F	C	L 1/5	5.00	+	M1-D	96	−	+	Dead
37	82	F	C	R 0/5	3.00	−	M1-D	120	−	−	Dead
38	65	F	C	R 0/5	5.00	+	M1-D	96	−	−	Dead
39	76	M	D	L 1/5	3.20	+	M1-D	90	−	−	Dead
40	65	M	B		4.00	+	PCA	24	+	−	Good

M, male; *F*, female; Cons.: level of consciousness: *A*, alert; *B*, lethargic; *C*, drowsy; *D*, semicoma; Motor symptom: *L*, Left; *R*, right hemiparesis (manual muscle testing); *AF*, atrial fibrillation; *ECG*, electrocardiogram; Site of occlusion (lower limit); *IC-C*, internal carotid artery (cervical portion); *IC-P*, internal carotid artery (petrous portion); *IC-S*, internal carotid artery (siphon); *M1-P*, proximal middle cerebral artery (M1); *M1-D*, distal middle cerebral artery (M1); *M2*, middle cerebral artery (M2); *PCA*, posterior cerebral artery; *UK*, urokinase; Recan., recanalization: −, none; +, partial; ++, complete; *HI*, hemorrhagic infarction: +, mild, ++, massive; Outcome: *Excellent*, complete recovery without deficit; *Good*, satisfactory recovery with minor deficit; *Fair*, improvement with major deficit; *Poor*, confined to bed vegetative.
[a] Preoperative anticoagulant medication.

Table 2. Summary of cases (BA occlusion)

Case	Age (years)	Sex	Consciousness	Operation timing (h)	AF (ECG)	Site of occlusion	Collateral PICA→SCA (AICA)	Circulation PcomA	UK dosis ($\times 10^4$ IU)	Recanalization	HI	Outcome Early	Outcome 2 months
Sudden onset group													
41	44	M	Semicoma	4	+	Distal	Good	Fair	96	Partial bilateral SCA	–	Bilateral IIIrd nerve palsy ataxia	Good
42	74	M	Semicoma	3	+	Distal	Good	None	96	Partial L SCA, PCA	–	Weber syndrome	Fair
43	57	M	Semicoma	5	+	Distal	Good	Fair	36	–	–	Locked-in syndrome	Poor
44	61	M	Semicoma	4	–	Middle	Good	Unknown	24	–	–	Brain death (day 4)	Dead (day 21)
45	76	F	Semicoma	4	+	Distal	Good	Fair	72	Partial R SCA, PCA L SCA	+ L thalamus	Weber syndrome	dead (day 10 MI)
Progressive stroke group													
46	67	M	Lethargic	6	–	Proximal	Good	Good	72	–	–	R hemiparesis ataxia	Good
47	69	M	Drowsy	6	+	Distal	Good	Fair	72	–	–	Weber syndrome	Good
48	72	M	Semicoma	10	–	Proximal	None	Fair	48	Partial BA	–	R hemiparesis	Good
49	58	M	Lethargic	24	–	Proximal	Good	Fair	24	–	–	R hemiparesis dysarthria	Fair
50	63	F	Drowsy	13	+	Middle	Good	Unknown	72	–	–	Brain death (day 2)	Dead (day 4)

BA, basilar artery; *AF*, atrial fibrillation; *ECG*, electrocardiogram; *PICA*, posterior inferior cerebellar artery; *SCA*, superior cerebellar artery; *AICA*, anterior inferior cerebellar artery; *PcomA*, posterior communicating artery; *UK*, urokinase; *PCA*, posterior cerebral artery; *R*, right; *L*, left; *HI*, hemorrhagic infarction; *MI*, myocardial infarction.

Results (Tables 1 and 2)

With ICA occlusion there were no cases of complete recanalization immediately after UK infusion. Although partial recanalization was noted in 10 of 19 cases, marked neurological improvement was only seen in 3 cases (cases 1, 2, 5). Atrial fibrillation was noted in 12 cases. The 2-month outcome was excellent in 2 cases, good in 2, fair in 6, poor in 3, and dead in 6. In the 20 cases of MCA occlusion, complete recanalization was seen in 12 cases. Atrial fibrillation was noted in eight cases. The 2-month outcome was excellent in four cases, good in one, fair in seven, poor in four, and dead in four. The cases of BA occlusion were divided into two groups: sudden onset and progressive stroke groups. Sudden onset cases deteriorated suddenly to a semicoma at the time of onset, and all but one had atrial fibrillation before the attack. Although there were no cases of complete recanalization immediately after UK infusion, four cases had partial recanalization and showed dramatic recovery from a life-threatening state to alertness within a few days. The 2-month outcome was good in four cases, fair in two, poor in one, and death in three.

Discussion

Recanalization was noted in 28 patients and marked neurological improvement in 10 patients, 2 in ICA, 4 in MCA, and 4 in BA occlusion. Of these, 8 patients had infusion therapy within 4 h after onset of symptoms. Early timing of the UK infusion seems to be one of the important factors necessary to obtain an excellent outcome.

Summary

Topical intraarterial UK infusion therapy may be first choice for the treatment for acute stroke with embolic occlusion of the major cerebral arteries. However, it is our impression that patients undergoing anticoagulant therapy should be carefully treated and some adjunctive intraarterial manipulations, for instance piercing of plug thrombus, would also be necessary to promote thrombolysis and to reduce the dosis of urokinase in selected patients.

References

1. Daniels L (1956) Muscle testing technique of manual examination. Saunders, Philadelphia
2. del Zoppo GJ, Zeumer H, Harker LA (1986) Thrombolytic therapy in stroke. Possibilities and hazards. Stroke 17:595–607
3. Mori E, Tabuchi M, Yoshida T, Yamadori A (1988) Intracarotid urokinase with thromboembolic occlusion of the middle cerebral artery. Stroke 19:802–812
4. Zeumer H, Freitag HJ, Grzyska U, Neunzig HP (1989) Local intraarterial fibrinolysis in acute vertebrobasilar occlusion. Neuroradiololgy 31:336–340

Local Thrombolytic Therapy in Acute Basilar Artery Occlusion: Experience with 18 Patients

E. Möbius[1], E. Berg-Dammer[1], D. Kühne[2], and H.C. Nahser[2]

Since the introduction of local thrombolytic therapy (LTT) in acute ischemia by Zeumer and colleagues in 1982 [3], it has been possible to rescue patients with basilar artery occlusion and progressive brain stem damage and to limit their neurological deficiencies [1, 2]. We have treated 18 patients with local intraarterial lysis who suffered from basilar artery occlusions at various sites (Fig. 1). LTT was used because the following prerequisites were fulfilled. Clinically the patients presented with progressive strokes in the vertebro-basilar territory. Digital subtraction angiography showed either an occlusion of the basilar artery or of both intracranial vertebral arteries and there were no contraindications of LTT, such as sustained coma or coma with lack of brain stem reflexes or major brain stem lesions. A microcatheter was positioned close to the occlusion, whenever possible, between the thrombus and arterial wall. Then fibrinolysis was instituted with continuous administration of streptokinase or urokinase through a perfusion system. The given range was 120 000–600 000 U streptokinase or 300 000–950 000 U urokinase within 2 h. Angiographic checks were made every ½ h. If then sufficient recanalization had been achieved, treatment was stopped and intravenous anticoagulation with heparin was started. If no reopening resulted within 2 h, the lysis therapy was terminated.

One patient is reported, to demonstrate that LTT may be a lifesaving method even in vertebral artery dissection and subsequent occlusion of the basilar artery.

Case Report

An obese, but otherwise healthy, 30-year-old woman experienced sudden loss of consciousness and left hemiplegia in her 3rd month of pregnancy. On arrival after a 4-h period of coma, the patient presented with ocular bobbing and decerebrate posturing. A CT scan showed no evidence of an ischemic or hemorrhagic brain stem lesion. The angiography revealed presumptive

[1] Neurologische Klinik und
[2] Neuroradiologische Abteilung des Alfried-Krupp-von-Bohlen-und-Halbach-Krankenhauses, Alfried-Krupp-Str. 21, W-4300 Essen 1, FRG.

Hacke et al (Eds)
Thrombolytic Therapy in Acute Ischemic Stroke
© Springer-Verlag Berlin Heidelberg 1991

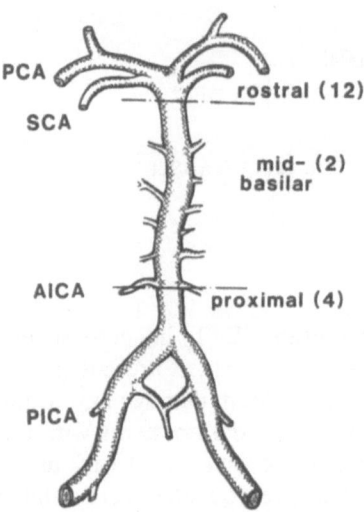

Fig. 1. Location of thromboembolic occlusions in the basilar artery in our patients. The number of patients is given in *parentheses*. *PCA*, posterior cerebral artery; *SCA*, superior cerebellar artery; *AICA*, anterior inferior cerebellar artery; *PICA*, posterior inferior cerebellar artery

spontaneous bilateral vertebral artery dissection. There was an elongated and irregular tapered 90% stenosis of the right vertebral artery and a thrombotic occlusion of the left vertebral artery in its midcervical segment. The mid portion of the basilar artery was occluded. Bilateral carotid angiograms were normal and showed no collateral circulation to the vertebrobasilar system via the posterior communicating arteries. Because of the life-threatening situation LTT was started despite the pregnancy. A microcatheter was positioned in the midbasilar thrombus and a 5-French catheter was placed close to the thrombus of the left vertebral artery. Thrombolytic therapy was given through both catheters, 500 000 U urokinase administered via the microcatheter, and 350 000 U urokinase administered via the 5-French catheter. After 1 h complete recanalization of the basilar artery was achieved but the left vertebral artery remained occluded. Then the fibrinolysis was stopped. Neurological examination the following day revealed a complete locked-in syndrome which gradually resolved during the anticoagulation with heparin. Upon hospital discharge after 3 months, the patient had a normal mental state, saccadic eye movements on smooth pursuit, moderate dysarthria, and discoordination of the upper limbs. Despite residual mild tetraparesis and slight gait ataxia the patient is able to walk with sticks. She recently delivered a healthy boy.

Our results are summarized in Table 1. The fact that all the patients in whom recanalization was not obtained died supports our belief that LTT is the treatment of choice in basilar artery occlusions combined with progressive

Table 1. Local thrombolytic therapy results

Total	18 patients
Recanalization (14)	1 complete recovery 5 minor deficits 4 moderate deficits 2 major deficits
No recanalization (4)	4 deaths

brain stem damage. In our experience rapid institution of high-dose LTT applied via microcatheters is essential for a successful outcome, and there have been no hemorrhagic complications in our patients.

References

1. Hacke W, Zeumer H, Ferbert A, Brückmann H, del Zoppo GJ (1988) Intraarterial fibrinolytic therapy improves outcome in patients with acute vertebrobasilar occlusive disease. Stroke 19:1216–1222
2. Möbius E, Berg-Dammer E, Kühne D, Kunitsch G, Nahser HC (1989) Lokale intraarterielle Fibrinolyse bei A. basilaris-Verschluß mit progredientem Hirnstamminfarkt. Akt Neurol 16:184–190
3. Zeumer H, Hacke W, Kolmann HL, Poeck K (1982) Lokale Fibrinolysetherapie bei Basilaris-Thrombose. Dtsch Med Wochenschr 107:728–731

Vertebrobasilar Occlusion: Outcome With and Without Local Intraarterial Fibrinolysis

G. Pfeiffer[1], G. Thayssen[1], A. Arlt[1], G. Siepmann[2], H. Zeumer, and K. Kunze[2]

Introduction

Previous studies have shown that about half of the patients treated with local intraarterial fibrinolysis (LIF) after vertebrobasilar occlusion survived without severe deficits [2, 3, 5, 6]. In one series, however, all patients had poor outcomes [4]. There may be subgroups of patients who do not benefit from LIF. We retrospectively analyzed 20 cases to delineate these subgroups. This might lead to more realistic expectations concerning LIF and to improved therapy studies.

Patients and Methods

Since 1987, 20 patients with acute progressing brain stem symptoms and vertebrobasilar occlusion demonstrated by early angiography have been treated in the Neurological Department. Sixteen patients received LIF (for protocol see [7]). Cases with suspected embolism and those with suspected local atherothrombosis were evaluated separately. An embolic occlusion was suspected if it could be bypassed with the microcatheter [7]. This was usually confirmed by the angiographic finding of smooth vessel walls after LIF. Clinical data were used for the classification of pathogenesis, if the angiographic criteria were insufficient after unsuccessful revascularization or impossible local microcatheter investigation. Outcome was evaluated after 6 months.

[1] Department of Neuroradiology and
[2] Department of Neurology, Univerity of Hamburg, Martinistr. 52, W-2000 Hamburg 20, FRG.

Hacke et al. (Eds.)
Thrombolytic Therapy in Acute Ischemic Stroke
© Springer-Verlag Berlin Heidelberg 1991

Results

All patients with embolic occlusion (upper part of Table 1) who were not tetraplegic or comatose at the time of LIF did well in contrast to patients who already had severe deficits. The clinical deficits at the time of LIF were an all or nothing indicator of outcome and prognostically superior to the timespan between onset of symptoms or deterioration and LIF. All patients with suspected artery-to-artery embolism ("Art. " in Table 1) had a poor outcome. However, all had severe deficits before LIF was begun. Recurrent embolism is threatening in these patients. Patient Wi (Table 1) improved after LIF but died unexpectedly 1 month later, 2 weeks after full-dose heparin had been gradually reduced. Angiography had suggested embolism from vertebral artery dissection in this patient, and a second artery-to-artery embolism might have been the cause of death.

Minor deficits at the time of LIF were a predictor for a favorable outcome after atherosclerotic thrombotic occlusion ("ath." in Table 1) with some notable exceptions. Deterioration from minor to severe deficits due to downstream embolism occurred in two patients after LIF and in one patient during LIF (patient Gl, Table 1). Patient Gl complained of dizziness and diplopia during the preceding weeks. Overnight he developed dysphagia and dysarthria. On angiography he had bilateral vertebral artery occlusion. During LIF he suddenly became comatose, and embolism to the top of the basilar artery was visualized by angiography. He never recovered from severe brain stem dysfunction. Prognosis was better if local thrombosis was caused by hypercoagulation (patient Bi, Table 1) or low flow (patient So, Table 1). Patient So is a young man who developed anarthria within hours after continued head retroflection when painting a ceiling. Revascularization of the occluded basilar artery was achieved 18 h after onset of stroke. He was tetraplegic and somnolent for 3 weeks, but after 6 months he was ambulatory and continued his studies 1 year later handicapped by moderate spastic tetraparesis. Four patients with atherothrombotic occlusion were not treated with LIF (lower part of Table 1). Good collateralization was demonstrated in those two patients who survived with minor deficits without LIF.

The deficit at the time of LIF (minor versus tetraplegic or comatose) was the only significant predictor of outcome after 6 months (minor deficits versus locked-in or dead; Fisher's exact test; $p = 0.02$). Age (below or above 60 years; $p = 0.51$) and time since onset of symptoms or deterioration (less or more than 10 h; $p = 0.51$) did not predict outcome. Fourteen patients received CT scans 1–10 days after LIF. All patients had infarctions within the vertebrobasilar territory, which were hemorrhagic in four cases. In only one case was the clinical course influenced by this hemorrhage (patient Mö), which involved the fourth ventricle. Massive bleeding did not occur.

Table 1. Results of LIF in verbebrobasilar occlusion

Patient	Preexisting disease	Prodromes	Vertebral artery	Basilar artery	Pathogenesis	LIF data	CT after LIF	Outcome
Kl 72 M	[a]	–		M. oc.	Car.	5 m +	I	+
Me 61 M	[b] CI	–		D. oc.	Car.	5 m +	I he.	+
Be 57 M	D, HT	Left HP	Right oc.	D. oc.	Art.	5 t (+)	?	–
Ma 64 M			Right oc.	D. oc.	Art.	8 t +	I	–
Mö 68 M		–	Right oc.	Oc.	Art.	13 t +	I he.	–
Sc 46 F	[c]	–		D. oc.	Art.	18 t +	I[a]	–
Wi 52 F	HT	DI	Left dissection	M. oc.	Art.	4 c +	I he.[a]	–
Bi 45 M		–	Right stenosis	Oc.	[c] ath.[d]	4 m (+)	(I)	+
So 27 M		–	Left oc.	Oc.		12 m +	I	+
Br 53 M	CI	DI, amnesia	Left hypoplast. PICA +	Oc.	Ath.	6 c +	I	–
Gl 63 M		DV DI	Right oc. PICA +	Oc.	Ath.	5 m +	?	–
He 66 F	HT	Syncope, Left HP	Left oc. Right thrombi	Coll. (CA)	Ath.	10 m (+)	I he.	–
Ob 61 M	MI	DI	Right oc. Left oc. PICA +	Coll. (PICA) P. oc.	Ath.	28 c –	I[e]	–
Oe 42 M	D	DI	Right oc. Left oc. PICA +	Coll. (CA) P. oc. Coll. (PICA) P. oc.	Ath.	48 t +	I	–

Patient	Preexisting disease	Prodromes	Angiography		Pathogenesis	LIF data			CT	Outcome
Tu 56 M	D, HT, MI	DI		P. oc.	Ath.	8 m (+)				–
Zu 70 M	MI	DI		Oc.	Ath.	8 t (+)				–
Sc 50 M	HT	DI, DA		Oc. / Coll. (PICA)	Ath.					+
We 54 F	HT, CI	Right HP, DA	Left oc. / Right oc. coll.	Stenosis	Ath.					+
Bi 68 F	TIAs	Anakusis DI	Left oc. / Right oc.	Oc. / Coll. (PICA)	Ath.					–
Ju 56 M	MI, CI	DI, DV	Right missing / Left oc.	Oc.	Ath.					–

Patient data (columns 1–3): patient, age (years), sex (male/female)

Preexisting disease (column 4): MI, myocardial infarction; CI cerebral infarction; D, diabetes; HT, hypertension

[a] atrial fibrillation; [b] aortic valve surgery; [c] surgical revascularization of occluded subclavian artery

Prodromes (column 5): DA, dysarthria; DI, dizziness; DV, double vision; HP, hemiparesis

Angiography (columns 6–7): oc., occluded; PICA +, occluded distal of posterior inferior cerebellar artery coll., collateralized, (CA), collateralized, via carotid artery; M, middle; D., distal; P., proximal

Pathogenesis (column 8): embolic (upper part): car., cardiac origin; art., artery origin; local thrombosis (middle and lower part): ath., atherothrombosis

[c] hypercoagulation after epistaxis; [d] low flow

LIF data (columns 9–11): hours between onset or deterioration and LIF (column 8); clinical state at LIF (m, minor deficits; c, coma; t, tetraplegia); success (+, revascularization; (+), partial; –, no revascularization)

CT after LIF (column 12):

[e] infarction already at LIF

I, infarction; he, hemorrhagic I

Outcome (Column 13): +, better than dead or locked in

Discussion

Revascularization was successful in all but two patients. This rate of success seems to favor local over systemic fibrinolysis (see other authors in this volume). A second advantage of LIF is the low rate of hemorrhage. In spite of successful revascularization, only 25% of our patients had a good outcome, which is low compared with previous studies [2, 3, 5, 6]. Patients with atherothrombosis are overrepresented in our series. They have an increased risk of reocclusion and downstream embolism during revascularization, which was the most dramatic complication in our series. Therefore, the prognosis of patients with atherothrombotic occlusion is doubtful even after successful LIF. Some of these patients had a good prognosis without LIF [7]. If collateralization of an atherothrombotic occlusion is demonstrated, conservative therapy with heparin might be preferable to LIF. The outcome of our patients might have been better if embolic occlusion had been as frequent as in previous series [5], and if the time limit of LIF had been observed more closely. However, our analysis shows that even older patients or patients with late LIF have a chance to recover if brain stem function is not severely impaired at the time of LIF. Because of its low rate of hemorrhagic complications, LIF may still be considered as the ultimate last hope if early treatment cannot be achieved or if coma or tetraplegia have already occurred. Future therapy studies, however, should account for the pathogenesis of vertebrobasilar occlusion and the severity of neurological deficits at the time of LIF as the most relevant prognostic factors.

References

1. Bogousslavsky J, Gates PC, Fox AJ, Barnett HJM (1986) Bilateral occlusion of vertebral artery. Neurology 36:1309–1315
2. Courtheaux J, Theon J, Derlon JM, Alakchar F, Casasco A (1986) In situ fibrinolysis in supra-aortic main vessels. J Neuroradiology 13:111–124
3. Hacke W, Zeumer H, Ferbert A, Brückmann H, del Zoppo GJ (1988) Intra-arterial thrombolytic therapy improves outcome in patients with acute vertebrobasilar occlusive disease. Stroke 19:1216–1222
4. Kollikowski H, Ewert T, Lehman HJ, Scharafinski HW, Schulz M (1986) Intraarterial local fibrinolysis of basilar artery thrombosis in elderly patients. Akt Neurol 13:201–206
5. Möbius E, Berg-Dammer E, Kühne D, Kunitsch G, Nahser HC (1989) Local intra-arterial fibrinolysis in acute basilar occlusion with progressive brainstem damage. Akt Neurol 16:184–190
6. Zeumer H (1985) Vascular recanalization techniques in interventional neuroradiology. J Neurol 231:287–294
7. Zeumer H, Freitag H-J, Grzyska U, Neunzig H-P (1989) Local intraarterial fibrinolysis in acute vertebrobasilar occlusion. Neuroradiology 31:336–340

Recanalization of Acute Middle Cerebral Artery Occlusion Monitored by Transcranial Doppler Sonography

R. Biniek, E.B. Ringelstein, H. Brückmann, G. Leonhardt, B. Ammeling, and P. Nolte

Between June 1988 and February 1990 we examined 44 patients who had suffered acute stroke due to an acute occlusion of the middle cerebral artery (MCA). Only patients who could be investigated within 24 h of the onset of stroke were included. All patients were examined by transcranial Doppler sonography (TCD) at fixed intervals six times during the first 24 h after stroke, and then on days 2, 3, 10, and 17. A simultaneous neurological examination was also carried out each time. Angiography was performed in 24 patients during the first 2 h after admission to the hospital.

Thus, 24 men with an average age of 59 years and 20 women (55 years) were examined. Of these patients, 15 were treated with recombinant tissue plasminogen activator (rt-PA) [1, 2]. The remaining 29 were either admitted 8 h after the stroke, or had other contraindications which prohibited rt-PA treatment, and most received full heparinization. From the initial neurological assessment on admission we calculated a modified neurological score ranging from 15 for a person without neurological deficit to 0 for death. The average scores on admission were 7.13 for rt-PA patients and 6.24 for the spontaneous course patients, indicating that the spontaneous course group contained more severely impaired patients.

Figure 1 shows the TCD course of a 52-year-old man who was admitted with global aphasia and right side hemiplegia. Lysis was not performed on account of contraindications and full heparinization was started. Sonography of the extracranial arteries revealed an occlusion of the internal carotid artery, so that arterioarterial embolism could be assumed. The graph presents the complete TCD findings for the 17 days. The x-axis shows the depth of examination, on the left side the normal right MCA and on the right side the affected left MCA. The y-axis plots the mean TCD velocities, and the z-axis the examination times. Partial recanalization started between 18 and 26 h after stroke and full recanalization within 50–74.. One phenomenon frequently observed in our patients is hyperperfusion after recanalization, which can be seen between days 3 and 10. The results from day 17 are not visible in this graph since they are hidden by the hyperperfusion on day 10.

Department of Neurology, RWTH Aachen, Pauwelsstr., W-5100 Aachen, FRG.

Hacke et al. (Eds)
Thrombolytic Therapy in Acute Ischemic Stroke
© Springer-Verlag Berlin Heidelberg 1991

222 R. Biniek et al.

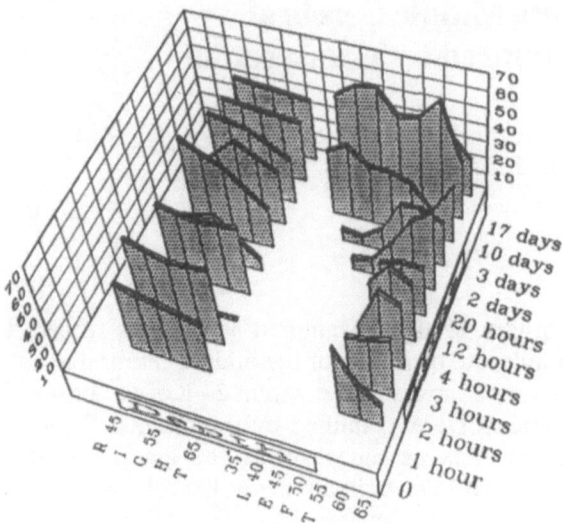

Fig. 1. Transcranial Doppler sonography course of a patient with acute occlusion of the MCA

Irrespective of the therapy, we have tried to examine the recanalization time by means of TCD and the size and number of computed tomography (CT) lesions. We have therefore calculated a simple score for the MCA territory ranging from 4 for a complete lesion of the full territory to 1 for only 1 lesion in one of the anterior, middle, posterior, or striatocapsular regions. A correlation between the CT score and recanalization time could be demonstrated, indicating that an early recanalization time is associated with minor lesions in CT.

There were some striking differences when we examined the purely striatocapsular infarctions. Excluding the two patients with recanalization times of over 150 h and those patients without recanalization, all purely striatocapsular infarctions ($n = 7$) showed recanalized MCAs after 3.86 h. All other infarct patterns ($n = 25$) displayed a recanalization time of 20.6 h. It can thus be concluded that purely striatocapsular infarctions are in most cases associated with a rapid recanalization of the occluded MCA. One explanation of this phenomenon may be a partial supply of the MCA territory in the cortex by leptomeningeal anastomosis, which may supply this region for a certain period. Since the capsulostriatal region does not have such an anastomosis, an infarction occurs despite early recanalization.

Summing up, it can be said that monitoring of occluded MCAs by TCD is a reliable method, which can be performed even on a busy intensive care unit and in the angiography room while lysis is performed. With rapid reexaminations we are able to detect the time of recanalization. This information has not been available until now. Recanalization of occluded MCAs has occurred in most of our 44 patients, whereby 93% of rt-PA-treated and 76% of heparin-treated patients have shown a recanalization. A difference in the size and pattern of CT lesions can be seen in a comparison of patients with later recanalization. These findings indicate that the patients have benefited from early recanalization.

References

1. Ringelstein EB, Ley-Pozo J (1990) Transcranial Doppler sonography for the carotid siphon and middle cerebral artery. Ann Neurol 28:758–765
2. rt-PA Acute Stroke Study Group (1990) An open multicenter study of the safety and efficacy of various doses of t-PA in patients with acute stroke: A progress report. Stroke 21:181

Neuropathological Findings
After Thrombolytic Therapy in Acute Ischemic Stroke

P. PILZ, G. LADURNER, and E. GRIEBNITZ

Thrombolytic therapy (TT) in acute ischemic stroke is a rather experimental form of treatment. Therefore it is desirable to gain as much as possible information about every individual patient. One source of information in patients with acute ischemic stroke is a detailed autopsy study. Twenty-two patients were submitted for TT from 1985 to 1989. A quantity of 100 mg intravenous recombinant tissue plasminogen activator (rt-PA) was administered within 3 h, and only one patient received urokinase (case 1). Seventeen patients presented with basilar artery (BA) occlusion. A postmortem was performed in 10 of 11 patients who died and in 2 who died after middle cerebral artery (MCA) occlusion. The clinical and postmortem findings from these 12 patients are summarized in Table 1.

Discussion

Of the ten patients presenting with BA occlusion five had recanalization of the vessel at autopsy. Two had a favorable neurological outcome, but died of extracranial causes. The remaining three displayed extensive hemorrhagic infarcts, while in contrast only one patient of the "nonrecanalized group" showed hemorrhagic transformation. Definite diagnosis of embolic or thrombotic occlusion can be difficult even on autopsy. A serial section must be made to reveal the embolic or thrombotic core in an apposition thrombus. The types of arterial occlusion shown in Table 1 and Fig. 1 were determined from clinical and postmortem findings. In four patients classified as having definite embolism, signs of embolic disease were found in only two (left atrial thrombi, case 9; renal infarct, case 6). An intimal tear at the top of the BA was found in two cases. This could either represent the focus for a thrombotic occlusion, but more likely results from the impact of an embolus in these cases. This finding seems not to have been previously reported [1–3]. In some cases arterial clots displayed a striking deficiency of fibrin (cases 2, 4, 6).

Landesnervenklinik, Departments of Neurology and Neuropathology, Ignaz-Harrer-Str. 79, 5020 Salzburg, Austria

Hacke et al. (Eds.)
Thrombolytic Therapy in Acute Ischemic Stroke
© Springer-Verlag Berlin Heidelberg 1991

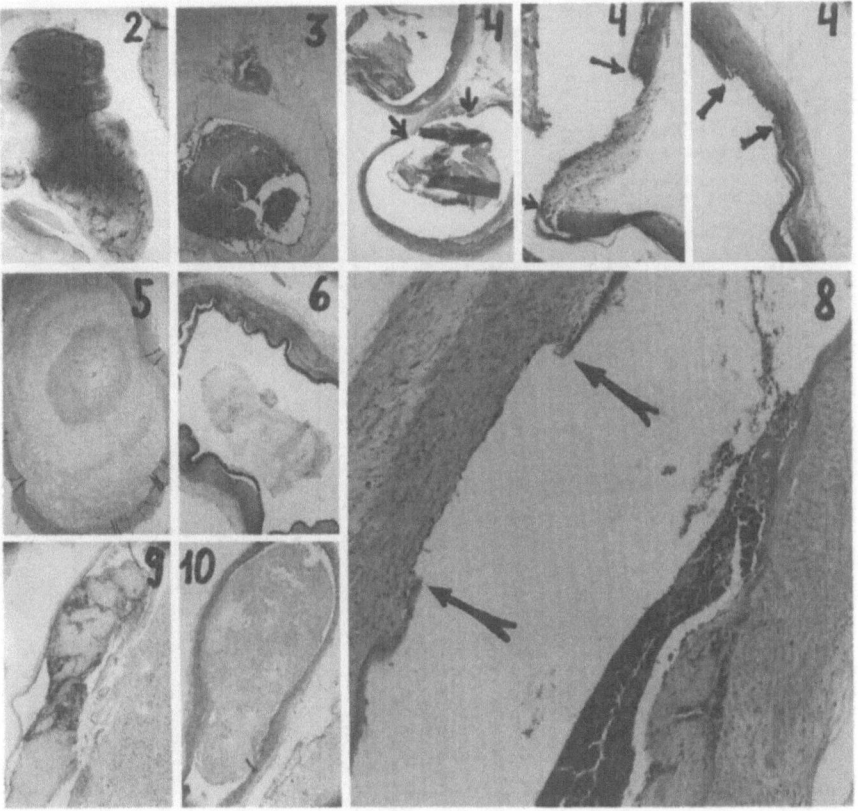

Fig. 1. *Numbers* correspond to the case numbers in Table 1 and the parts show the cerebral blood vessel pathological findings in Table 1. In addition: (*4*) BA top, embolic occlusion? intimal tear (*arrows*) followed in serial sections. (*8*) BA top, intimal tear (*arrows*), parietal thrombus and intimal hemorrhage on the opposite side

Detailed investigations on clot morphology of cerebral artery occlusion are lacking in the literature.

In the MCA group, the patient in case 11 displayed hemorrhagic transformation the 2nd day after TT associated with clinical deterioration, while the patient received heparin (thrombin time >100s). This infarct had been pale on the 1st day; the MCA was recanalized at autopsy. Case 12 is an example of myxomatous emboli detached from a cardiac myxoma nonsusceptible to TT. Hemorrhagic complications after TT occurred (gastrointestinal, one case; nasopharyngeal, one case; local hematoma at angiography site, four cases) but were never severe.

In conclusion recanalization occurred in half of the patients after TT who died, but in no case of definite atherothrombosis. Hemorrhagic infarcts predominantly were found in recanalized vascular territories. Intimal tears

Table 1. Clinical and postmortem findings in patients receiving thrombolytic therapy after acute ischemic stroke

Case No.	1	2	3	4	5	6	7	8	9	10	11	12
Occluded artery	Basilar artery										Middle cerebral artery	
Age (years)/sex	72 M	75 F	58 M	78 F	76 M	53 M	66 M	73 M	59 F	59 M	69 F	29 M
Onset	Progressive	Acute	Progressive	Acute	Progressive	Acute	Progressive	Progressive	Acute	Acute	Acute	Acute
Neurological findings	Diplopia hemiparesis convulsions	Tetraparesis	Prosis, tetraparesis, convulsions	Mydriasis, tetraparesis	Tetraparesis	Tetraparesis	Action myoclonus	Diplopia tetraparesis	Mydriasis, tetraparesis	Tetraparesis, convulsions	Hemiparesis	Hemiparesis
Duration of coma before TT	8 h	7 h	3 h	4 h	5 h	4 h	–	3 h	5 h	–	6 h	4 h
Angiography	Proximal BA occlusion	Proximal BA occlusion	TCD only	BA and distal VA	BA and distal VA	BA top occlusion	TCD only	TCD only	Distal BA occlusion	BA top occlusion	MCA trunk	TCD only
Survival time	5 days	12 h	5 days	1 day	20 days	8 days	33 days	4 days	3 days	1 day	9 days	16 h
Cause of death	High ICP	Cardiac arrest	High ICP	High ICP	Pneumonia	Cardiac failure	Septic shock	High ICP	High ICP	High ICP	Pneumonia	HIgh ICP
Nature of occlusion	Athero-thrombus	Embolus	Athero-thrombus	Embolus?	Athero-thrombus	Embolus	?	Embolus?	Embolus	Embolus	Embolus	Embolus[a]

Post mortem findings

	Basilar artery occluded					Basilar artery recanalized				Recanalized	Occluded	
Case No.	1	2	3	4	5	6	7	8	9	10	11	12
Infarcts	PCA bl, TH bl, CB bl, BST bl	BST, CB bl	BST, CB	TH (HT), BST (HT), CB	BST	BST (microscopic)	BST (microscopic)	PCA bl (HT), TH bl (HT), CB bl (HT), BST (HT)	PCA bl (HT), TH bl (HT), CB bl (HT)	CB (HT)	MCA (HT)	ACA bl, MCA
Cerebral blood vessel pathological findings	Severe atheroma of BA, plaque rupture thrombosis	Embolus, occlusion of BA top, low clot fibrin content	Severe atheroma of proximal BA, plaque, hemorrhage, thrombosis	Embolus occlusion? of distal BA, intimal tear, low fibrin content	Atheromatous occlusion of proximal BA	Moderate Atheromatous parietal thrombus, low fibrin cont	Moderate Atheromatous cartilage cells	intimal tear, parietal thrombous, digital BA, no atheroma	No Atheroma, fragmented embolus PCA and SCA	No Atheroma, fragmented Embolus PCA	No Atheroma recanalized	Myxomatous[a], emboli, cardiac myxoma

ACA, anterior cerebral artery; *BA,* basilar artery; *bl,* bilateral; *BST,* brain stem; *CB,* cerebellum; *HT,* hemorrhagic transformation; *ICP,* intracranial pressure; *MCA,* middle cerebral artery; *PCA,* posterior cerebral artery; *TCD,* transcranial Doppler; *TH,* thalamus.

can result from the impact of an embolus (hypothesis). Time course and extensive atheromas are critical factors determining outcome after TT. Severe complications contributing to death and unequivocally resulting from TT did not occur.

References

1. Camilleri JP, Berry CL, Fiessinger JN, Bariély J (eds) (1989) Diseases of the arterial wall. Springer, Berlin Heidelberg New York
2. Krauland W (1982) Verletzungen der intrakraniellen Schlagadern. Springer, Berlin Heidelberg New York
3. Stehbens WE (1972) Pathology of cerebral blood vessels. Mosby, St. Louis

How Many Stroke Patients Are Candidates for Thrombolysis?

M. KAPS, C.R. HORNIG, M. NÜCKEL, and I. SINGER

Thrombolytic therapy needs special skills as well as considerable effort concerning staff disposition and technical equipment. All these requirements must be available immediately, 24 h a day. The questions we have addressed are:

1. How many patients are generally candidates for therapeutic thrombolysis? (assuming clinical admission without delay after stroke)?
2. What is the clinical course of these patients without thrombolysis (with "conservative" therapy)?

Patients and Method

Two hundred consecutive patients suffering from acute stroke were analyzed retrospectively over a period of 1 year (March 1988 to March 1989). Exclusion criteria were applied according to the study protocols now generally accepted:

```
Age >75 years
Minor neurological deficit
Regressive symptoms
Lacunar syndromes
Recurrent stroke
Hypertension (>200/100 mmHg)
Others (gastic ulcer, surgery, urogenital
   bleeding, malignancy)
```

Neurological deficit was evaluated on admission and after 2 weeks of inpatient treatment, using a noncomplex and nonambiguous neurological scale focussing on patients' quality of life:

Department of Neurology, Justus-Liebig University, Am Steg 14, W-6300 Giessen, FRG.

Hacke et al. (Eds)
Thrombolytic Therapy in Acute Ischemic Stroke
© Springer-Verlag Berlin Heidelberg 1991

1 = no neurological deficit
2 = minimal deficit, normal daily activities
3 = mild deficit, restricted daily activities, needs no help
4 = moderate deficit, needs occasional help
5 = severe deficit, totally dependent
6 = death

The data obtained were analyzed using a flow diagram (Fig. 1) applying the different exclusion criteria in a stepwise mode.

Results

Of 200 stroke patients, 161 (80.5%) did not meet the requirements for thrombolytic therapy (Fig. 1). Age was the most common cause of exclusion. Since minor neurological deficits do not justify thrombolytic therapy at present, according to our protocol 35 patients had to be excluded for this reason. Of the patients less than 75 years of age, 22 stroke victims showed

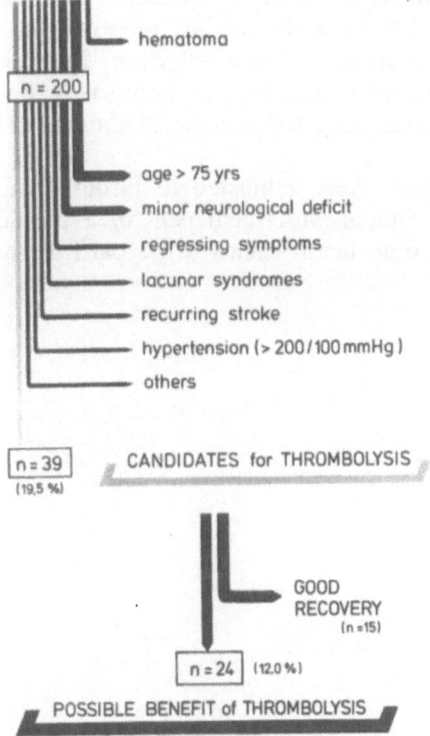

n = 200

hematoma

age > 75 yrs
minor neurological deficit
regressing symptoms
lacunar syndromes
recurring stroke
hypertension (> 200/100 mmHg)
others

n = 39
(19,5 %)   CANDIDATES for THROMBOLYSIS

GOOD
RECOVERY
(n = 15)

n = 24   (12,0 %)

POSSIBLE BENEFIT of THROMBOLYSIS

Fig. 1. Flow chart showing use of the exclusion criteria

lacunar syndromes or showed spontaneous improvement within 6 h after onset of clinical symptoms. In the remaining group, recurrent stroke and uncontrolled hypertension occurred in 21 cases. Exceptional contraindications (stomach ulcer, gastrointestinal or urogenital bleeding, surgery within the previous 10 days) were found in 7 cases.

The remaining 39 candidates met the current criteria for thrombolytic therapy with a disability score of 4 or 5 (moderate or severe deficit) on admission. Cerebral ischemia was attributed to the carotid territory in 23 (11.5%) and to the vertebrobasilar circulation in 16 (8%).

Analysis of the further clinical course showed satisfactory resolution of clinical deficits without pharmacologically induced thrombolysis in 15 patients improving to disability scale 1 or 2. Retrospectively 24 (12%) patients remained moderately or severely disabled, and might have had some benefit from early therapeutic thrombolysis.

Conclusion

One out of five stroke patients admitted to our neurological department was placed on thrombolytic therapy on the basis of currently applied inclusion and exclusion criteria. Without thrombolytic therapy one-third of these patients improved satisfactorily. The considerable rate of recovery in a subgroup of our stroke patients can be seen as a result of selection. The rate of clinical deterioration due to thrombolysis cannot be estimated so far, but must be taken into account when considering the benefit of therapeutic thrombolysis.

De facto, only 2 out of 200 patients were subjected to thrombolytic medication mainly due to delays. These data of course do depend on a specific referral pattern, but nevertheless the time factor seems to be particularly critical.

Spontaneous Recanalization in Middle Cerebral Artery Occlusion

M. KAPS and U. TESCHENDORF

The threat to life and the catastrophic deficits caused by occlusion of the middle cerebral artery (MCA) underline the clinical significance of this particular entity, in which young patients with cardiogenic cerebral embolism constitute a special subgroup. In many cases, clinical data in combination with typical infarction patterns in computed tomography (CT) suggest the diagnosis of MCA occlusion. Until now, angiography of the cerebral arteries has been necessary for final confirmation. However, this procedure is unfortunately seldom indicated in the acute phase of stroke. As patients cannot be subjected to repeated angiography shortly after stroke, our knowledge as to frequency and time of spontaneous recanalization remains incomplete. The percentage of occlusions recanalizing during the first days and weeks is estimated to be 30%–50% [1, 3, 4, 7] or even up to 95% [8]. Knowledge of the factors determining persistence or lysis of thrombembolic material is also incomplete, as is the influence of recanalization on outcome. Such basic data are, however, of major significance regarding therapeutic strategies such as thrombolysis.

Patients and Methods

The results comprise transcranial Doppler ultrasound (TCD) recordings of 23 patients suffering from acute MCA occlusion. All cases were subjected to complete clinical and CT workup. CT was repeated to discover the possibility of hemorrhage into the infarcted brain tissue in cases undergoing recanalization. The investigations of the basal cerebral arteries were conducted with a standard pulsed 2-MHz Doppler device (TC 2–64 B, EME, D-7770 Überlingen, FRG). Diagnosis of MCA occlusion was established according to criteria published elsewhere [5].

Department of Neurology, Justus-Liebig University, Am Steg 14, W-6300 Giessen, FRG.

Hacke et al. (Eds.)
Thrombolytic Therapy in Acute Ischemic Stroke
© Springer-Verlag Berlin Heidelberg 1991

Results

Transcranial Doppler ultrasound follow-up studies were conducted repeatedly in the acute period after occlusion; recanalization of the MCA could be monitored in 16 cases (Table 1). Recanalization occurred gradually: A high-frequency stenotic signal indicating partially reopened lumen was discrete at first. In later stages the TCD signs of MCA stenosis became more obvious. A further increase in vascular lumen led to a decrease in flow velocity in the M1 segment; finally, turbulent signal irregularities disappeared (Fig. 1). Recanalization was seen in this collective until the 17th day after stroke onset. Augmented flow velocity in the M1 segment disappeared between 11 days or 4 weeks. Three patients (Table 1, nos. 14, 15, 17) died after recanalization of the MCA secondary to temporal herniation after developing extensive postischemic edema. In three patients blood flow velocity enhancement persisted for weeks (Table 1, nos. 5, 8, 10). Unfortunately it was not possible to repeat angiography, to demonstrate a residual MCA stenosis in these cases. Differentiation between postischemic hyperemia and residual MCA stenosis during the process of recanalization caused considerable problems.

Hemorrhagic transformation causing clinical deterioration in relation to artery recanalization was not observed (under hemodilution therapy and 300 mg/day aspirin).

Discussion

Patients with MCA occlusion persisting at least 1 day revealed very variable clinical courses as well as CT lesion patterns. This was independent of spontaneous recanalization later on, indicating the crucial importance of early collateral blood supply by leptomeningeal anastomoses [2]. Five cases featured typical "deep" subcortical CT infarctions which are considered to be the result of proximal MCA trunk occlusion and blockade of lenticulostriate end arteries.

Shortly after ischemic stroke, increased or diminished blood flow velocity can be observed frequently in the affected MCA compared with the opposite side. As normal ranges of blood flow velocity in cerebral arteries are wide and differences between sides of up to 20% are not necessarily pathological, clear-cut limits of physiological and pathological flow velocity values are hard to establish. Follow-up studies are especially helpful in this respect, since reactive hyperemia decreases with time, enabling accurate diagnosis by TCD retrospectively. In this study, a more than 50% increase in flow velocity was classified as abnormal.

Our TCD findings elucidate more complicated intracerebral hemodynamics after acute stroke than simply "ischemia." Hyperemia was shown to

Table 1. Transcranial Doppler ultrasound follow-up studies in patients with MCA occlusion

No./age (years)/sex	Confirmed by	Recanalization After	Increased velocity[a]	MCA lesion pattern	Neurological deficit
1/44/M	Angiogram	7 days	No increase	Multiple branches	Severe
2/24/F	Angiogram	No recanalization		LSA	Moderate
3/56/M	Angiogram	No follow-up		Multiple branches	Severe
4/50/M[b]	Angiogram	2 days	11 days	Multiple branches	Severe
5/40/F[b]	Angiogram	1 day	>7 weeks (stenosis?)	Branch	Mild
6/44/M[b]	Angiogram	4 days	No increase	LSA	Severe
7/49/M	Angiogram	No recanalization (within 4 weeks)		LSA	Moderate
8/49/M	Angiogram	17 days	>4 weeks (stenosis?)		Moderate
9/34/F	Angiogram	2 days	28 days	LSA + branch	Moderate
10/34/F	Angiogram	12 days	Persistent (stenosis?)	LSA	Moderate
11/45/M	Angiogram	2 weeks	No increase	Branch	Mild
12/74/M	Necropsy	No recanalization		Complete	Death
13/81/M	Necropsy	No recanalization		Complete	Death
14/73/M	TCD follow-up	7 days		No classification	Death
15/67/M	TCD follow-up	1 day		Complete	Death
16/63/M	TCD follow-up	1 day	33 days	LSA	Severe
17/82/M	TCD follow-up	1 day		Complete	Exitus
18/68/M[b]	TCD follow-up	4 days		LSA	Moderate
19/78/M[b]	TCD follow-up	7 days	25 days	LSA	Severe
20/77/F	TCD follow up	3 days	No increase	Branch	Severe
21/77/F	TCD follow-up	9 days	8 days	LSA	Severe
22/55/F	Multiple embolism	No recanalization		LSA	Moderate
23/67/M	Multiple embolism	No recanalization		Complete	Exitus

LSA, supply area of lenticulostriate arteries.
[a] More than 50% increase of flow velocity compared with opposite site (duration not determined when patient died).
[b] Additional ipsilateral carotid occlusion.

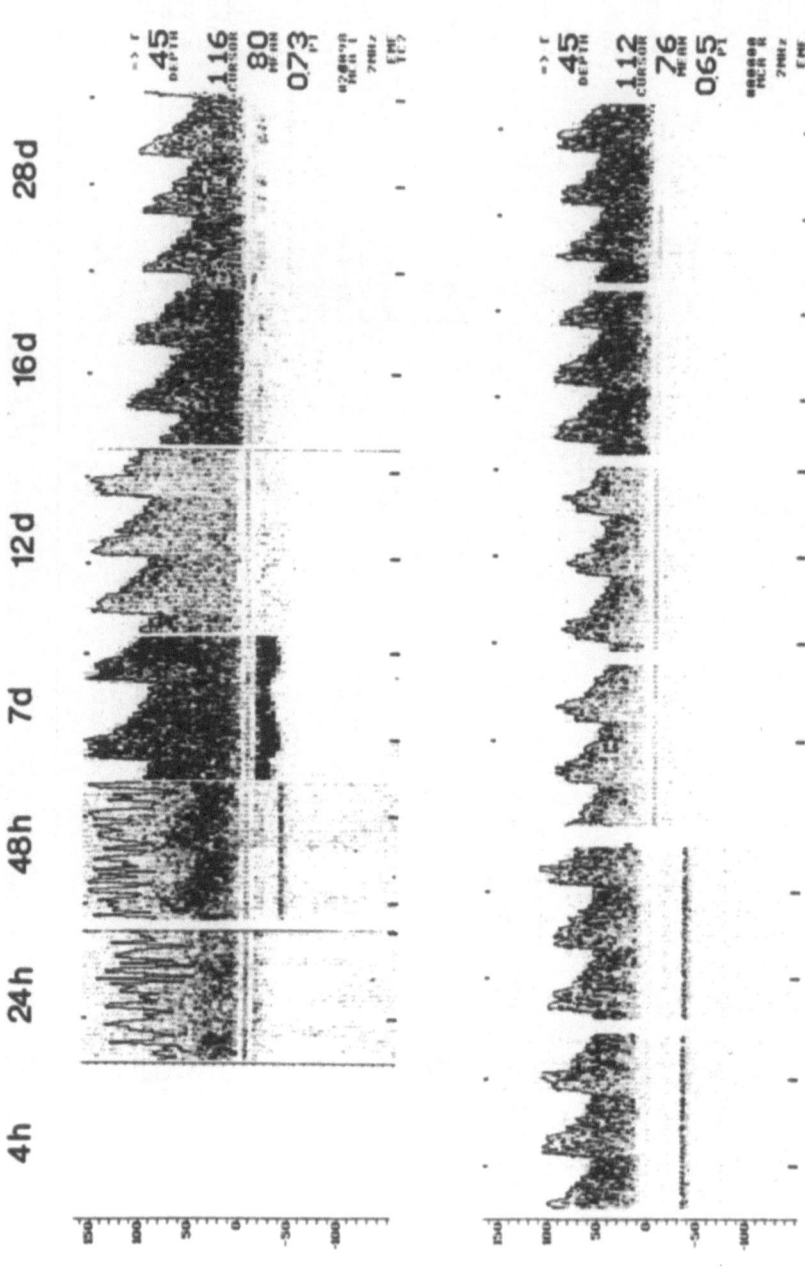

Fig. 1. Thirty-four-year-old patient suffering from cardiac embolism. *Above*, Recanalization of the MCA beginning 24 h after clinical onset. Initially a stenotic signal is prominent; 4 weeks later the TCD signal is symmetrical and normal on both sides. Differentiation between stenosis and postischemic hyperemia is difficult. *Below*, contralateral MCA serving as reference

be due to migration of embolic material to the periphery [6]. Exact localization of the MCA obstruction (proximal or distal main stem) is not possible. Distal MCA branch occlusions cannot be diagnosed as well, since there is no reliable method of investigating these segments of the artery by ultrasound. TCD may nevertheless provide important individual information regarding embolus migration uncovering pathophysiological mechanisms underlying cerebral ischemia. Immediate exclusion of an MCA occlusion can provide important information as well, influencing further diagnostic and therapeutic strategies. This information is generally obtained by TCD with minimal delay and considerable accuracy.

Angiography remains the "gold standard" for verification of MCA occlusions diagnosed by TCD. However, it can deliver only snapshot information, initially showing MCA occlusion, later possibly stenosis. After completed resolution of symptoms, angiography is of no diagnostic value.

References

1. Allock JM (1967) Occlusion of the middle cerebral artery: serial angiography as a guide to conservative therapy. J Neurosurg 27:353–363
2. Bozzao L, Fantozzi LM, Bastianello S, Bozzao A, Fieschi C (1989) Early collateral supply and late parenchymal brain damage in patients with middle cerebral artery occlusion. Stroke 20:735–740
3. Dalal PM (1965) Cerebral embolism. Angiographic observation on spontaneous clot lysis. Lancet 1:61–64
4. Irino T, Taneda M, Minami T (1977) Angiographic manifestation in postrecanalized cerebral infarction. Neurology 27:471–475
5. Kaps M, Damian MS, Teschendorf U, Dorndorf W (1990) Transcranial Doppler ultrasound findings in middle cerebral artery occlusion. Stroke 21:532–537
6. Olsen TS, Lassen NA (1984) A dynamic concept of middle cerebral artery occlusion and cerebral infarction in the acute state based on interpreting severe hyperemia as a sign of embolic migration. Stroke 15:458–468
7. Olsen TS (1986) Regional cerebral blood flow after occlusion of the middle cerebral artery. Acta Neurol Scand 73:321–337
8. Okada Y, Yamaguchi T, Minematsu K, Sawada T, Sadoshima S, Fujishima M, Omae T (1989) Hemorrhagic transformation in cerebral embolism. Stroke 20:598–603

In Vitro Thrombus Lysis by Urokinase in Preparation for Patient Studies

K. Matsumoto and K. Satoh

As a modern approach to the treatment of acute ischemic stroke caused by major or principal cerebral arterial occlusion, local intraarterial thrombolytic therapy has recently attracted much interest. In this treatment, a urokinase (UK) solution is administered through an angiographic catheter at a site proximal to the occlusion immediately after diagnostic angiography. The purpose of this paper is to reconfirm and evaluate the thrombolytic action of a UK solution by in vitro experiments in preparation for patient studies of intraarterial UK infusion therapy [1–3].

Materials and Methods

Arterial blood was obtained by femoral tap from a dog under ketamine anesthesia. The arterial blood was poured into a straight glass tube. The tube was rotated horizontally along its long axis for 10 min in order to form a homogeneous plug thrombus inside the tube. This was then incubated for several hours at 37°C. The clotted plug thrombus adhered tightly to the inside of the glass tube, and the lumen of the glass tube was obstructed by the thrombus in the middle. The tube was placed perpendicularly and a UK solution was poured from the top of the tube onto the plug thrombus. A saline solution was used as a control. The half-time ($T_{1/2}$), that is the time required for the height of the solution on top of the plug thrombus to decrease to half of the initial level, was measured as an indicator of thrombolytic action of the test solution (Fig. 1).

Department of Neurological Surgery, School of Medicine, University of Tokushima, 2-chome, Kuramoto-Cho, Tokushima 770, Japan.

Hacke et al. (Eds.)
Thrombolytic Therapy in Acute Ischemic Stroke
© Springer-Verlag Berlin Heidelberg 1991

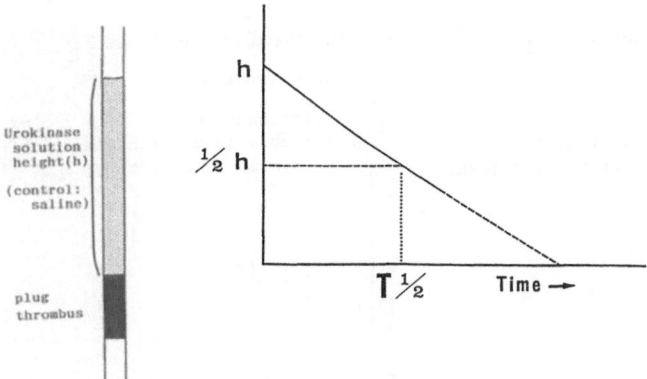

Fig. 1. Measurement of a half-time $(T_{1/2})$

Results

The saline solution placed on the thrombus to a height of 5 cm in a 2.7-mm-diameter glass tube gradually passed down through the thrombus by infiltration without recanalization. The $T_{1/2}$ value was 70 min in the case of a 1-cm plug thrombus, 90 min for a 2-cm thrombus, and 280 min for a 5-cm thrombus. In contrast, a UK solution (1000 IU/ml) placed on the thrombus to a height of 5 cm fell through a recanalized channel in the center of thrombus, and the $T_{1/2}$ value was 8 min in the case of a 1-cm plug thrombus, 25 min for a 2-cm thrombus, 70 min for a 5-cm plug thrombus, and 300 min for a 10-cm thrombus (Fig. 2A). $T_{1/2}$ in the case of the plug thrombus in 4-mm-diameter glass tubes was smaller than that in the case of 2.7-mm-diameter tubes (Fig. 2B). However, there was no apparent difference in the $T_{1/2}$ value as a function of the height (5, 10, 25, 50, and 100 cm) of the test solution (UK or saline) on top of the 2-cm plug thrombus (Fig. 2C).

The $T_{1/2}$ values were also compared for the plug thrombus, which had had various incubation times of 1, 1.5, 3, 12, 24, and 48 h. The $T_{1/2}$ value was reduced for thrombi with an incubation time of up to 3 h. Thrombi which had been incubated for 3–24 h showed practically the same $T_{1/2}$ value with the UK solution; a similar tendency was observed with saline solution (Fig. 2D). With regard to the effect of the concentration of the UK solution, $T_{1/2}$ values reached a plateau at 1000 IU/ml and over.

Finally as an additional test, piercing the plug thrombus with a 0.038-in. (0.96-mm) guide wire was attempted. In the case of the control, the saline solution passed down through the pierced channel with no other macroscopic change in the thrombus, whereas the center of the plug thrombus started to melt away after the UK solution passed down the channel.

A. Plug thrombus length and $T\frac{1}{2}$

(Inner diameter 2.7 mm)

Solution height   : 5 cm
Thrombus incubation time: 2 h
Urokinase concentration : 10^3 IU/ml

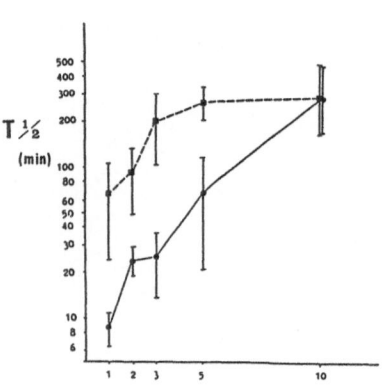

B. Plug thrombus length and $T\frac{1}{2}$

(Inner diameter 4.0 mm)

Solution height   · 5 cm
Thrombus incubation time: 2 h
Urokinase concentration : 10^3 IU/ml

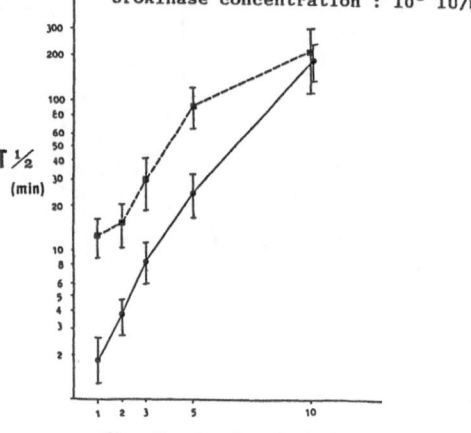

C. Solution height (h) and $T\frac{1}{2}$

Inner diameter   : 2.7 mm
Plug thrombus length   : 2 cm
Thrombus incubation time: 2 h
Urokinase concentration : 10^3 IU/ml

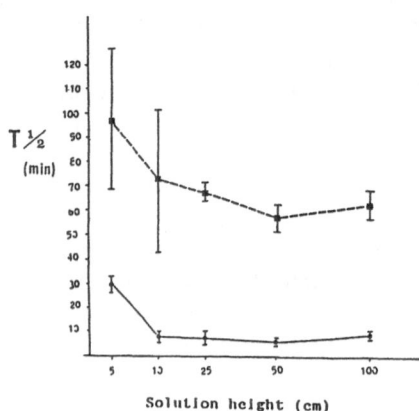

D. Plug thrombus incubation time and $T\frac{1}{2}$

Inner diameter   : 2.7 mm
Plug thrombus length   : 2 cm
Solution height   : 5 cm
Urokinase concentration : 10^3 IU/ml

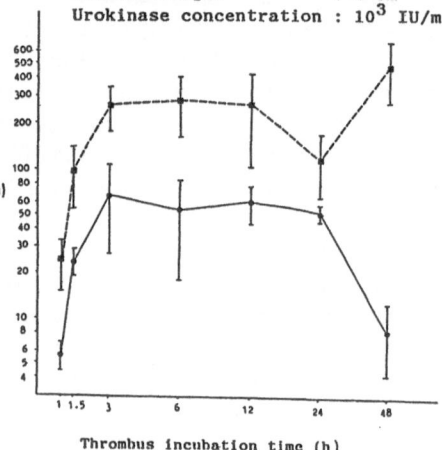

Fig. 2A-D. Half-times ($T_{1/2}$) in various situations. ■—■ Control; ●—● Urokinase

Discussion

A logical approach to therapy for acute thromboembolic arterial obstruction would seem to be infusion of a UK solution to the site of the lesion through an angiographic catheter. However, the thrombolytic action of UK may be limited to the bottom surface of the thrombus obstructing an artery. Moreover, the UK solution is also soon diluted and diverted by the systemic blood circulation.

In this in vitro experiment, the basic conditions for the thrombolytic action of UK were tested with regard to the length of the plug thrombus, the diameter of the plug thrombus, the static pressure of the UK solution on the plug thrombus, the freshness of the plug thrombus, and the concentration of the UK solution. The most fruitful findings were that fresh clots responded well to the thrombolytic action of UK, and piercing of the plug thrombus markedly promoted thrombolysis after the UK solution passed through the pierced channel of the thrombus.

Summary

The following findings were obtained in relation to the thrombolytic action of a UK solution:

1. A plug thrombus with a larger diameter showed a shorter recanalization time.
2. The thrombolytic action may be limited by the length of the plug thrombus.
3. The pressure of the UK solution on the plug thrombus had little recanalization effect.
4. Fresh clots (an incubation time of less than 3 h) responded well to the thrombolytic action of UK.
5. In a series of UK concentrations up to 30 000 IU/ml, the recanalization time reached a plateau at 1000 IU/ml or more.
6. Piercing of the plug thrombus showed marked promotion of the thrombolytic action of UK.

References

1. Chandler AB (1958) In vitro thrombotic coagulation of blood: a method for producing a thrombus. Lab Invest 7:110–114
2. McNicol GP, Bain WH, Walker F, Rifkind BM, Douglas AS (1965) Thrombolysis studied in an artificial circulation. Lancet 1:838–842
3. Ogston CM, Ogston D, Fullerton HW (1968) Observations on the lysis of artificial thrombi by urokinase. Thromb Diath Hemorrh 19:107–116

Local Intraarterial Fibrinolysis in Acute Middle Cerebral Artery Occlusion

G. SIEPMANN[1], M. MÜLLER-JENSEN[1], H. GOOSSENS-MERKT[2], L. LACHENMAYER[2], and H. ZEUMER[1]

Introduction

The technical equipment for performing local intraarterial fibrinolysis (LIF) such as digital subtraction angiography (DSA), microcatheters, and contrast media has been improved significantly in recent years. New microcatheter systems such as the Tracker catheter offer not only the opportunity to administer fibrinolytic agents very close to an embolus within the middle cerebral artery (MCA), but superselective catheterization also permits angiography distal to the occlusion site [5, 6]. In our experience, it is usually possible to bypass occluding MCA emboli in order to contrast the downstream vessels. Afterwards we have been able to place the tip of the catheter between the wall of the MCA and the embolus to perform fibrinolysis.

We have demonstrated four major types of embolic occlusion within the carotid system. *Type I* is an occlusion in the internal carotid artery at the level of the anterior chorioidal artery leading to hemiplegia. *Type II* is an embolic occlusion in front of the trifurcation occluding the lenticulostriate arteries. The bifurcating vessels, however, are not occluded by thrombembolic material. *Type III* is an occlusion not only at the trifurcation of the MCA but also at least one main branch of the MCA. *Type IV* shows only a peripheral branch occlusion of the MCA. This type of occlusion has never been treated with our technique.

With the "M" type of carotid territory stroke, multiple occlusions within the middle and the anterior cerebral artery territories are demonstrable [1−4].

---

[1] Department of Neuroradiology, University of Hamburg, Martinistr. 52, W-2000 Hamburg 20, FRG.

[2] Department of Neurology, University of Hamburg, Martinistr. 52, W-2000 Hamburg 20, FRG.

Hacke et al (Eds.)
Thrombolytic Therapy in Acute Ischemic Stroke
© Springer-Verlag Berlin Heidelberg 1991

Case Reports

The 50-year-old patient R.L. experienced a left-sided hemiplegia during coronary angiography. CT on admission was normal. Cerebral angiography performed within 3 h after onset of stroke showed occlusion of the MCA. Good leptomeningeal collateralization of the distal vessels was observed. Superselective angiography demonstrated a type II MCA occlusion with an embolus lodging in front of the MCA trifurcation but with patent distal vessels. The catheter tip was positioned close to the trifurcation between the embolus and the vessel wall. A quantity of 750 000 units urokinase were infused over 2 h. The postfibrinolysis angiogram showed complete revascularization of the previously occluded MCA and demonstrated all the peripheral vessels. Clinical improvement occurred rapidly within the subsequent week. Finally only minimal deficits were observed.

The 60-year-old female patient P.M. had suffered from hypertension and atrial fibrillation over a long period. She was admitted 4 h after the onset of a left complete hemiplegia. The cerebral angiography showed a complete occlusion of the MCA with collaterals from leptomeningeal anastomoses arising from the anterior cerebral artery. After microcatheterization had demonstrated type II MCA occlusion, the tip of the microcatheter was positioned at the embolus surface. Only 575 000 units of urokinase administered over a period of 1.5 h were necessary to recanalize the vessel. The postfibrinolysis angiogram showed complete revascularization. Restoration of normal neurological status was obtained in this patient, and some of the mild hemiparesis disappeared during the 1st week. Post-LIFCT showed no infarction or hemorrhage.

The 53-year-old male patient M.H. suffered from aortic valve stenosis and arterial hypertension. Cerebral angiography could be performed 4 h after the onset of complete left hemiplegia and aphasia. Clot material was seen in the carotid siphon, the A1 segment of the anterior cerebral artery, and the M1 segment of the MCA. Multiple thrombi were demonstrated within the peripheral vessels. After fibrinolysis only an incomplete recanalization was demonstrated in the trifurcational area. Revascularization of the peripheral vessels was not achieved. Post-LIFCT 1 day later showed complete infarction of the MCA and parts of the anterior cerebral artery territory. The patient died from brain swelling and final herniation.

Results

Eleven patients were treated during the period from April 1989 until April 1990. Initially all patients presented with complete hemiplegia. The patients were classified corresponding to their initial angiographic findings as well as in four groups related to the persisting neurological deficits after fibrinolysis (Table 1).

Table 1. Local intraarterial fibrinolysis for carotid territory stroke

Outcome with neurological deficits	No.	Type of occlusion				Recanalization		
		I	II	III	M	Complete	Incomplete	None
Mild	5	1	4			5		
Moderate	2			1	1		2	
Severe	1			1			1	
Death	3				3		1	2

The first group, containing five patients, left the hospital with no or minor neurological deficits. All these patients had shown type I or II occlusion, i.e., carotid siphon or M1 occlusion. In the group with moderate and severe neurological outcome, angiography had demonstrated "M" type vascular occlusion in one and type III occlusion in the other patients. In three cases with multiple occluded vessels, this condition led to severe brain swelling, herniation, and finally death.

Conclusions

1. Arterial recanalization after embolic stroke is usually possible using microcatheter-guided superselective angiography in circumscribed vascular occlusion.
2. No severe complications have occurred yet.
3. The thesis to be tested after these preliminary results is: The benefit from LIF is probably better the more proximal the embolus is sited. Branch occlusion leads to greater or lesser neurological deficits, depending on which vessel could not be recanalized.
4. Multiple emboli lead to extended infarction and due to poor collateralization to severe brain edema.

References

1. Adams HP, Damasio HC, Putman SF, Damasio AR (1983) Middle cerebral artery occlusion as a cause of isolated subcortical infarction. Stroke 14:948–951
2. Bozzao L, Fantozzi LM, Bastianello S, Bozzao A, Fieschi C (1989) Early collateral blood supply and late parenchymal brain damage in patients with middle cerebral artery occlusion. Stroke 20:735–740
3. Saito I, Serugawa H, Shiokawa S, Tsutsumi K (1987) Middle cerebral artery occlusion: correlation of computed tomography and angiography with clinical outcome. Stroke 18:863–868

4. Taneda M, Shimada N, Tsuchiya T (1985) Transient neurological deficits due to embolic occlusion and reopening of the cerebral arteries. Stroke 16:522–524
5. Theron J, Courtheoux P, Casasco A, Alachkar F, Notari F, Ganem F, Maiza D (1989) Local intraarterial fibrinolysis in carotid territory. AJNR 10:753–756
6. Zeumer H, Hündgen R, Ferbert A, Ringelstein EB (1984) Local intraarterial fibrinolytic therapy in inaccessible internal carotid occlusion. Neuroradiology 26:315–317

Treatment of Acute Ischemic Stroke with Recombinant Tissue Plasminogen Activator: Evaluation with Regional Cerebral Blood Flow Single Photon Emission Computed Tomography

D. Herderschee[1], M. Limburg[1], A. Hijdra[1], E.A. van Royen[3], and P.A. Koster[3]

Introduction

The objectives of the study described in this contribution were to run a pilot study on the efficacy and safety of recombinant tissue plasminogen activator (rt-PA) treatment in patients with intermediate MCA ischemic lesions and to assess the efficacy of perfusion with noninvasive neuroimaging with technetium-99 m hexamethyl propyleneamine oxime (TcHMPAO) regional cerebral blood flow (rCBF) single photon emission computed tomography (SPECT).

Methods

Patients were eligible when they had at least a hemiparesis, but not a typical lacunar syndrome, were previously activities of daily living (ADL) independent, were between 18 and 75 years old, and were not on anticoagulants. CT scanning excluded nonischemic pathology. SPECT had to show a compatible incomplete MCA flow deficit. Treatment with 100 mg recombinant-type tissue plasminogen activator (rt-PA) (Boehringer) was given intravenously within 6 h, followed by heparin for 5 days. Assessment was carried out clinically and with repeat rCBF-SPECT after 24 h.

Results

The results are summarized in Table 1.

[1] Department of Neurology and
[2] Department of Nuclear Medicine and
[3] Department of Diagnostic Radiology, Academisch Medisch Centrum, 1105 AZ Amsterdam, The Netherlands.

Hacke et al (Eds.)
Thrombolytic Therapy in Acute Ischemic Stroke
© Springer-Verlag Berlin Heidelberg 1991

Table 1. Summary of clinical and laboratory data of five patients treated with rt-PA

	Cases				
	1	2	3	4	5
Delay stroke onset treatment	3 h	5 h 30 min	5 h 50 min	4 h 30 min	3 h 30 min
Initial deficit	Lethargy, aphasia, hemianopia, hemiparalysis	Aphasia, hemiparesis	Aphasia, hemianopia, hemiparalysis	Somnolence, aphasia, hemianopia, hemiparalysis, incontinence	Neglect, hemianopia, hemiparesis, forced deviation
Clinical change	None	Recovered completely	None	None	None
Complications	None	None	Hematuria after 3 days	None	Rebleeding of wounds, transfusion
One month outcome	Severely disabled, bedridden	Normal function	Severely disabled, wheelchair, constant help	Dead after 5 days	Moderately disabled, walks without help, ADL dependent
Plasminogen (percentage of control) before/12 h after	130/67	93/52	115/62	106/61	85/56
α-2-Anti plasmin (percentage of control) before/12 h after	115/31	90/32	98/35	93/38	84/34
SPECT defect (semiquantitative scale; see text) before/24 h after	41/35	11/0	29/71	45/54	39/14

Conclusion

A possible explanation for treatment failure in patients 1, 3, 4, and 5 is that they had no reperfusion or were given reperfusion too late. In patient 1, repeat transcranial Doppler scan suggested reperfusion which did not result in clinical or SPECT improvement. Patient 2, with moderate deficit, normalized during rt-PA infusion and repeat SPECT was normal. SPECT is superior to angiography in that imaging represents a tight coupling between flow and viable tissue and in the finding that a complete MCA deficit on initial SPECT is predictive of transtentorial herniation [2]. Reviewing the SPECT of patient 4, a natural course with death due to transtentorial herniation was highly probable, irrespective of therapy. The results suggest that in patients with large and complete SPECT deficits even reperfusion after 3 h is too late for recovery. On the other hand, reperfusion might not have been achieved [1]. Complications in these patients were minor. Important points for future studies are early treatment, grading of extent of ischemia, and choice of ancillary investigations.

References

1. Jang IK, Gold HK, Ziskind AA, Fallon JT, Holt RE, Leinbach RC, May JW, Collen D (1989) Differential sensitivity of erythrocyte-rich and platelet-rich arterial thrombi to lysis with rTPA. Circulation 79:920–928
2. Limburg M, van Royen EA, Hijdra A, de Bruine JF, Verbeeten BWJ (1990) Regional cerebral blood flow, single photon emission computed tomography and early death in acute ischemic stroke. Stroke 21:1150–1155

Thrombolytic Therapy in Acute Ischemic Stroke: The Copenhagen Multicenter Study

K. Overgaard[1], H. Pedersen[2], and G. Boysen[1]

Introduction

In most cases of acute stroke the underlying pathoanatomical etiology is a vascular occlusion. Most of these occlusions tend to disappear as a natural process of thrombus disintegration and endogenous thrombolysis, but often this happens too late to be of benefit. In acute occlusion of the middle cerebral artery trunk, mortality is about 30% [2]. In the ISIS-2 and ASSET [1, 4], mortality in acute myocardial infarction was reduced about 25% by thrombolytic therapy. These results have renewed the hope that early thrombolytic therapy in acute ischemic stroke could reopen occluded arteries, thereby reducing ischemic damage, neurological deficits, and mortality. The problems in verifying the possible benefits of this treatment are:

1. Older studies with poor design (no CT scan, inclusion of patients with symptoms lasting several days, poor quality and dose regimen of thrombolytic agent).
2. Uncertainty as to which thrombolytic agent and which dose regimen will give the optimal efficacy and safety.
3. Results of controlled clinical trials have not yet been published.

Material and Methods

We have just started an open pilot study among the neurological departments in Copenhagen; hopefully we will include 20 patients within 1 year. The study design is as follows:

---

[1] Department of Neurology and
[2] Department of Neuroradiology, University Hospital, Rigshospitalet, Copenhagen, Denmark.

Hacke et al. (Eds.)
Thrombolytic Therapy in Acute Ischemic Stroke
© Springer-Verlag Berlin Heidelberg 1991

Inclusion Criteria

1. Patients with neurological deficits with acute onset due to a presumed vascular occlusion. The symptoms should be of a certain severity.
2. The interval from symptom onset to start of thrombolytic therapy should be less than 6 h.
3. Age between 18 and 75 years.
4. Informed consent from patient or/and relatives.

Exclusion Criteria

1. Former intracranial disease [with the exception of transient ischemia attack (TIA)].
2. Moderate to severe impairment of consciousness.
3. Remission of the neurological deficits during the observation period.
4. Patients with malignant disease or other serious, disabling disease.
5. Known bleeding tendency.
6. High blood pressure.
7. Pregnancy.
8. Computed tomography scan with hypodense areas or even slight edema, with other parenchymatous abnormalities, aneurysms, arterial venous malformations, or bleeding.

Included patients are then treated with Actilyse (rt-PA, Boehringer, Ingelheim). A bolus of 15 mg is given i.v. in 2 min, followed by 85 mg i.v. during the subsequent hour. The total dose was 100 mg.

Treatment Evaluation

Within the first 24 h a CT scan and angiography are performed. A CT scan is also performed on the 4th day and after 1 month. The patients are followed clinically with neurological scoring [3] (Table 1) and recording of side effects, both hemorrhagic and other serious events and causes of death. With this protocol we expect to obtain data for vascular patency, infarct size, and neurological outcome, which will give us some idea of efficacy. Concerning safety we will obtain data concerning bleeding risk, morbidity, and mortality.

This protocol is approved by the Danish Health and Drug Administration and by the Ethical Committee.

Table 1. Initial prognostic and long-term functional scores used for the multicenter hemo-dilution trial

	Score	Prognostic score	Long-term score
Consciousness			
Fully conscious	6		
Somnolent, can be awakened to full consciousness	4	□	
Reacts to verbal command, but is not fully conscious	2		
Eye movements			
No gaze palsy	4		
Gaze palsy present	2	□	
Conjugate eye deviation	0		
Arm, motor power[a]			
Raises arm with normal strength	6		
Raises arm with reduced strength	5		
Raises arm with flexion in elbow	4	□	□
Can move, but not against gravity	2		
Paralysis	0		
Hand, motor power[a]			
Normal strength	6		
Reduced strength in full range	4		□
Some movement, fingertips do not reach palm	2		
Paralysis	0		
Leg, motor power			
Normal strength	6		
Raises straight leg with reduced strength	5		
Raises leg with flexion of knee	4	□	□
Can move, but not against gravity	2		
Paralysis	0		
Orientation			
Correct for time, place, and person	6		
Two of these	4		□
One of these	2		
Completely disorientated	0		
Speech			
No aphasia	10		
Limited vocabulary or incoherent speech	6		□
More than yes/no, but not longer sentences	3		
Only yes/no or less	0		
Facial palsy			
None/dubious	2		□
Present	0		
Gait			
Walks 5 m without aids	12		
Walks with aids	9		
Walks with help of another person	6		□
Sits without support	3		
Bedridden/wheelchair	0		
Maximal score		22	48

[a] Motor power is assessed only on the affected side.

References

1. ISIS-2 (Second International Study of Infarct Survival) Collaborative Group (1988) Randomised trial of intravenous streptokinase, oral aspirin, both, or neither among 17 187 cases of suspected acute myocardial infarction: ISIS-2. Lancet 2:349–360
2. Saito I, Segawa H, Shiokawa Y, Taniguchi M, Tsutsumi K (1987) Middle cerebral artery occlusion: correlation of computed tomography and angiography with clinical outcome. Stroke 18:863–868
3. Scandinavian Stroke Study Group (1985) Multicenter trial of hemodilution in ischemic stroke–background and study protocol. Stroke 16:885–889
4. Wilcox RG, Lippe G von der, Olsson CG, Jensen G, Skene AM, Hampton JR (1988) Trial of tissue plasminogen activator for mortality reduction in acute myocardial infarction. Anglo-Scandinavian Study of Early Thrombolysis (ASSET). Lancet 2:525–530

Thrombolytic Therapy in Cerebral Sinus Thrombosis: A Case Report

K. Spitzer, J. Freitag, A. Thie, L. Lachenmayer, and G. Siepmann

Introduction

Venous sinus thrombosis (VST) is a grave neurologic disorder that may be associated with otologic infection, head trauma, neoplasm, or coagulopathy. Systemic anticoagulation with heparin has been the mainstay of treatment during the early course. Experience with thrombolytic therapy is still scanty.

Case Report

History

A 43-year-old man was admitted after sudden occurrence of weakness of the left extremities. He had been in good health until 3 days earlier when diffuse headache developed. There was no history of trauma or neurologic or medical illness. On the way to the hospital, two generalized tonic-clonic seizures were observed.

Clinical Findings

On admission, the patient was comatose with oral automatisms and severe respiratory depression. There was a conjugate deviation to the right. Pupil size was equal with sluggish reaction to light. The corneal response was negative on the left, and oculocephalic and ciliospinal reflexes were sluggishly positive. There were no spontaneous movements of the extremities, but decorticate posturing on the right and no response on the left to painful stimuli. The muscle stretch reflexes were symmetric. The plantar response was flexor on the right and extensor on the left.

Neurologische Universitätsklinik Eppendorf, Martinistr. 52, W-2000 Hamburg 20, FRG.

Hacke et al. (Eds.)
Thrombolytic Therapy in Acute Ischemic Stroke
© Springer-Verlag Berlin Heidelberg 1991

Radiology

Computed tomography scan showed a right parietal intracerebral hematoma measuring 0.5 × 1 cm, but no other abnormalities were detected.

Cerebral angiography disclosed thrombosis of the superior sagittal sinus, and the left sigmoid and transverse sinus distal to Labbé's vein. Due to severe stasis the bridging veins were not visualized (Fig. 1, *top*).

Therapy

Urokinase 500 000 IU was administered into the right carotid siphon over a 1-h period with concomitant i.v. administration of 7000 IU heparin. Heparin

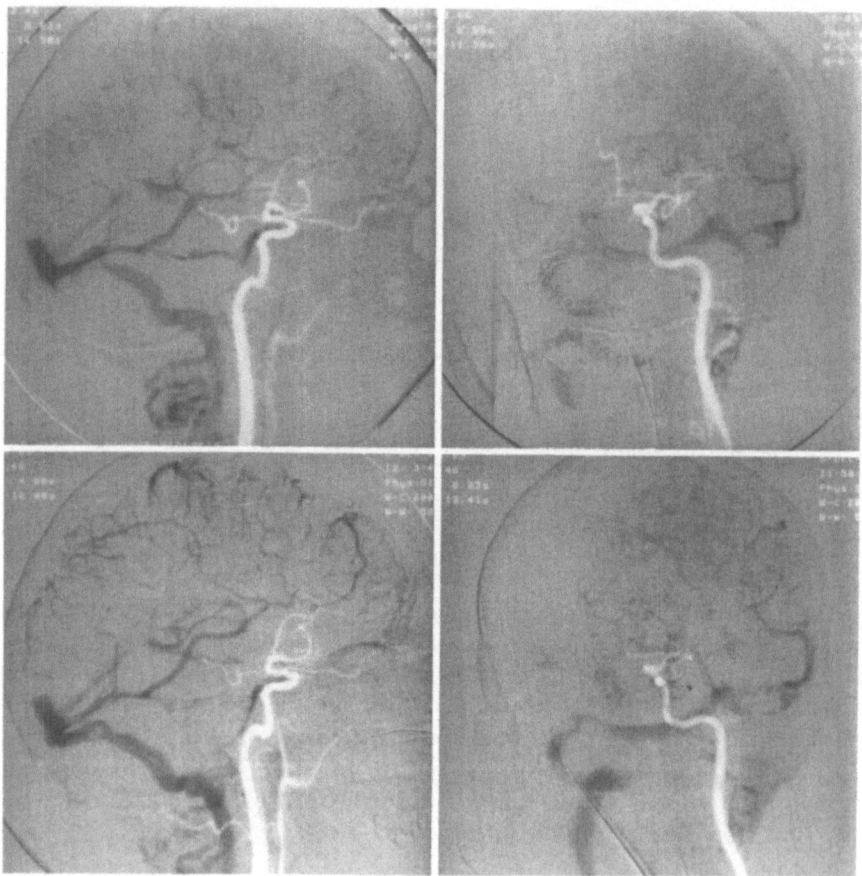

Fig. 1. *Top*, lateral (*left*) and anteroposterior (*right*) projections of first angiography. *Bottom*, lateral (*left*), and anteroposterior (*right*) projections of repeat angiography 20 h after urokinase bolus

was continued by i.v. infusion of 10 000 IU during the subsequent 12 h, and 25 000 IU/day for 3 days.

Course

On repeat angiography 20 h later, the bridging veins were visualized indicating improved perfusion, but the superior sagittal sinus remained occluded (Fig. 1, *bottom*). Clinically, the patient regained consciousness on day 2. Left hemiparesis markedly improved over the subsequent few days, although another angiography session on day 8 still failed to visualize the superior sagittal sinus. The patient was discharged on day 16 with only mild left hemiparesis on sodium warfarin (Coumadin) for a period of 3 months. Repeat CT scan before discharge revealed resolution of intracerebral bleeding. No cause of VST was detected.

Discussion

Early anticoagulation with heparin has been established in the management of VST [1]. Other forms of treatment have been sporadically successful [2]. Local thrombolytic therapy has been reported in only a few patients [3–5].

In our patient, poor clinical condition with coma and focal neurologic deficits has prompted administration of urokinase in the acute phase. Due to the small number of patients successfully treated by thrombolytic therapy, no definite conclusions can be drawn with regard to its true value in VST. Yet, our experience in this patient in conjunction with other reported cases demonstrates that dramatic improvement may occur after a single dose of urokinase. It should be noted that the favorable clinical course in our patient contrasted with the angiographic findings of incomplete resolution of venous occlusion. Apparently, improvement of venous congestion was sufficient for clinical recovery.

Conclusions

Our limited experience suggests that local thrombolysis can be safe and should be considered in selected patients with VST and poor neurologic condition. For monitoring purposes, clinical course may be more reliable, in assessing efficacy of treatment than angiography demonstrating resolution of venous occlusion.

References

1. del Zoppo GJ (1988) Thrombolytic therapy in cerebrovascular disease. Stroke 19: 1174–1179
2. Hanley DF, Feldman E (1988) Treatment of sagittal sinus thrombosis associated with cerebral hemorrhage and intracranial pressure. Stroke 19:903–909
3. Higashida RT, Helmer E, Van Halbach V, Hieshima GB (1989) Direct thrombolytic therapy for superior sagittal sinus thrombosis. AJNR 10:4–6
4. Scott JA, Pascuzzi RM, Hall PV, Becker GJ (1988) Treatment of dural sinus thrombosis with local urokinase infusion. Case report. J Neurosurg 68:284–287
5. Zeumer H, Ringelstein EB, Hacke W (1983) Gefäßrekanalisierende Verfahren der interventionellen Neuroradiologie. RÖFO 139:467–475

Basilar Artery Occlusion Associated with Protein C Deficiency: Successful Treatment Using Recombinant Tissue Plasminogen Activator Infusion

B. WILDEMANN[1], R. VON KUMMER[2], M. HUTSCHENREUTER[1],
D. KRIEGER[1], and W. HACKE[1]

Introduction

Protein C is a vitamin K-dependent serine protease with both anticoagulant and fibrinolytic properties. Its absence or reduced concentration is frequently associated with an increased risk for venous thrombosis, but only rarely with arterial thrombotic disorders. We describe a young woman with partial protein C deficiency who developed acute basilar artery occlusion associated with progressive, life-threatening brain stem dysfunction. Recanalization was safely achieved by intravenous use of clot-selective fibrinolytic agents.

Case Report

A 44-year-old woman presented with acute left-sided deafness, intermittent dysarthria, and a slight right-sided sensorimotor hemiparesis and hemiataxia. Within hours she became comatose and required artificial ventilation. The patient had suffered from thrombophlebitis of the left leg 10 years earlier. Her father had a history of several deep venous thromboses and had died of recurrent pulmonary embolism.

Transfemoral arterial digital subtraction angiography performed 3½ h after the onset of symptoms showed a mid basilar artery occlusion (Fig. 1a). The initial cranial CT scan was normal. With informed consent the patient was treated with 100 mg recombinant tissue plasminogen activator (rt-PA) (Genentech material, Thomae, Biberach, FRG) given continuously over 90 min. The rt-PA infusion was preceded by a heparin bolus (3000 IU i.v.) and followed by 35 000 IU heparin i.v./24 h. Within several hours the neurological deficit gradually improved to normal except for a moderate spontaneous right horizontal nystagmus and a right-sided accentuation of the deep

[1] Department of Neurology and
[2] Department of Neuroradiology, University Hospital, W-6900 Heidelberg, FRG.

Hacke et al (Eds)
Thrombolytic Therapy in Acute Ischemic Stroke
© Springer-Verlag Berlin Heidelberg 1991

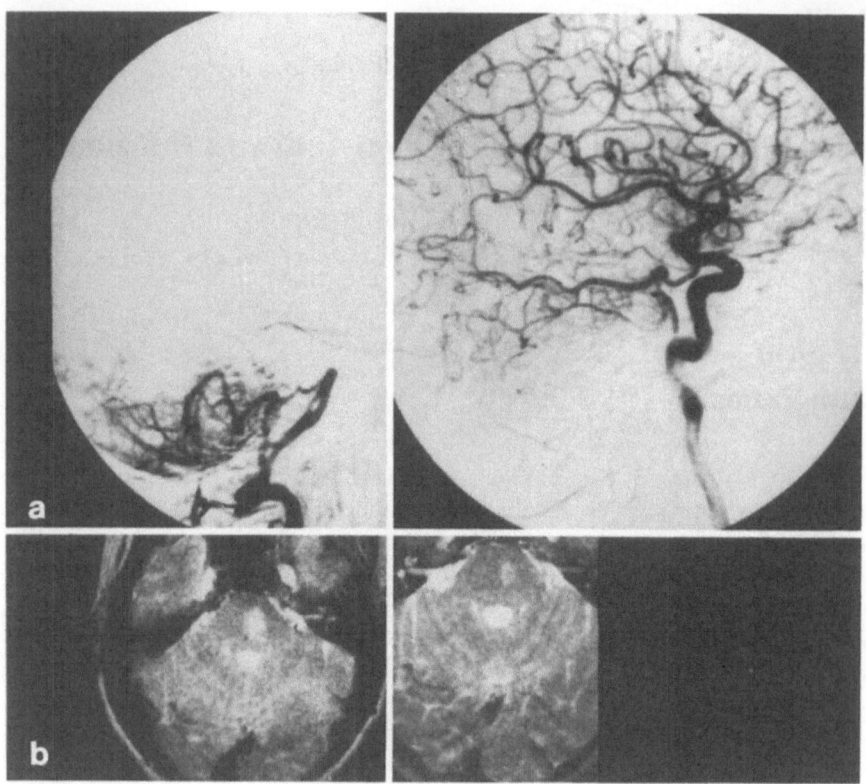

Fig. 1. a Mid basilar artery occlusion demonstrated by digital subtraction angiography 3½ h after onset of symptoms. **b** Paramedian pontine infarction revealed 10 days (*left*) and 4 weeks (*right*) after stroke by magnetic resonance imaging

tendon reflexes. Twenty-four hours after treatment transcranial Doppler ultrasound showed patency of the basilar artery; a repeat cranial CT and electrophysiological studies including brain stem auditory evoked potential (BAEP), median nerve somatosensory evoked potential (SEP), and blink reflex were normal. MRI scanning performed 10 days after the acute event showed an area of abnormal signal intensity in the territory of the left para-median perforating pontine arteries, which was significantly reduced 4 weeks later (Fig. 1b). The patient was put on warfarin and was discharged with no neurological sequelae.

Routine laboratory studies and antinuclear, VDRL, and anti-cardiolipin antibodies were unremarkable. The results of the coagulation tests including activated partial thromboplastin time (PTT), prothrombin time, antithrombin III, fibrinogen, and fibrin degradation products were all within the normal ranges. All antigen levels of vitamin-K-dependent clotting factors were normal except for protein C. The protein C antigen level was determined to be 55% of normal (70%–140%) and 22% after stable warfarin anticoagulation was achieved. Functional protein C activity was not assessed. Cardiac investigation was negative.

Discussion

Protein C regulates blood coagulation by inactivating circulating factors Va and VIIIa as well as platelet-bound factor Va. Furthermore, protein C promotes fibrinolysis by inhibition of tissue plasminogen activator-inhibitors. Its anticoagulant effect is enhanced by endothelial-derived thrombomodulin and protein S, its fibrinolytic effect by thrombomodulin only (review in [2]). Protein C deficiency can result from acquired or hereditary disorders [1, 2]. Several authors have described an increased risk of venous thrombosis in individuals with heterozygote affection and either reduced levels of protein C or the presence of a functionally abnormal protein C molecule (review in [2]). An association of protein C deficiency with arterial thrombosis has rarely been reported [3, 5].

In our case the clinical features together with the individual and family history of recurrent venous thromboses are consistent with a congenital type of partial protein C deficiency. Low protein C levels were found to be the only laboratory abnormality eventually predisposing to stroke. No cardiac dysfunction was detected. We suggest that the laboratory assessment of patients with cerebral ischemia, especially in young adults, should include a protein C analysis. Protein-C-deficient patients with stroke might more easily be proposed for long-term anticoagulation and might be candidates for thrombolytic therapy. The good clinical outcome in our patient following systemic rt-PA infusion agrees well with the recently published positive results in patients with basilar artery occlusion receiving local intraarterial fibrinolytic therapy [4].

References

1. Bertina RM, Broekmans AW, Krommenhoek-van Es C, Wijngaarden A van (1984) The use of a functional and immunologic assay for plasma protein C in the study of the heterogeneity of congenital protein C deficiency. Thromb Haemost 51:1–5
2. Clouse LH, Comp PC (1986) The regulation of hemostasis: the protein C system. N Engl J Med 314:1298–1304
3. Coller BS, Owen J, Jesty J, Horowitz D, Reitman MJ, Spear J, Yeh T, Comp PC (1987) Deficiency of plasma protein S, protein C, or antithrombin III and arterial thrombosis. Arteriosclerosis 7:456–462

4. Hacke W, Zeumer H, Ferbert A, Brückmann H, del Zoppo GJ (1988) Intraarterial thrombolytic therapy improves outcome in patients with acute vertebrobasilar occlusive disease. Stroke 19:1216–1222
5. Israels SJ, Seshia SS (1987) Childhood stroke associated with protein C or S deficiency. J Pediatr 111:562–5641

Intracerebral Hemorrhage and Infarction Volume Following Recombinant Tissue Plasminogen Activator in an Acute Stroke Model*

G.J. del Zoppo[1], K.E. Anderchek[2], J.A. Koziol[1], B.R. Copeland[2], and W. Hacke[3]

Introduction

Early studies of fibrin nonselective thrombolytic agents in patients with nonacute stroke raised concerns regarding the possible risks of intracerebral hemorrhage that might accompany the use of those agents. Although hemorrhagic transformation following local intraarterial infusion of urokinase (u-PA) and streptokinase for acute carotid territory thrombolytic stroke has been reported [3, 5, 7], the risk of hemorrhagic transformation and symptomatic parenchymatous hemorrhage following intravenous infusion of the fibrin-selective agent, recombinant tissue plasminogen activator (rt-PA), is unknown. More specifically, the incidence of local cerebral hemorrhage attributable to a thrombolytic agent following focal ischemia and reperfusion in the carotid territory is unknown. We report the results of a study to assess the contribution of ischemia (and reperfusion) to hemorrhagic transformation following early intravenous infusion of rt-PA in an awake nonhuman primate model of acute focal middle cerebral artery (MCA) stroke.

Materials

Thirty adolescent male baboons (*Papio cynocephalus/anubis*), 11-13 kg in weight, were employed for the present study. All procedures were approved by the Institution Animal Research Committee and were in accord with the National Institutes of Health Guide for the Care and Use of Laboratory Animals. The procedures for implantation of the right (MCA) inflatable balloon device, characteristics of anesthesia, and recovery at early functional outcome have been described elsewhere [1, 2]. The long-term (14-day)

* Supported in part by grant 1-R01-NS26945 of the National Institutes of Health.

[1] Department of Molecular and Experimental Medicine, BCR-8 and
[2] Department of Neurosurgery, Scripps Clinic and Research Foundation, 10666 North Torrey Pines Road, La Jolla, CA 92037, USA.
[3] Karl-Ruprechts-Universität Heidelberg, Im Neuenheimer Feld 400, W-6900 Heidelberg, FRG.

Hacke et al. (Eds.)
Thrombolytic Therapy in Acute Ischemic Stroke
© Springer-Verlag Berlin Heidelberg 1991

experimental format was similar to that employed in previous studies [2]. Following 3 h of MCA occlusion and 30 min of reperfusion, all animals received a 60-min intravenous infusion of rt-PA or placebo:

I.   Open Study: rt-PA = 0.3 mg/kg (group A, n = 6), rt-PA = 10.0 mg/kg (group C, n = 6), and saline placebo (group A/C placebo, n = 6)
II. Randomized study: rt-PA = 1.5 mg/kg (group b, n = 6) versus saline placebo (group B placebo, n = 6)

No anticoagulants or antiplatelet agents were employed. The following outcome measurements were used: (a) neurological function according to a quantitative scale [6], (b) volume of infarction by neuropathology at 14 days, by summation of defects from serial 2-mm coronal slices, (c) intracerebral hemorrhage on the rostral surface of each respective coronal slice, (d) peripheral (noncerebral) hemorrhage, and (e) region of low attenuation on serial cerebral CT scans (GE9800 scanner).

The experiments were terminated by pressure perfusion-fixation at 14 days. Serial t-PA antigen levels and circulating fibrinogen levels were determined by immunoradiometric assay (IRMA) and the method of Jacobson, respectively. The rt-PA preparations were predominantly two-chain and were obtained as gifts from Genentech, Inc. (group A), and the Wellcome Research laboratories (groups B, C). The dose rates employed were based on the manufacturer's labeling only.

Results

The neurologic scores for rt-PA groups B and C did not differ significantly from those of the respective placebo cohorts, despite an apparent significant improvement in the group A treated cohort. No neurologic deterioration was evident in any subject during or after infusion of rt-PA. A significant dose-dependent increase in the incidence of venepuncture site and other peripheral hemorrhages was noted among groups B and C compared with group A and both placebo cohorts.

While most rt-PA- and placebo-treated subjects displayed petechial hemorrhages in the region of cerebral infarction, confluent petechial hemorrhages were unusual, and parenchymatous hemorrhage did not occur. No relation between the volume of hemorrhage and the rt-PA dose, or the peak level of plasma t-PA, was found. Furthermore, no significant difference in the mean volume of infarction was apparent between the rt-PA-treated and the respective placebo-treated groups at any dose. A dose-rate dependence of volume of infarction could not be established. When the data were pooled, no relation between the presence or volume of infarction-related hemorrhage and the volume of infarction (independent of treatment) was apparent.

Discussion

This study was designed to evaluate the contribution of territorial ischemia alone to the incidence of hemorrhage following intravenous rt-PA in acute stroke. Hemorrhagic transformation with clinically significant extension of hemorrhage associated with focal ischemia and reperfusion did not differ between rt-PA-treated and placebo-treated animals. Sample sizes in this study were sufficient to detect a hemorrhage volume difference of $0.004\,\text{cm}^3$ between groups with the power of 0.5, $\alpha = 0.05$, in a one-sided test.

While the thrombolytic effect of the rt-PA at the doses employed could not directly be determined, a dose dependence between measured plasma t-PA antigen levels and the respective increase in the incidence of peripheral hemorrhages suggests such a relationship. The disparity between the incidence of venepuncture hemorrhage and the absence of ischemia-related hemorrhagic transformation probably reflects differences in the responses of different vascular beds to differing injuries in the presence of rt-PA. Vascular structure, the presence of tissue factor, and local inhibitors may contribute further to this difference.

Experience with fibrin-selective and nonselective agents in thrombotic stroke has demonstrated hemorrhagic transformation and symptomatic hemorrhage in a limited number of patients when the agents were given in the acute setting. We suggest that, in patients receiving thrombolytic agents for acute thrombotic stroke, ischemia per se does not add substantially to the incidence of hemorrhage, suggesting that additional undefined factors may contribute to hemorrhagic risk [4].

References

1. del Zoppo GJ, Copeland BR, Waltz TA, Zyroff J, Plow EF, Harker LA (1986) The beneficial effect of intracarotid urokinase of acute stroke in a baboon model. Stroke 17:638–643
2. del Zoppo GJ, Copeland BR, Harker LA, Waltz TA, Zyroff J, Hanson SR, Battenberg E (1986) Experimental acute thrombotic stroke in baboons. Stroke 17:1254–1265
3. del Zoppo GJ, Ferbert A, Otis S, Bruckmann H, Hacke W, Zyroff J, Harker LA, Zeumer H (1988) Local intra-arterial fibrinolytic therapy in acute carotid territory stroke: a pilot study. Stroke 19:307–313
4. del Zoppo GJ, Copeland BR, Anderchek K, Hacke W, Koziol JA (1990) Hemorrhagic transformation following tissue plasminogen activator in experimental cerebral infarction. Stroke 21:596–601
5. Hacke W, Zeumer H, Ferbert A, Bruckmann H, del Zoppo GJ (1988) Intraarterial thrombolytic therapy improves outcome in patients with acute vertebrobasilar occlusive disease. Stroke 19:1216–1222
6. Spetzler RF, Selman WR, Weinstein P, Townsend J, Mehdoric M, Telks D, Crummine RC, Macko R (1980) Chronic reversible cerebral ischemia: evaluation of a new baboon model. J Neurosurg 7:257–261
7. Zeumer H (1985) Survey of progress: vascular recanalizing techniques in interventional neuroradiology. J Neurol 231:287–294

Prourokinase Therapy in Stroke

G. Hamann[1], A. Haass[1], G. Pindur[2], E. Wenzel[2], and K. Schimrigk[1]

Introduction and Objective

Local fibrinolytic therapy using interventional neuroradiological techniques give a new chance in therapy in acute stroke [8]. In particular, vertebrobasilar disturbances are important indications [7]. Local lysis, however, is often difficult, time-consuming, and needs permanent attention by specially trained staff. Thus the positive results of systemic fibrinolytic therapy in myocardial infarction (e.g., [6]) have resulted in new studies using clot-specific agents, particularly recombinant tissue plasminoge activator (rt-PA) in stroke. Experience gained in treating acute myocardial infarction (AMI), with prourokinase (PUK), and especially the low incidence of bleeding complications (e.g., [2]), led to the use of PUK in stroke therapy. In this contribution, results from five patients treated with PUK as a clot-specific agent are presented. Target points were the clinical time-course and the monitoring of fibrinolytic effects.

Patients and Methods

Five patients, one woman and four men, aged between 26 and 63 years were included in this pilot trial. Two patients suffered from a basilar thrombosis and three from a MCA stroke. The main selection criteria were: (a) therapy starting within 6 h after the onset of acute stroke; (b) thrombosis in a cerebral vessel demonstrated by digital subtraction angiograpy (DSA); (c) a negative cranial computerized tomography (CCT) scan; and (d) absence of any stenosis or occlusion in the carotid system shown by Doppler sonography.

Bleeding, infarction, or any sign of a cerebral microangiopathy on the CCT scan, any contraindications to DSA or fibrinolysis, and a severe hypertension were considered as negative selection criteria.

[1] Department of Neurology and
[2] Department of Clinical Haemostasiology and Transfusion Medicine, University of the Saarland, W-6650 Homburg/Saar, FRG.

Hacke et al (Eds)
Thrombolytic Therapy in Acute Ischemic Stroke
© Springer-Verlag Berlin Heidelberg 1991

Having started on a programme of intensive care, the patients fulfilling the above-mentioned criteria were first treated with 15 IU heparin/kg per hour i.v. Fibrinolysis was started by injecting a bolus of 250 000 IU urokinase (UK), followed by infusion of 4.5×10^6 IU PUK (Sandoz, Nuremberg) over 40 min.

Blood was drawn (0.11 M citrate as anticoagulant) before and 5 min, 1h, 2h, 3h, 6h, 9h, 12h, and 24h after the beginning of therapy. The fibrinolytic monitoring was done by checking the following selected parameters: (a) partial thromboplastin time, (b) prothrombin time, (c) plasminogen, (d) α_2-antiplasmin, (e) fibrinogen, (f) reptilase time, (g) fibrinolytic activity, and (h) D-dimer.

Results

Both patients with basilar thrombosis were, clinically, a complete success; angiographic follow-up failed due to technical problems. One of the three patients with MCA infarction showed total recovery, both clinically and on angiography; in another patient, angiography showed that treatment had not been successful and a small infarction developed in the MCA region, and the third patient had a total MCA infarction with slight bleeding in the region of the reopened striate arteries, followed by secondary midbrain signs, and finally death.

The fibrinolytic monitoring showed that there were no changes in platelet counts and reptilase time, there was an anticoagulant effect of heparin shown by a rise in the partial thromboplastin time, and there were no significant deviations of prothrombin time and fibrinogen. The fibrinolytic effect was reflected by a rise in fibrinolytic activity 5 min after the beginning of treatment and its subsequent decrease over the following 2 h (see Fig. 1). Plasminogen activity and α_2-antiplasmin showed a simultaneous decrease while a variable increase was seen in D-dimer.

Conclusions

Different studies using rt-PA in stroke have shown that fibrinolytic therapy with clot-selective agents can be successful in ischemic cerebrovascular disease [9]. PUK is not commonly used in stroke [1, 5]. The good results in AMI [2–4] provide a rationale for using PUK in stroke patients. For this reason, UK and PUK were administered in a similiar manner to AMI with respect to dosage and duration of treatment (e.g. [2]). Bleeding complications were rarely seen in AMI patients using PUK. The following conclusions may be drawn:

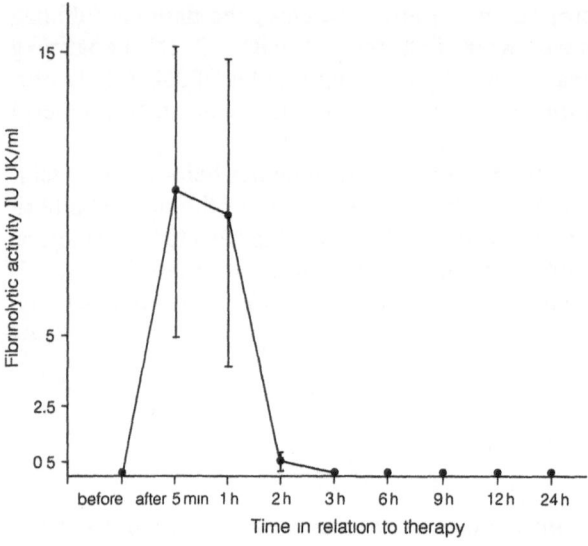

Fig. 1. Time-course of fibrinolytic activity with UK/PUK fibrinolysis in five patients with acute stroke

1. PUK increases the chance of successful fibrinolysis in stroke patients.
2. Fibrinolytic monitoring is an important tool for detecting problems arising in the course of fibrinolysis.
3. Fibrinolytic effects are low, but detectable in plasma, at a maximum within 5–60 min, and decrease over the next 2 h.
4. The complication rate seems to be as low as described in AMI.
5. PUK is a possible alternative to rt-PA in fibrinolysis.

The systemic fibrinolytic activity which is explained by initial low-dose UK bolus was moderate and did not cause a marked decrease in fibrinogen. The combination of UK and PUK is effective in stroke and should encourage further investigations.

References

1. Del Zoppo GJ, Zeumer H, Harker LA (1986) Thrombolytic therapy in stroke: possibilities and hazards. Stroke 17:595–607
2. Gulba DCL, Fischer K, Barthels M et al. (1989) Low dose urokinase preactivated natural prourokinase for thrombolysis in acute myocardial infarction. Am J Cardiol 63:1025–1031
3. Loscalzo J, Wharton TP, Kirshenbaum JM et al. (1989) Clot-selective coronary thrombolysis with prourokinase. Circulation 79:776–782
4. PRIMI-Trial-Study-Group (1989) Randomized double-blind trial of recombinant prourokinase against streptokinase in acute myocardial infarction. Lancet I 8643:863–868

5. Sloan MA (1987) Thrombolysis and stroke. Arch Neurol 44:748–768
6. TIMI Study Group (1985) Special report: "The thrombolysis in myocardial infarction (TIMI) trial". N Engl J Med 312:932–936
7. Zeumer H, Hacke W, Kolmann HL, Poeck K (1982) Lokale Fibrinolysetherapie bei Basilaristhrombose. Dtsch Med Wochenschr 107:728–731
8. Zeumer H, Ringelstein EB, Hacke W (1983) Rekanalisierende Verfahren der interventionellen Neuroradiologie. Fortschr Roentgen 139:467–475
9. Zivin JA, Fisher M, DeGirolami U (1985) Tissue plasmin activator reduces neurological damage after cerebral embolism. Science 320:1289–1292

Subject Index